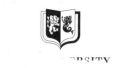

RSITY

CHILDREN OF CHOICE

CHILDREN OF CHOICE

FREEDOM AND THE
NEW REPRODUCTIVE TECHNOLOGIES

John A. Robertson

PRINCETON UNIVERSITY PRESS   PRINCETON, NEW JERSEY

Library of Congress Cataloging-in-Publication Data

Robertson, John A. (John Ancona), 1943–
Children of choice : freedom and the new reproductive technologies
/ John A. Robertson.
p.   cm.
Includes bibliographical references and index.
ISBN 0-691-03353-6
ISBN 0-691-03665-9 (pbk.)
1. Human reproductive technology—Moral and ethical aspects.
2. Contraception—Moral and ethical aspects.   3. Abortion—Moral
and ethical aspects.   I. Title.
RG133.5.R63   1994
176—dc20   93-35880

Be fruitful and multiply.
—Genesis

Blood is thicker than water.
—Old Proverb

Your body is a battleground.
—Barbara Kruger

Contents

Preface   ix

Chapter 1
Introduction: Technology, Liberty, and the Reproductive
Revolution   3

Chapter 2
The Presumptive Primacy of Procreative Liberty   22

ABORTION AND CONTRACEPTION

Chapter 3
Abortion, Contragestion, and the Resuscitation of *Roe v. Wade*   45

Chapter 4
Norplant, Forced Contraception, and Irresponsible Reproduction   69

ASSISTED REPRODUCTION

Chapter 5
IVF, Infertility, and the Status of Embryos   97

Chapter 6
Collaborative Reproduction: Donors and Surrogates   119

QUALITY CONTROL

Chapter 7
Selection and Shaping of Offspring Characteristics: Genetic
Screening and Manipulation   149

Chapter 8
Preventing Prenatal Harm to Offspring   173

EXTENSIONS AND LIMITATIONS

Chapter 9
Farming the Uterus: Nonreproductive Uses of Reproductive
Capacity   197

Chapter 10
Class, Feminist, and Communitarian Critiques of Procreative
Liberty   220

Notes   237

Index   279

Preface

ONE SUMMER day in 1984 a newspaper headline caught my attention: "Test Tube Orphans: Frozen Embryos Might Inherit $8 Million Fortune." The story was about a wealthy American couple who had died in a plane crash with frozen embryos in storage in Australia.

The headline was both familiar and shocking. Novel issues of technology at the edge of life had been staple fare since I had begun teaching in the Law School and the Program in Medical Ethics of the University of Wisconsin in 1973. My colleagues and I dealt daily with theoretic and clinical issues of treatment of handicapped newborns, human experimentation, organ transplantation, death and dying, genetic screening, and the other issues that medical technology presented. Another technology, another headline.

"Test Tube Orphans" was shocking, however, because of what it conveyed about how little we knew about our technological control of reproduction. Although I had written on procreative liberty and was aware of in vitro fertilization, I, a purported "expert" in bioethics, had no idea what legal rules, ethical guidelines, and social practices should apply to human embryos. I resolved, almost on the spot, to work out the legal and ethical rules that should govern their use.

This book is the result of my continuing fascination with extracorporeal embryos and the questions they raise. Since other new reproductive technologies also needed attention, the scope of inquiry has been expanded to include seven technologies of importance to individuals, couples, families, physicians, and others involved with using—or not using—the latest scientific techniques to satisfy procreative needs.

My efforts to understand those issues were helped immensely by attending, for several months in 1985, the weekly clinical meetings of the St. David's Hospital In Vitro Fertilization Program, which taught me much about the medical and technical aspects of infertility treatment. At the same time, I became a member of the Ethics Committee of the American Fertility Society as it began drafting an influential report entitled "Ethical Considerations of the New Reproductive Technologies." Membership on the National Institutes of Health Advisory Panel on Fetal Tissue Transplantation Research, and participation in numerous other conferences and symposia also helped me gain insight and gather information.

This book has been long in conception and gestation. It could not have been completed without the generous support of the Gender Roles

Program of the Rockefeller Foundation and Dean Mark Yudof of the University of Texas School of Law. Rockefeller enabled me to take a semester of research leave in 1988 on the basis of my proposal to write this book. Mark Yudof, dean extraordinaire of an outstanding law school, has been very generous with research leaves and summer support. This book could not have been born without his help or without the example that he and my Texas colleagues set for scholarly achievement. Law School colleagues also gave me the benefit of their wisdom at two colloquia, and students in my 1993 Law and Bioethics Seminar kindly read and criticized an earlier draft. I am greatly indebted to Roy Mersky, Dave Gunn, Marlyn Robinson, and other members of the Tarlton Law Library's excellent staff for their research help.

Many other persons have enabled me to complete this project through their inspiration, their example, their conversation, their comments, their research assistance, and their nuture, care, and support. I am grateful to George Annas, Norman Fost, Rebecca Dresser, Dan Wikler, Ted Schneyer, Joel Handler, Lori Andrews, Ed Wallach, Howard Jones, Leroy Walters, Clifford Grobstein, Tom Vaughn, Richard Marrs, Ruby Fisher, Ryan Anderson, Jackie Johnson, Dan Callahan, Richard Markovits, Leonard Glantz, Alta Charo, and Jim Childress. James Shultz's spiritual guidance persuaded me to "just do it." I am especially grateful to Carlota Smith for her example, her encouragement, and her understanding of all the pitfalls along the way.

CHILDREN OF CHOICE

CHAPTER 1

Introduction

TECHNOLOGY, LIBERTY, AND THE
REPRODUCTIVE REVOLUTION

UNTIL recently, all human reproduction resulted from sexual intercourse, and couples had to be prepared for the luck of the natural lottery. Now powerful new technologies are changing the reproductive landscape and challenging basic notions about procreation, parenthood, family, and children.

These developments excite both huzzas of approval and homilies of despair. On the one hand, they are eagerly sought by persons who suffer from infertility, who risk offspring with genetic disease, or who wish greater control over the timing of children. But others decry their use as unnatural interventions into reproduction, and fear their effect on children, families, women, and society.

Indeed, there is something profoundly frightening about technological control over the beginning of human life. Anxiety over these techniques abounds, even as a growing number of persons seek them out. We are both fascinated and repelled by surrogate motherhood, in utero fetal surgery, prenatal genetic manipulation, the latest frozen embryo case, and the other technologies now on the menu of reproductive choice. They present a series of dilemmas. Individuals must decide whether to use novel means to achieve their reproductive goals despite the ethical and social uncertainties involved. If so, they must also learn to use them in responsible, constructive ways that minimize harmful effects on participants and offspring. In some cases, they will have to resist technologies that partners, physicians, or governments try to foist on them.

At the same time, society must decide whether to permit these techniques to be developed and used. It must identify the circumstances in which use should be restricted or regulated, and devise a framework for respecting individual desires for access while maintaining ethical values, protecting offspring and participants, and preventing injustice and oppression in their use. This is no small task. The deepest needs of individuals must be reconciled with community values in a setting where the rules are still unwritten and subject to change.

The goal of this book is to show the importance of procreative liberty—the freedom to decide whether or not to have offspring—in devising the framework for resolving the controversies that reproductive technology creates. It views the issues presented by reproductive technology as first and foremost a question of the scope and limits of procreative freedom, and assesses reproductive technologies in that light.

The lens of procreative liberty is essential because reproductive technologies are necessarily bound up with procreative choice. They are means to achieve or avoid the reproductive experiences that are central to personal conceptions of meaning and identity. To deny procreative choice is to deny or impose a crucial self-defining experience, thus denying persons respect and dignity at the most basic level.

The scope of procreative liberty, however, has never been fully elaborated. Past controversies about contraception and abortion have concerned the avoidance of reproduction. With the exception of eugenic sterilization and overpopulation in the Third World, limitations on procreation itself have been rarely discussed. New reproductive technologies, by changing the landscape of conflict and choice, force us to inquire into the meaning and scope of procreative liberty.

This inquiry will show that procreative liberty is a deeply held moral and legal value that deserves a strong measure of respect in all reproductive activities. While this value is widely acknowledged when reproduction occurs *au naturel*, this book will show that it should be equally honored when reproduction requires technological assistance. As a result, individuals should be free to use these techniques or not as they choose, without governmental restriction, unless strong justification for limiting them can be established. As I will demonstrate with seven major reproductive technologies, the strong justification needed for restricting reproductive choice is seldom present. Thus decisions about reproductive technology should, in almost all cases, be left to the individuals directly involved.

Before I describe the value conflicts that reproductive technology generates and explaining why procreative liberty holds the solution for resolving them, it is essential for the reader to understand the scope of the reproductive revolution that technological change has now wrought.

TECHNOLOGY AND THE REPRODUCTIVE REVOLUTION

The birth in December 1978 of Louise Brown, the first child conceived in a petri dish in a laboratory, is the most visible marker of the technological reproductive revolution that is the subject of this book. However, that revolution encompasses far more than high-tech laboratory conceptions, and began long before in vitro fertilization became a practical reality.

The term "reproductive revolution" is not mere hyperbole. Most human reproduction will, of course, continue to occur as the result of sexual intercourse with only the technology of modern obstetrics involved. The major issues of human reproduction will remain access to prenatal and postnatal care, reduction of infant mortality, provision of adequate child care, and access to contraception and abortion.

What is revolutionary, however, is the unprecedented technical control that medical science now brings to the entire reproductive enterprise, thereby creating a fertile source of options for individuals facing reproductive decisions. Consider the reproductive topics that have have been the focus of media attention since the 1978 birth of Louise Brown: frozen embryos, surrogate motherhood, genetic screening, manipulation of embryos, forced cesarean section, criminal punishment of pregnant drug users, Norplant and RU486, in utero fetal surgery, and fetal tissue transplants. In years to come, other technologies will cascade out of medical laboratories and into social practice, as micromanipulation of embryos, nuclear transplantation, egg fusion, cloning, interspecies gestation, ectogenesis, and gene therapy are developed.

The conclusion is unavoidable that the character and nature of human reproduction have irreversibly changed, even if only a small percentage of persons ever use those techniques. Like Caesar crossing the Rubicon, there is no turning back from the technical control that we now have over human reproduction. The decision to have or not have children is, at some important level, no longer a matter of God or nature, but has been made subject to human will and technical expertise. It has become a matter of choice whether persons reproduce now or later, whether they overcome infertility, whether their children have certain genetic characteristics, or whether they use their reproductive capacity to produce tissue for transplant or embryos and fetuses for research.

In fact these technologies do affect a significant number of persons. While only 30,000 to 40,000 of the 3 million births that occur annually in the United States are the direct result of technological conception, the number of persons directly touched by reproductive technology is substantial when contraception, abortion, and prenatal screening are factored in.[1] As infertility increases, genetic screening grows, and as new technologies develop, more people will face these issues. Prenatal screening, for example, will become routine in most cases of coital conception, and noncoital means will take over some areas of coital reproduction. Government efforts to prevent prenatal harm to offspring or to discourage irresponsible reproduction may also increase the number of persons directly affected, as will new contraceptive and abortion techniques.

Thus millions of people will face decisions about whether to use or not to use a reproductive technology, if only in the techniques of contraception or abortion that are chosen, and in the use of some method of prenatal screening to check the health of expected offspring. For individuals who are infertile, who are at risk for genetic disease, or who have some other need that a reproductive technology can satisfy, additional decisions will have to be faced. In many cases these decisions will have a dilemmatic quality. Although they offer options for real benefit, they also present problems, ranging from cost to the uncertainties of laboratory conception and the use of gamete donors and surrogates to form families. These choices will unfold against a backdrop of state and private regulatory policies, which encourage, inhibit, or prohibit use of these technologies.

The value clashes and social practices that develop over these techniques will inevitably color how all reproduction is viewed. Once coital conception ceases to monopolize the field, noncoital means of conception and the emphasis on quality will loop back to influence how we view "normal" reproduction itself. Thus both the conditions of access to powerful technologies and their impact on "normal" reproduction are at stake in the controversies and conflicts that attend these developments.

While it is important to see the broad sweep of issues, it is also essential to paint with a finer brush, for public policies to resolve these conflicts should be fashioned in light of the particular problems and benefits of each technique. Several concerns cut across the whole array of new techniques, but each technology presents its own variation on these themes and requires separate scrutiny. To appreciate the breadth and depth of the reproductive revolution, four aspects of that revolution are separately considered: (1) contraception and abortion; (2) treating infertility; (3) controlling the quality of offspring; and (4) using reproductive capacity for nonreproductive ends.

Avoiding Reproduction: Contraception and Abortion

If the reproductive revolution is marked by the technical control of a person's reproductive life, then that revolution, like so much else in our lives in the 1990s, began in the 1960s with the development of the birth control pill and the willingness to use it. First approved by the FDA in 1962, oral contraceptive technology was an important contributor to the sexual loosening and personal-rights consciousness that arose in the 1960s, though many other factors also played a role. When the Supreme Court recognized a right to abortion in 1973, the development of dilation and evacuation techniques of abortion made abortion an easy out-patient procedure and gave further impetus to the drive for control of reproduction.

The technological separation of sex from reproduction was not immediately accepted either in the United States or in the rest of the world. The war over control of one's sexual and reproductive life continues as a major public issue, even as the battles and skirmishes of that war have moved from total prohibition of contraception and abortion to issues of public funding, teenager access, and the circumstances of abortion. The issues of liberty vs. license, freedom vs. responsibility, and individual vs. community that were fought out in the 1960s and 1970s continue in current battles over access to abortion and contraception, and reappear in controversies over the use of noncoital methods of conception and prenatal screening techniques. Many of the issues faced today are an outgrowth of the recognition that first occurred in the 1960s that a person has the right to control his or her reproductive life—to separate sex and reproduction when they find it convenient to do so.

Because contraception and abortion continue to be contested issues, technological developments will continue to influence their status. With regard to abortion, techniques that avoid surgery and act before or shortly after pregnancy has begun are now becoming available. The most important will be contragestive agents such as RU486, which prevent implantation of the embryo in the walls of the uterus or interrupt implantation shortly after it has occurred by means of a pill taken in the privacy of a doctor's office or one's home. Because termination occurs before a fetus is fully formed, it has the potential of reducing some of the heat surrounding the abortion controversy.

New contraceptive technologies will increase the ability to prevent conception or pregnancy. A significant development in this regard is the Norplant system. It consists of six flexible matchstick-sized capsules inserted under the skin in the upper arm that contain a synthetic progestin widely used in oral contraceptives. The capsules, which can be removed at any time, remain effective for five years, slowly releasing progestin, which interferes with fertility in much the same way as oral contraceptives.

Because they are convenient, effective, and have tolerable side-effects, long-lasting contraceptives such as Norplant increase reproductive choice. Norplant will have special appeal to subgroups of women who want a reliable method of contraception without the burden of daily action. As an easily reversible technique, however, it also opens the door to governmental actions to impose it on women whose reproduction is viewed as irresponsible or undesirable, such as those with AIDS or those on welfare. In this case a technology intended to expand contraceptive choice has the potential effect of reducing a woman's ability to reproduce.

Assisted Reproductive Techniques for Relieving Infertility

While issues concerning contraception and abortion have been with us for many years, the most visible aspect of the reproductive revolution is the treatment of infertility. In 1980 the field of assisted reproduction was unnamed and largely unknown. Today, it is a billion dollar industry and a main contributor to the revolution in the control of fertility.

Artificial insemination (AI) is the oldest and most widely used of assisted reproductive techniques. An estimated 20,000 to 30,000 children are born each year in the United States with donor sperm, and thousands more from AI with husband sperm.[2] Although basically a low-tech procedure accomplished with a syringe (some women eschew medical help and inseminate themselves with turkey basters), AI has several important medical components. With infertile couples, the male factor in infertility must be identified, a safe and reliable source of donor sperm procured, and inseminations timed to achieve fertility. AI also occurs frequently with the male partner's sperm to by-pass barriers to conception in the cervical mucous. AI is the least controversial of the assisted reproductive techniques, though unethical practitioners, such as Dr. Cecil B. Jacobsen, who substituted his own sperm for that of anonymous donors in over sixty instances, occasionally bring it into the public eye.[3]

AI is more controversial when it is used, as it increasingly is, by single women and lesbian couples. Due to discriminatory access to the medicalized system of sperm procurement, an unknown amount of AI occurs outside doctors offices with privately procured sperm and self-administration via turkey basters or syringes.[4] It has become an important avenue to pregnancy and child rearing for women who lack a male partner and wish to reproduce.

AI is also used to impregnate a surrogate mother—a woman who agrees to relinquish the child at birth to the father and his infertile wife for rearing. Despite legislation and court cases that discourage these arrangements, surrogate motherhood continues to be sought by infertile couples. Several for-profit surrogacy brokers are now in business, and a few hundred paid surrogacy births occur annually. While most such arrangements have been concluded without problems, some cases of surrogate mothers refusing to relinquish their child to the hiring couple have been highly publicized—most notably the Baby M case, which was front-page news for months in 1987 and 1988.

By far the most visibile, dramatic, and important assisted reproductive technique has been in vitro fertilization (IVF). First developed in Great Britain and perfected in Australia, IVF depends on the medical ability to stimulate the ovaries, remove multiple eggs, fertilize them in vitro, and place them in the uterus so that they may implant and come to term as any other infant. Initially a treatment for blocked fallopian tubes, it is now used for many other indications, including unexplained infertility and very low sperm count. More than 40,000 children have been born world-wide from IVF. There are more than 250 IVF programs in the United States alone, and 31,000 or more IVF treatment cycles occur in this country annually, though less than 20 percent of treatment cycles lead to a live birth.[5] IVF has become a mainstay of modern infertility practice.

The hyperstimulation techniques that underlie basic IVF offer several alternative ways to assist reproduction. Fertilized eggs can be placed at different stages of development directly into the fallopian tube rather than the uterus. Egg and sperm can be inserted prior to fertilization into the fallopian tube, in a procedure known as "gamete intrafallopian transfer" or GIFT. Retrieval and fertilization of multiple eggs allows extra embryos to be frozen, discarded, used in research, or donated to others. Microsurgery on the egg before or after fertilization may increase the chances that conception and implantation will occur. Intentional twinning, by splitting the embryos, and cloning may eventually be possible.

IVF also makes possible the separation of female genetic and gestational motherhood through egg and embryo donation, and gestational surrogacy. In egg donation, women have their ovaries stimulated with hormones so that they may provide eggs for fertilization with the sperm of an infertile woman's partner. The fertilized egg or embryo is then implanted in the infertile wife, who carries the child to term and becomes the rearing mother. As the latest and fastest-growing assisted reproductive procedure, it is now offered by most American IVF clinics to treat premature menopause and other ovarian dysfunctions.

IVF also makes it possible for an embryo created by the egg and sperm of one couple to be donated to another couple. The gestating woman and her partner who rear the child have no genetic connection with the offspring. Because both partners will seldom lack gametes, demand for embryo donation may be lower than for other techniques, but cases will inevitably arise. Embryo donation is also a way to dispose of unwanted or extra embryos without destroying them.

IVF also makes possible the practice of gestational surrogacy, in which one woman carries or "gestates" the embryo of another couple. Women who have functioning ovaries but no uterus or who cannot safely bear children might seek such an arrangement. Unlike situations in which the surrogate mother also provides the egg, the child has a genetic tie with her rearing mother but no genetic or rearing relationship with the gestational mother. However, sisters or even mothers of the egg source or her partner might serve as the gestational surrogate.

Technologies to Control the Quality of Offspring

A third aspect of the reproductive revolution is the greatly increased control now being exercised over the quality of offspring. Fueled both by technological developments and by a couple's desire for a healthy baby, there is a growing demand for—and development of—techniques to assure that healthy children will be born. The term "quality control" sounds perjorative, but it is the parents' interest in healthy offspring that has spurred these developments.

This development is especially significant because it has a reach as potentially wide as reproduction itself. Quality control technologies are not dependent on the mode of conception. Indeed, the most widespread form of quality control occurs through prenatal screening of coitally conceived fetuses by means of amniocentesis, chorion villus sampling, ultrasound, or maternal alphafetal protein testing. Sixty to 70 percent of pregnancies in the United States are now screened in one form or another.[6] The expected development of a maternal blood test of the fetus is likely to make prenatal screening for a wide range of diseases a routine part of prenatal care. Advances in genetics, resulting from the Human Genome Initiative, will also increase demand for prenatal screening, as well as lead to routine preconceptual screening for cystic fibrosis, Duchenne's muscular dystrophy, and other common genetic diseases.

Technology will also push prenatal screening back to the preimplantation or embryonic stage of development. By externalizing the embryo at its preimplantation stages, cells can be removed from early embryos and their genetic structure diagnosed before implantation. Those embryos with the genetic defect in question can be discarded, thus obviating the need for later prenatal diagnosis and abortion. In the future, therapeutic genetic alteration may be possible to treat the affected embryo. Such a development will open the door to other genetic interventions, including nontherapeutic enhancement of offspring characteristics.

Another aspect of quality control grows out of screening techniques that identify a problem in the embryo or fetus. While termination of the pregnancy might occur in such cases, medical or surgical procedures to treat the problem in utero are increasingly possible. Increased attention to the health of fetuses has also focused attention on environmental and behavioral factors that affect the well-being of offspring in utero. Workplace toxins, smoking, drugs, and other actions are now seen to have deleterious prenatal effects on offspring, raising in turn the question of what actions may or should be taken to prevent such avoidable harm.

Nonreproductive Use of Reproductive Capacity

The reproductive revolution is also marked by an increasing tendency to use one's reproductive capacity for nonreproductive purposes, such as producing embryos and fetuses as a source of tissue for transplant or research. It is also evident in the creation of more embryos than may be needed to have IVF children, which can lead to selective reduction of the resulting multifetal pregnancies and to donations for research.

The most publicized aspect of this issue has arisen over the use of fetal tissue cells to treat Parkinson's and Alzheimer's disease, diabetes, and other conditions. Because fetuses must be aborted to get the needed tissue, the technology is controversial. Even use of tissue from abortions occurring for family planning reasons is contested because of the incentives to abort that it might offer. In the future the need to conceive and abort fetuses to get tissue could arise. Other controversies, exemplified by the widely publicized 1990 Ayala case in California, have arisen when parents deliberately conceive and carry to term a child in order to obtain bone marrow for an existing child with leukemia.

THE CONTROVERSIES AND THE CONFLICTS

This brief survey of the revolution in control and use of reproductive capacity illustrates the range of choices that now confront individuals, couples, physicians, and governments. While some of the techniques are firmly established and others are still on the drawing board, some degree of controversy or conflict surrounds all of them. Resolution of these controversies will determine how available these techniques become, and what their ultimate effect on society will be.

The controversy arises from the dual nature of the techniques. While these technologies offer important benefits for many people, none of them come without some significant personal or societal price tag. IVF, for example, is physically onerous, expensive, and manipulates early embryos. Contragestion, genetic screening, and conception of children to serve as tissue donors conflict with respect for prenatal human life. Collaborative reproductive techniques muddy notions of family and genetic lineage and may lead to family-wrenching disputes, such as occurred in the Baby M case. Quality control measures may in practice not be optional for many women, and may place unrealistic expectations on children who are born after prenatal screening.

All of these techniques seem to serve some basic need, while at the same time violating some other important value. This poses difficult questions for individuals, for professionals, for the law and ethics, and ultimately for society. To resolve these conflicts in an ethically acceptable and socially sound way, we must first acknowledge the value clashes that underlie them. Six possible ethical problems arise with each set of technologies.

Interference with Nature

A major source of controversy surrounding the new reproductive technologies is their artificial, interventionist character. Natural conception by sexual intercourse has been replaced by the bright glare of the laboratory. Outcomes of the genetic lottery are now altered by prenatal screening of pregnancies to make sure that the fetus meets predetermined standards of acceptability. Fetuses are removed from the uterus, subjected to surgery, and replaced. Embryos are discarded or implanted, depending on the outcome of genetic analysis. The mystery of conception and pregnancy is thus technologized and diminished, if not altogether denied.

The substitution of technological for natural reproduction raises deep fears about technological power running amok and robbing us of essential human characteristics. Images from Mary Shelley's *Frankenstein* and Aldous Huxley's *Brave New World* abound in discussions of these techniques. Even though technology pervades our lives in countless ways, its extension to the reproductive realm strikes an ominous chord, and in the minds of some persons justifies strict controls on their use.

Respect for Prenatal Life

Another source of ethical controversy is the cavalier attitude these technologies are perceived as taking toward prenatal forms of human life—an attitude thought to diminish respect for human life generally. Many technologies threaten this value. IVF, for example, externalizes embryos and then freezes, discards, researches, and biopsies them, treating them like objects of property, as was evident in the *Davis v. Davis* divorce dispute over seven frozen embryos. Prenatal screening often functions like a "search and destroy" mission aimed at imperfect fetuses, rejecting them simply because they lack acceptable characteristics. Contragestive drugs like RU486 make abortion easier and routine, to the detriment of embryos and early fetuses. Transplant technologies may also devalue prenatal life by causing deliberately conceived fetuses to be aborted in order to get tissue or organs for transplant. Maintaining respect for prenatal human life is a major factor in many conflicts that arise with the new reproductive technologies.

Welfare of Offspring

Radically new reproductive techniques also pose risks to offspring. Laboratory manipulation of embryos, the splitting of gestational and genetic parenthood, and prenatal screening risk producing children who are physically or psychologically injured by the techniques in question. Of special concern is the impact on children of several sets of genetic and social parents, some of whom the child will never know, which arise in the collaborative use of gamete donors and surrogates. Efforts to assure healthy offspring by prenatal genetic certification may create unrealistic parental expectations and set the stage for disappointment. Compulsory use of Norplant by women with HIV disease has been proposed to protect children who might be born with AIDS or be orphaned at an early age. Many conflicts concerning new technologies will concern whether they help or harm offspring who would not have been born but for use of the technology in question.

Impact on Family

New reproductive technologies are also often seen as a further cause of the disintegration and breakdown of the nuclear family, even as they serve family interests by allowing infertile or at-risk couples to have healthy, biologically related offspring. New abortion and contraception techniques are said to encourage promiscuity and high rates of teenage pregnancy, which lead to single-parent, fatherless households. The most often cited threat to family integrity arises from the collaborative reproductive techniques that separate genetic, gestational, and rearing parenthood through the use of gamete donors and surrogates, which have the potential to undermine traditional notions of paternity and motherhood. The wife-husband dyad may be altered in significant ways, either imploding under the extra pressure or expanding into a novel kind of blended family with multiple rearing partners whose precise relation to children and each other is unknown or bitterly disputed. Relations to each other, to the donor and surrogate, to the relatives of each, and to the child must all be negotiated without clear models or guides. Secrecy and nondisclosure may add further pressures, as would use of siblings and parents as donors or surrogates. With the nuclear family so battered by illegitimacy, divorce, and single and gay life-styles, the feared effect of reproductive technology on the family is a recurring ethical theme in the reception of these technologies.

Effect on Women

Reproductive technologies are particularly controversial because of their effect on women. While they open up liberating options for some women, they may also act as agents of further oppression. For most of the technologies operate on a woman's body in some way, turning it into a battleground of competing interests. Often they treat the woman as a reproductive vessel to produce or serve the interests of males and the state in healthy offspring. Some technologies may be imposed on women without their consent; with others, women may have no real chance to refuse.

It should thus be no surprise that feminists are wary of the new reproductive technologies and often oppose them. What strikes some as a revolution in control of reproduction is for feminists just business as usual—reproductive benefits secured through the bodies of women who often have few other real options. This is most evident with assisted reproductive technologies, which entail major intrusions into a woman's body while the man merely has to provide sperm through masturbation. Quality control techniques also involve physical burdens for the woman, not the man, and women, not men, are prosecuted for prenatal actions that harm offspring, or are made the subjects of coerced contraception. Because of inevitable inequalities in the distribution of reproductive burdens, the chance that new reproductive technologies will diminish rather than enhance justice for women is a major ethical concern.

Costs, Access, and Consumer Protection

A final source of ethical controversy arises after all the previous objections are overcome. Most technologies are quite expensive, and are available only to those who can pay. The result is to increase the disparities in access to health care that already plague American medical care—the rich get the benefits, the poor get a few crumbs or nothing. In addition, the high cost of reproductive technology creates opportunities for exploitation and profiteering by the professionals who control its use.

Disparity in access is most evident with assisted reproductive techniques such as IVF. The average cost of one IVF cycle is $8,000, and several cycles may be necessary to achieve pregnancy. Egg donation and surrogacy are even more expensive. Cost will also be a barrier to some forms of prenatal screening, to in utero surgery, and to fetal tissue transplants. In addition, many women will not be able to pay the $365 up-front cost of five years of Norplant contraception and additional physician charges for insertion and removal.

Discrimination by wealth, however, seems inevitable if reproductive technologies are to be available at all. While some persons would argue that access to reproductive technology should be a mandated benefit in any health insurance program, the high cost of universal health care for the uninsured makes it unlikely that most reproductive technologies will be covered. Other than contraception, abortion, and some prenatal screening, it is likely that access to most reproductive technologies will remain dependent on wealth.

Exploitation of infertile couples and other consumers of reproductive technology is also a problem. Many assisted reproductive techniques have a low success rate and do not deliver the child that is expected. Huge profits can be made selling or providing reproductive services, and the field is marked by a tendency of professionals to exaggerate success rates and benefits to couples who are vulnerable because of their strong desire to reproduce.[7] As these techniques proliferate, the need for regulation to protect consumers from fraud, misrepresentation, and incompetent practitioners will increase.

PROCREATIVE LIBERTY AND THE RESOLUTION OF REPRODUCTIVE CONFLICT

With so many important values at stake, it is not surprising that reproductive technologies generate controversy, bewilderment, and fears of larger social effects. Initial wonder at their marvels is usually followed by a nagging sense of discomfort because of the way in which they change nature and could harm children, family, women, and society.

The social and historical context also contributes to the ambivalence that marks their use. Reproductive technology has become available in an era of rapid change in sexual practices, gender roles, divorce rates, family structure, and economic life. One need think only of the great increase in single-parent families, the emergence of a gay rights movement, and the ongoing fight for equal rights for women to be reminded of how traditional roles and practices have changed. Yet before these changes have been fully assimilated into the social fabric, a set of technologies that calls into question the very basis of conception, family, and parenthood has appeared on the scene, marking a further stage in the disintegration of basic traditions. Whether a symptom or a cause of this perceived break-down, the new reproductive technologies cannot escape being tagged with the emotions and allegiances that attend those other issues.

Given these conflicting values, coming to terms with new reproductive technologies will not be an easy task for individuals or for the medical, legal, and social institutions involved. The dilemmas they present will not go away, but will become more acute as new technologies proliferate.

How then might individuals and society resolve questions of use and regulation of reproductive technology? Are some techniques so danger-ous that they should be prohibited altogether? What regulations are in order? Who will set these rules? Are there principles that can guide us safely through the minefield of ethical problems to the oasis of benefits at the other side?

I think there is such a principle, and I argue for it in this book. A central value implicated in each reproductive technology but not listed in the above catalog of issues is procreative liberty—the freedom to decide whether or not to have offspring and to control the use of one's reproduc-tive capacity. Indeed, all the problems of the new reproductive technologies arise from the fact that they appear to involve the exercise of procreative choice. Any restriction, regulation, or imposition of these technologies necessarily interferes with or limits procreative freedom.[8] The overarching moral and policy question thus concerns the scope of procreative liberty in an age of technology.

Determining the scope of procreative liberty requires some standard or method for balancing reproductive choice with the competing interests that it affects. A strong commitment to procreative liberty is the best can-didate for the job. I propose that procreative liberty be given presumptive priority in all conflicts, with the burden on opponents of any particular technique to show that harmful effects from its use justify limiting procre-ative choice. With this presumption as a standard, there is a consistent way for resolving the conflicts and controversies that arise with new re-productive technologies.

What justifies such a high regard for procreative choice? As chapter 2 will show, procreative liberty deserves presumptive respect because of its central importance to individual meaning, dignity, and identity. Al-though contested in some respects and never fully articulated in others, there is a well-developed social, ethical, and legal tradition of procreative freedom. While there have always been restrictions on who may marry and who may have sex, the freedom to have children within the marital relation has always been widely recognized. Since the 1960s, the right not to procreate through the use of birth control has been firmly established. The right to abortion at early stages of pregnancy, though still hotly con-tested, is also a fixed part of our social and legal landscape. Even if one opposes the legal availability of abortion, a strong commitment to procreative choice in other areas remains, despite disagreement and controversy over particular issues.

The challenge is to determine whether the high respect traditionally granted to reproductive choice should be extended to the use of new reproductive technologies. Does freedom of reproduction mean that any new technology must be used? Are any prohibitions, limits, or regulations possible?

To resolve these questions we must first analyze the various components of procreative freedom and the values and interests that justify its protection (see chapter 2). We must then evaluate the reproductive technologies at issue to see whether those values and interests are centrally implicated, for example, whether issues of procreative freedom are truly present. This is a novel enterprise since the concept of procreative liberty has rarely been analyzed beyond birth control and abortion.[9] Moreover, it will involve evaluation of procreative practices that differ in crucial ways from the prevailing norm of coital reproduction, thus requiring construction of the reproductive meaning inherent in new situations.

By the same token, questions of when the effects of reproduction are sufficient grounds for limiting it have never been adequately analyzed. General conceptions of reproductive responsibility have not, with the exception of abortion and the overpopulation debates of the 1960s and 1970s, had to be tested in the crucible of actual policies that limit procreative choice. The issues that count as sufficient justification for limiting such choice—that is, what impacts and costs are sufficient—raise even tougher questions when the technologies affect interests that have not previously been assessed in the particular way presented. A central question in this enterprise is to determine whether effects on embryos, families, women, and other participants rise to the level of severity necessary to justify infringing a basic right.

A stance strongly in favor of procreative liberty does not mean that procreative choice will always triumph. A strong presumption is not an absolute. In some cases a substantial procreative interest in use of the technology may be missing, or the danger to offspring or others from a particular activity may be patently obvious. In other situations, however, the analysis will identify both core procreative interests that deserve protection and competing concerns that are too speculative or symbolic to justify intrusion on procreative choice.

This approach will show that the reproductive interests claimed under the canopy of procreative liberty are not monolithic or unitary, but consist of a congeries of interests in procreating, avoiding procreation, having or not having a genetic connnection, using one's reproductive apparatus, selecting or controlling offspring traits, and the like.

By the same token, the opposing interests that make reproductive technology problematic also involve a complex of different interests, some consequentialist and others deontological. They concern varying notions of the right and the proper, the natural order, respect for fetuses and embryos, the role of women, the needs of offspring, and the structure of family. In each case the opposing interests need close scrutiny to determine their force and legitimacy in any given reproductive conflict. The task is to determine what value these different aspects of reproduction have in light of competing ethical and social concerns in the different contexts in which they appear.

In my view, this method of analysis is the best way to come to terms with the new reproductive technologies. By asking what procreative freedom demands, we can see how much presumptive choice individuals should have over the use of these techniques. By asking what is really at stake in the objections raised, we can see what value should be assigned to competing ethical and social concerns. This requires a careful analysis of both the asserted procreative interest and the asserted harms, so that procreative choice will be limited only when truly weighty concerns are present. The ultimate scope of both procreative liberty and societal regulation will thus be determined as we examine the various conflicts that new reproductive technology presents.

The result of this inquiry will be to show that in almost all instances an individual or couple's choice to use technology to achieve reproductive goals should be respected as a central aspect of people's freedom to define themselves through reproduction. Even if all readers do not agree with my strong normative commitment to procreative liberty, by examining reproductive technology through the lens of liberty they should at least be able to clear away the underbrush that now obscures this terrain and focus their attention on the core value issues that remain.

THE PLAN OF THE BOOK

To show the importance of procreative liberty in evaluating ethical, legal, and social issues in the new reproduction, chapter 2 addresses the moral and legal basis for respecting procreative liberty and discusses its scope and its limits. Basic distinctions about what procreative liberty does and does not involve must be drawn. These include distinctions between the liberty right to avoid and the liberty right to engage in reproduction, and distinctions between negative and positive procreative rights. The chapter also develops the constitutional basis for presumptive legal protection of procreative choice.

Once the presumptive importance of procreative liberty is established in chapter 2, I will examine the particular issues of reproductive technology that comprise the reproductive revolution described at the outset of this chapter. Chapters 3 and 4 apply my conception of procreative liberty to issues of avoiding reproduction as they arise with the new technologies of abortion and contraception.

Chapter 3 describes and assesses the debate and controversy over abortion, and argues for a strong moral and legal right based on a woman's interests in avoiding unwanted reproduction and on the lack of sufficiently strong countervailing state interests in protection of embryos and fetuses to overwhelm that right. It concludes by showing how new contragestive technologies such as RU486, which operate very early in gestation, have the potential to modulate or soften the abortion debate.

Chapter 4 concentrates on the long-lasting, reversible contraceptive Norplant as a technology that increases contraceptive options while it also carries the possibility of greater governmental control over contraceptive decisions. Because contraception is now so widely accepted, the chapter will focus on how contraceptive technologies can be misused by governmental attempts to prevent or discourage reproduction by women on welfare or those who have HIV, and by others whose reproduction is viewed as irresponsible. The chapter addresses limitations on the right to reproduce, and considers when governmental actions to educate, persuade, or coerce women not to reproduce are acceptable.

Chapters 5 and 6 deal with assisted reproductive techniques for treating infertility. Chapter 5 focuses on the ethical, legal, and policy issues that arise with in vitro fertilization and conception outside of the body. It analyzes the need for limits on IVF based on respect for embryos, and argues that deontological claims to protect embryos are insufficient to justify state limitation on use of this technique. It concludes that infertile couples have the right to control the disposition of embryos created in the process of treating infertility, and that consumer protection and regulatory measures to protect their choices are justified.

Chapter 6 addresses the consequentialist and deontological concerns that arise from using third-party gamete donors and surrogates to treat infertility. It analyzes the interests of the various participants, including the impact on offspring, and argues that the preconception intentions of reproductive collaborators concerning rearing of the resulting children should be honored. It also situates these techniques in ongoing debates over adoption and the breakdown of the family.

The next two chapters switch from assisted reproduction to issues in control of the quality or characteristics of offspring—a major source of reproductive innovation and controversy. Chapter 7 focuses on controlling offspring quality through genetic screening and techniques of genetic manipulation. Despite some potential dangers, these techniques clearly fall within prevailing conceptions of procreative choice. However, quality control efforts can be limited when prenatal manipulations serve purposes other than offspring welfare, as might occur with enhancement, cloning, or intentional diminishment of a child's characteristics.

Chapter 8 deals with control of offspring welfare from a different perspective—that of the obligation of parents to take steps to avoid prenatal harm to offspring from conduct during pregnancy. The chapter argues that prenatal conduct of mothers or fathers that unreasonably harms offspring is not part of procreative liberty and is subject to state restriction. However, policy considerations generally preclude resort to coercive sanctions to avoid such harm. Whenever measures are taken to prevent such harm, they should apply to men and women alike.

The last two chapters deal with possible extensions and limitations of a procreative liberty approach to reproductive technology. Chapter 9 examines extensions of reproductive choice to situations in which reproductive capacity is used for nonreproductive purposes, such as producing tissue for transplant, for research, and the like. The chapter shows that while certain practices—for example, generation of surplus embryos or fetuses (and the need for selective reduction of multifetal pregnancy)— may fall within procreative liberty, other practices, such as producing embryos and fetuses for research or as a source of tissue for transplant, do not directly involve procreative choice. The acceptability of those practices will then depend on whether the underlying personal interests they serve have independent, protected status. The answer varies with the technology under discussion.

Chapter 10 confronts several critiques of the rights-based, procreative liberty approach to reproductive technology. It evaluates a class, a feminist, and a communitarian assessment of a rights-based, liberty approach and concludes that none of the critiques provide persuasive reasons for abandoning the presumptive priority of procreative liberty in assessing reproductive technology. The chapter ends with a reminder of the ambivalence that results when one honors procreative liberty under controversial circumstances.

Throughout the book there is a recognition that respect for liberty has its costs. Although I conclude that few ethical or legal limits on the use of reproductive technology can be justified, I never deny the profound ambivalence that may attend recognition of procreative autonomy.

Ambivalence about the use of reproductive technology is inevitable at both the personal and the societal level. Even when respect for procreative liberty permits individuals to use or refuse particular reproductive techniques, many persons will eschew the technology even as others enthusiastically embrace it. Others will proceed more reluctantly, torn between their need for technologic assistance and their hope for a more natural solution.

Similarly, social acceptance of some new reproductive practices will be conflicted and hesitant. Because direct prohibition is rarely possible, social acceptance of reproductive technology may occur as a second-best solution in an imperfect world. Such divergent and ambivalent responses should not be surprising, given the potentially far-reaching effects of the technology and the importance of the liberty interests involved. The price of this liberty is ambivalence about how it is used. In the end, this is the dilemma of rights in liberal democracies, as the freedom to use new reproductive technologies makes excruciatingly clear.

The Presumptive Primacy of
Procreative Liberty

PROCREATIVE liberty has wide appeal but its scope has never been fully
elaborated and often is contested. The concept has several meanings that
must be clarified if it is to serve as a reliable guide for moral debate and
public policy regarding new reproductive technologies.

WHAT IS PROCREATIVE LIBERTY?

At the most general level, procreative liberty is the freedom either to have
children or to avoid having them. Although often expressed or realized in
the context of a couple, it is first and foremost an individual interest. It is
to be distinguished from freedom in the ancillary aspects of reproduction,
such as liberty in the conduct of pregnancy or choice of place or mode of
childbirth.

The concept of reproduction, however, has a certain ambiguity contained within it. In a strict sense, reproduction is always genetic. It occurs
by provision of one's gametes to a new person, and thus includes having
or producing offspring. While female reproduction has traditionally included gestation, in vitro fertilization (IVF) now allows female genetic
and gestational reproduction to be separated. Thus a woman who has
provided the egg that is carried by another has reproduced, even if she has
not gestated and does not rear resulting offspring. Because of the close
link between gestation and female reproduction, a woman who gestates
the embryo of another may also reasonably be viewed as having a reproductive experience, even though she does not reproduce genetically.[1]

In any case, reproduction in the genetic or gestational sense is to be
distinguished from child rearing. Although reproduction is highly valued
in part because it usually leads to child rearing, one can produce offspring
without rearing them and rear children without reproduction. One who
rears an adopted child has not reproduced, while one who has genetic
progeny but does not rear them has.

In this book the terms "procreative liberty" and "reproductive freedom" will mean the freedom to reproduce or not to reproduce in the

genetic sense, which may also include rearing or not, as intended by the parties. Those terms will also include female gestation whether or not there is a genetic connection to the resulting child.

Often the reproduction at issue will be important because it is intended to lead to child rearing. In cases where rearing is not intended, the value to be assigned to reproduction *tout court* will have to be determined. Similarly, when there is rearing without genetic or gestational involvement, the value of nonreproductive child rearing will also have to be assessed. In both cases the value assigned may depend on the proximity to reproduction where rearing is intended.

Two further qualifications on the meaning of procreative liberty should be noted. One is that "liberty" as used in procreative liberty is a negative right. It means that a person violates no moral duty in making a procreative choice, and that other persons have a duty not to interfere with that choice.[2] However, the negative right to procreate or not does not imply the duty of others to provide the resources or services necessary to exercise one's procreative liberty despite plausible moral arguments for governmental assistance.

As a matter of constitutional law, procreative liberty is a negative right against state interference with choices to procreate or to avoid procreation. It is not a right against private interference, though other laws might provide that protection. Nor is it a positive right to have the state or particular persons provide the means or resources necessary to have or avoid having children.[3] The exercise of procreative liberty may be severely constrained by social and economic circumstances. Access to medical care, child care, employment, housing, and other services may significantly affect whether one is able to exercise procreative liberty. However, the state presently has no constitutional obligation to provide those services. Whether the state should alleviate those conditions is a separate issue of social justice.[4]

The second qualification is that not everything that occurs in and around procreation falls within liberty interests that are distinctively procreative. Thus whether the father may be present during childbirth, whether midwives may assist birth, or whether childbirth may occur at home rather than in a hospital may be important for the parties involved, but they do not implicate the freedom to reproduce (unless one could show that the place or mode of birth would determine whether birth occurs at all). Similarly, questions about a pregnant woman's drug use or other conduct during pregnancy, a controversial topic treated in chapter 8, implicates liberty in the course of reproduction but not procreative liberty in the basic sense. Questions about whether the use of a technology is distinctively procreative recur throughout this book.

THE IMPORTANCE OF PROCREATIVE LIBERTY

Procreative liberty should enjoy presumptive primacy when conflicts about its exercise arise because control over whether one reproduces or not is central to personal identity, to dignity, and to the meaning of one's life. For example, deprivation of the ability to avoid reproduction determines one's self-definition in the most basic sense. It affects women's bodies in a direct and substantial way. It also centrally affects one's psychological and social identity and one's social and moral responsibilities. The resulting burdens are especially onerous for women, but they affect men in significant ways as well.

On the other hand, being deprived of the ability to reproduce prevents one from an experience that is central to individual identity and meaning in life. Although the desire to reproduce is in part socially constructed, at the most basic level transmission of one's genes through reproduction is an animal or species urge closely linked to the sex drive. In connecting us with nature and future generations, reproduction gives solace in the face of death. As Shakespeare noted, "nothing 'gainst Time's scythe can make defense/save breed."[5] For many people "breed"—reproduction and the parenting that usually accompanies it—is a central part of their life plan, and the most satisfying and meaningful experience they have. It also has primary importance as an expression of a couple's love or unity. For many persons, reproduction also has religious significance and is experienced as a "gift from God." Its denial—through infertility or governmental restriction—is experienced as a great loss, even if one has already had children or will have little or no rearing role with them.

Decisions to have or to avoid having children are thus personal decisions of great import that determine the shape and meaning of one's life. The person directly involved is best situated to determine whether that meaning should or should not occur. An ethic of personal autonomy as well as ethics of community or family should then recognize a presumption in favor of most personal reproductive choices. Such a presumption does not mean that reproductive choices are without consequence to others, nor that they should never be limited. Rather, it means that those who would limit procreative choice have the burden of showing that the reproductive actions at issue would create such substantial harm that they could justifiably be limited. Of course, what counts as the "substantial harm" that justifies interference with procreative choice may often be contested, as the discussion of reproductive technologies in this book will show.

A closely related reason for protecting reproductive choice is to avoid the highly intrusive measures that governmental control of reproduction usually entails. State interference with reproductive choice may extend beyond exhortation and penalties to gestapo and police state tactics. Margaret Atwood's powerful futuristic novel *The Handmaid's Tale* expresses this danger by creating a world where fertile women are forcibly impregnated by the ruling powers and their pregnancies monitored to replenish a decimated population.[6]

Equally frightening scenarios have occurred in recent years when repressive governments have interfered with reproductive choice. In Romania and China, men and women have had their most private activities scrutinized in the service of state reproductive goals. In Ceauşescu's Romania, where contraception and abortion were strictly forbidden, women's menstrual cycles were routinely monitored to see if they were pregnant.[7] Women who did not become pregnant or who had abortions were severely punished. Many women nevertheless sought illegal abortions and died, leaving their children orphaned and subject to sale to Westerners seeking children for adoption.[8]

In China, forcible abortion and sterilization have occurred in the service of a one-child-per-family population policy. Village cadres have seized pregnant women in their homes and forced them to have abortions.[9] A campaign of forcible sterilization in India in 1977 was seen as an "attack on women and children" and brought Indira Ghandi's government down.[10] In the United States, state-imposed sterilization of "mental defectives," sanctioned in 1927 by the United States Supreme Court in *Buck v. Bell*, resulted in 60,000 sterilizations over a forty-year period.[11] Many mentally normal people were sterilized by mistake, and mentally retarded persons who posed little risk of harm to others were subjected to surgery.[12] It is no surprise that current proposals for compulsory use of contraceptives such as Norplant are viewed with great suspicion.

TWO TYPES OF PROCREATIVE LIBERTY

To see how values of procreative liberty affect the ethical and public policy evaluation of new reproductive technologies, we must determine whether the interests that underlie the high value accorded procreative liberty are implicated in their use. This is not a simple task because procreative liberty is not unitary, but consists of strands of varying interests in the conception and gestation of offspring. The different strands implicate different interests, have different legal and constitutional status, and are differently affected by technology.

An essential distinction is between the freedom to avoid reproduction and the freedom to reproduce. When people talk of reproductive rights, they usually have one or the other aspect in mind. Because different inter-

ests and justifications underlie each and countervailing interests for limiting each aspect vary, recognition of one aspect does not necessarily mean
that the other will also be respected; nor does limitation of one mean that
the other can also be denied.

However, there is a mirroring or reciprocal relationship here. Denial of
one type of reproductive liberty necessarily implicates the other. If a
woman is not able to avoid reproduction through contraception or abortion, she may end up reproducing, with all the burdens that unwanted
reproduction entails. Similarly, if one is denied the liberty to reproduce
through forcible sterilization, one is forced to avoid reproduction, thus
experiencing the loss that absence of progeny brings. By extending reproductive options, new reproductive technologies present challenges to
both aspects of procreative choice.

AVOIDING REPRODUCTION: THE LIBERTY
NOT TO REPRODUCE

One sense in which people commonly understand procreative liberty is as
the freedom to avoid reproduction—to avoid begetting or bearing offspring and the rearing demands they make.[13] Procreative liberty in this
sense could involve several different choices, because decisions to avoid
procreation arise at several different stages. A decision not to procreate
could occur prior to conception through sexual abstinence, contraceptive
use, or refusal to seek treatment for infertility. At this stage, the main
issues concern freedom to refrain from sexual intercourse, the freedom to
use contraceptives, and the freedom to withhold gametes for use in noncoital conception. Countervailing interests concern societal interests in
increasing population, a partner's interest in sexual intimacy and progeny, and moral views about the unity of sex and reproduction.

Once pregnancy has occurred, reproduction can be avoided only by
termination of pregnancy. Procreative freedom here would involve the
freedom to abort the pregnancy. Competing interests are protection of
embryos and fetuses and respect for human life generally, the most heated
issue of reproductive rights. They may also include moral or social beliefs
about the connectedness of sex and reproduction, or views about a
woman's reproductive and work roles.

Once a child is born, procreation has occurred, and the procreators
ordinarily have parenting obligations. Freeing oneself from rearing obligations is not strictly speaking a matter of procreative liberty, though it is
an important personal interest. Even if parents relinquish the child for
adoption, the psychological reality that one has reproduced remains. Opposing interests at this stage involve the need to provide parenting, nur-

turing, and financial support to offspring. The right to be free of those obligations, as well as the right to assume them after birth occurs, is not directly addressed in this book except to the extent that those rights affect reproductive decisions.[14]

Technology and the Avoidance of Reproduction

Many reproductive technologies raise questions about the scope of the liberty interest in avoiding reproduction. New contraceptive, contragestive, and abortion technologies raise avoidance issues directly, though the issues raised are not always novel. For example, an important issue in voluntary use of long-lasting contraceptives concerns access by minors and the poor, an issue of justice in the distribution of medical resources that currently exists with other contraceptives. The more publicized issue of whether the state may require child abusers or women on welfare to use Norplant implicates the target group's right to procreate, not their liberty interest in avoiding reproduction.[15]

Contragestive agents such as RU486, which prevent reproduction after conception has occurred, raise many of the current issues of the abortion debate. Because RU486 operates so early in pregnancy, however, it focuses attention on the moral status of very early abortions and the moral differences, if any, between postcoital contraceptives and abortifacients. Ethical assessment and legal rights to use contragestives will depend on the ethical and legal status of early prenatal stages of human life.

More novel avoidance issues will arise with IVF and embryo cryopreservation technology. IVF often produces more embryos than can be safely implanted in the uterus. If couples must donate rather than discard unwanted embryos, they will become biologic parents against their will. This prospect raises the question of whether the liberty interest in avoiding reproduction includes avoiding genetic offspring when no rearing obligations will attach—reproduction *tout court*. Is one's fundamental interest in avoiding reproduction seriously implicated if one will never know or have contact with one's offspring? The resulting moral and policy issue is how to balance the interest in avoiding genetic offspring *tout court* with respect for preimplantation stages of human life.

Technologies of quality control and selection through genetic screening and manipulation will also raise novel questions about the right to avoid reproduction. Prenatal screening enables couples to avoid reproduction because of the genetic characteristics of expected offspring. Are the interests that support protecting the freedom to avoid reproduction present when that freedom is exercised selectively? Because some reasons for rejecting fetuses are more appealing than others, would devising criteria for such choices violate the right not to procreate? For example, should law or morality permit abortion of a fetus with Tay-Sachs disease or Down's syndrome but not female fetuses or fetuses with a disease of varying expressivity such as cystic fibrosis?

Legal Status of Avoiding Reproduction

Legally, the negative freedom to avoid reproduction is widely recognized, though great controversy over abortion persists, and there is no positive constitutional right to contraception and abortion.[16] The freedom to avoid reproduction is clearest for men and women prior to conception. In the United States and most developed countries, marriage and sexual intercourse are a matter of choice. However, rape laws do not always effectively protect women, and some jurisdictions do not criminalize marital rape.[17] Legal access to contraception and sterilization is firmly established, though controversy exists over providing contraception to adolescents because of fears that it would encourage nonmarital sexual intercourse.

Constitutional recognition of the right to use contraceptives—to have sex and not reproduce—occurred in the 1965 landmark case of *Griswold v. Connecticut*.[18] A doctor and a married couple challenged a Connecticut law that made it a crime to use or distribute contraceptives. The United States Supreme Court found that the law violated a fundamental liberty right of married couples, which it later extended to unmarried persons, to use contraceptives as a matter of personal liberty or privacy.[19] Although the Court alluded to the unsavory prospect of police searching the marital bedroom for evidence of the crime as a reason for invalidating the law, it is clear that the Court was protecting the right of persons who engage in sexual intimacy to avoid unwanted reproduction.[20] The right to avoid reproduction through contraception is thus firmly protected, even where fornication laws remain in effect.

Legal protection also exists for other activities tied to avoiding reproduction prior to pregnancy. Thus both men and women are deemed owners of gametes within or outside their bodies, so that they may prevent them from being used for reproduction without their permission. Men and women also have rights to prevent extracorporeal embryos formed from their gametes from being placed in women and brought to term without their consent.[21]

Once conception has occurred, the right to avoid reproduction differs for the woman and man involved. In the United States and most of Western Europe, abortion in early stages of the pregnancy is widely permitted.

Under *Roe v. Wade*, whose central holding was reaffirmed in 1992 in *Planned Parenthood v. Casey*, women, whether single or married, adult or minor, have a right to terminate pregnancy up to viability.[22] However, the state may inform them of its views concerning the worth of the fetus and require them to wait 24 hours before obtaining an abortion.[23] Parental consent or notification requirements can be imposed on minors, as long as a judicial bypass is provided in cases in which the minor does not wish to inform her parents.[24] Also, because the right to abortion is a negative right, the state has no obligation to fund abortions for indigent women.[25]

Although pregnancy termination usually kills the fetus, the right to end pregnancy does not protect the right to cause the death of a fetus that has emerged alive from the abortion process, or even to choose a method of abortion that is most likely to cause fetal demise.[26] Nor does it give a woman the right to engage in prenatal conduct that poses unreasonable risks to the health of future offspring when she is choosing to go to term.[27] After birth occurs, the mother and father have obligations to the child until custody is formally relinquished or transferred to others.

The father, once conception through sexual intercourse has occurred, has no right to require or prevent abortion, and cannot avoid rearing duties of financial support once birth occurs.[28] This is true even if the woman has misled him about her fertility or her use of contraceptives.[29] However, he is free to relinquish custody and give up for adoption. He is also free to determine whether IVF embryos formed from his sperm should be implanted in the uterus.[30]

The law's recognition of a right to avoid reproduction both prior to and after conception provides the legal framework for resolving conflicts presented by new reproductive technologies that affect interests in avoiding reproduction. While many technologies raise the same issues confronted in *Griswold* and *Roe*, new twists will arise that directly challenge the scope of that right. To resolve those conflicts, the separate elements that comprise the interest in avoiding reproduction must be analyzed and evaluated against the competing interests affected by those technologies.

THE FREEDOM TO PROCREATE

In addition to freedom to avoid procreation, procreative liberty also includes the freedom to procreate—the freedom to beget and bear children if one chooses. As with avoiding reproduction, the right to reproduce is a negative right against public or private interference, not a positive right to the services or the resources needed to reproduce. It is an important freedom that is widely accepted as a basic, human right.[31] But its various components and dimensions have never been fully analyzed, as technologies of conception and selection now force us to do.

As with avoiding reproduction, the freedom to procreate involves the freedom to engage in a series of actions that eventuate in reproduction and usually in child rearing. One must be free to marry or find a willing partner, engage in sexual intercourse, achieve conception and pregnancy, carry a pregnancy to term, and rear offspring. Social and natural barriers to reproduction would involve the unavailability of willing or suitable partners, impotence or infertility, and lack of medical and child-care resources. State barriers to marriage, to sexual intercourse, to conception, to infertility treatment, to carrying pregnancies to term, and to certain child-rearing arrangements would also limit the freedom to procreate. The most commonly asserted reasons for limiting coital reproduction are overpopulation, unfitness of parents, harm to offspring, and costs to the state or others. Technologies that treat infertility raise additional concerns that are discussed below.

The moral right to reproduce is respected because of the centrality of reproduction to personal identity, meaning, and dignity. This importance makes the liberty to procreate an important moral right, both for an ethic of individual autonomy and for ethics of community or family that view the purpose of marriage and sexual union as the reproduction and rearing of offspring. Because of this importance, the right to reproduce is widely recognized as a prima facie moral right that cannot be limited except for very good reason.

Recognition of the primacy of procreation does not mean that all reproduction is morally blameless, much less that reproduction is always responsible and praiseworthy and can never be limited. However, the presumptive primacy of procreative liberty sets a very high standard for limiting those rights, tilting the balance in favor of reproducing but not totally determining its acceptability. A two-step process of analysis is envisaged here. The first question is whether a distinctively procreative interest is involved. If so, the question then is whether the harm threatened by reproduction satisfies the strict standard for overriding this liberty interest.

The personal importance of procreation helps answer questions about who holds procreative rights and about the circumstances under which the right to reproduce may be limited. A person's capacity to find signficance in reproduction should determine whether one holds the presumptive right, though this question is often discussed in terms of whether persons with such a capacity are fit parents. To have a liberty interest in procreating, one should at a minimum have the mental capacity to understand or appreciate the meanings associated with reproduction. This minimum would exclude severely retarded persons from having reproductive

interests, though it would not remove their right to bodily integrity. However, being unmarried, homosexual, physically disabled, infected with
HIV, or imprisoned would not disqualify one from having reproductive
interests, though some of those conditions might affect one's ability to
rear offspring. Whether those characteristics justify limitations on reproduction is discussed later.[32] Nor would already having reproduced negate
a person's interest in reproducing again, though at a certain point the
marginal value to a person of additional offspring diminishes.[33]

What kinds of interests or harms make reproduction unduly selfish or
irresponsible and thus could justifiably limit the presumptive right to procreate? To answer this question, we must distinguish coital and noncoital
reproduction. Surprisingly, there is a widespread reluctance to speak of
coital reproduction as irresponsible, much less to urge public action to
prevent irresponsible coital reproduction from occurring. If such a conversation did occur, reasons for limiting coital reproduction would involve the heavy costs that it imposed on others—costs that outweighed
whatever personal meaning or satisfaction the person(s) reproducing experienced. With coital reproduction, such costs might arise if there were
severe overpopulation, if the persons reproducing were unfit parents, if
reproduction would harm offspring, or if significant medical or social
costs were imposed on others.

Because the United States does not face the severe overpopulation of
some countries, the main grounds for claiming that reproduction is irresponsible is where the person(s) reproducing lack the financial means to
raise offspring or will otherwise harm their children. As later discussions
will show, both grounds are seriously inadequate as justifications for interfering with procreative choice. Imposing rearing costs on others may
not rise to the level of harm that justifies depriving a person of a fundamental moral right. Moreover, protection of offspring from unfit parenting requires that unfit parents not rear, not that they not reproduce. Offspring could be protected by having others rear them without interfering
with parental reproduction.

A further problem, if coital reproduction were found to be unjustified,
concerns what action should then be taken. Exhortation or moral condemnation might be acceptable, but more stringent or coercive measures
would act on the body of the person deemed irresponsible. Past experience with forced sterilization of retarded persons and the inevitable focus
on the poor and minorities as targets of coercive policies make such proposals highly unappealing. Because of these doubts, there have been surprisingly few attempts to restrict coital reproduction in the United States
since the era of eugenic sterilization, even though some instances of reproduction—for example, teenage pregnancy, inability to care for offspring—appear to be socially irresponsible.

An entirely different set of concerns arises with noncoital reproductive techniques. Charges that noncoital reproduction is unethical or irresponsible arise because of its expense, its highly technological character, its decomposition of parenthood into genetic, gestational, and social components, and its potential effects on embryos, women, and offspring. To assess whether these effects justify moral condemnation or public limitation, we must first determine whether noncoital reproduction implicates important aspects of procreative liberty.

The Right to Reproduce and Noncoital Technology

If the moral right to reproduce presumptively protects coital reproduction, then it should protect noncoital reproduction as well. The moral right of the coitally infertile to reproduce is based on the same desire for offspring that the coitally fertile have. They too wish to replicate themselves, transmit genes, gestate, and rear children biologically related to them. Their infertility should no more disqualify them from reproductive experiences than physical disability should disqualify persons from moving about with mechanical assistance. The unique risks posed by noncoital reproduction may provide independent justifications for limiting its use, but neither the noncoital nature of the means used nor the infertility of their beneficiaries mean that the presumptively protected moral interest in reproduction is not present.

A major question about this position, however, is whether the noncoital or collaborative nature of the means used truly implicates reproductive interests. For example, what if only one aspect of reproduction—genetic transfer, gestation, or rearing—occurs, as happens with gamete donors or surrogates who play no rearing role? Is a person's procreative liberty substantially implicated in such partial reproductive roles? The answer will depend on the value attributed to the particular collaborative contribution and on whether the collaborative enterprise is viewed from the donor's or recipient's perspective.

Gamete donors and surrogates are clearly reproducing even though they have no intention to rear. Because reproduction *tout court* may seem less important than reproduction with intent to rear, the donor's reproductive interest may appear less important. However, more experience with these practices is needed to determine the inherent value of "partial" reproductive experiences to donors and surrogates.[34] Experience may show that it is independently meaningful, regardless of their contact with offspring. If not, then countervailing interests would more easily override their right to enter these roles.

Viewed from the recipient's perspective, however, the donor or surrogate's reproduction *tout court* does not lessen the reproductive impor-

tance of her contribution. A woman who receives an egg or embryo donation has no genetic connection with offspring but has a gestational
relation of great personal significance. In addition, gamete donors and
surrogates enable one or both rearing partners to have a biological relation with offspring. If one of them has no biological connection at all,
they will still have a strong interest in rearing their partner's biologic
offspring. Whether viewed singly through the eyes of the partner who is
reproducing, or jointly as an endeavor of a couple seeking to rear children
who are biologically related to at least one of the two, a significant reproductive interest is at stake. If so, noncoital, collaborative treatments for
infertility should be respected to the same extent as coital reproduction is.

Questions about the core meaning of reproduction will also arise in the
temporal dislocations that cryopreservation of sperm and embryos make
possible. For example, embryo freezing allows siblings to be conceived at
the same time, but born years apart and to different gestational mothers.
Twins could be created by splitting one embryo into two. If one half is
frozen for later use, identical twins could be born at widely different
times. Sperm, egg, and embryo freezing also make posthumous reproduction possible.

Such temporally dislocative practices clearly implicate core reproductive interests when the ultimate recipient has no alternative means of reproduction. However, if the procreative interests of the recipient couple
are not directly implicated, we must ask whether those whose gametes are
used have an independent procreative interest, as might occur if they directed that gametes or embryos be thawed after their death for purposes
of posthumous reproduction. In that case the question is whether the ex-
pectancy of posthumous reproduction is so central to an individual's procreative identity or life-plan that it should receive the same respect that
one's reproduction when alive receives.[35] The answer to such a question
will be important in devising policy for storing and posthumously dispos-
ing of gametes and embryos. The answer will also affect inheritance questions and have implications for management of pregnant women who are
irreversibly comatose or brain dead.

The problem of determining whether technology implicates a major
reproductive interest also arises with technologies that select offspring
characteristics, a topic addressed in chapter 7. Some degree of quality
control would seem logically to fall within the realm of procreative liberty. For many couples the decision whether to procreate depends on the
ability to have healthy children. Without some guarantee or protection
against the risk of handicapped children, they might not reproduce at all.

Thus viewed, quality control devices become part of the liberty interest
in procreating or in avoiding procreation, and arguably should receive
the same degree of protection. If so, genetic screening and selective abortion, as well as the right to select a mate or a source for donated eggs,

sperm, or embryos should be protected as part of procreative liberty. The same arguments would apply to positive interventions to cure disease at the fetal or embryo stage. However, futuristic practices such as non-therapeutic enhancement, cloning, or intentional diminishment of offspring characteristics may so deviate from the core interests that make reproduction meaningful as to fall outside the protective canopy of procreative liberty.[36]

Finally, technology will present questions of whether one may use one's reproductive capacity to produce gametes, embryos, and fetuses for nonreproductive uses in research or therapy. Here the purpose is not to have children to rear, but to get material for research or transplant. Are such uses of reproductive capacity tied closely enough to the values and interests that underlie procreative freedom to warrant similar respect? Even if procreative choice is not directly involved, other liberties may protect the activity.

Are Noncoital Technologies Unethical?

If this analysis is accepted, then procreative liberty would include the right to use noncoital and other technologies to form a family and shape the characteristics of offspring. Neither infertility nor the fact that one will only partially reproduce eliminates the existence of a prima facie reproductive experience for someone. However, judgments about the proximity of these partial reproductive experiences to the core meanings of reproduction will be required in balancing those claims against competing moral concerns.

Judgment about the reproductive importance of noncoital technologies is crucial because many people have serious ethical reservations about them, and are more than willing to restrict their use. The concerns here are not the fears of overpopulation, parental unfitness, and societal costs that arise with allegedly irresponsible coital reproduction. Instead, they include reduction of demand for hard-to-adopt children, the coercive or exploitive bargains that will be offered to poor women, the commodification of both children and reproductive collaborators, the objectification of women as reproductive vessels, and the undermining of the nuclear family.

However, often the harms feared are deontological in character. In some cases they stem from a religious or moral conception of the unity of sex and reproduction or the definition of family. Such a view characterizes the Vatican's strong opposition to IVF, donor sperm, and other noncoital and collaborative techniques.[37] Other deontological concerns derive from a particular conception of the proper reproductive role of women. Many persons, for example, oppose paid surrogate motherhood because of a judgment about the wrongness of a woman's willingness to sever the mother-child bond for the sake of money.[38] They also insist that the gestational mother is always morally entitled to rear, despite her pre-conception promise to the contrary. Closely related are dignitary objections to allowing any reproductive factors to be purchased, or to having offspring selected on the basis of their genes.

Finally, there is a broader concern that noncoital reproduction will undermine the deeper community interest in having a clear social framework to define boundaries of families, sexuality, and reproduction. The traditional family provides a container for the narcissism and irrationality that often drives human reproduction. This container assures commitments to the identifications and taboos that protect children from various types of abuse. The technical ability to disaggregate and recombine genetic, gestational, and rearing connections and to control the genes of offspring may thus undermine essential protections for offspring, couples, families, and society.

These criticisms are powerful ones that explain much of the ambivalence that surrounds the use of certain reproductive technologies. They call into question the wisdom of individual decisions to use them, and the willingness of society to promote or facilitate their use. Unless one is operating out of a specific religious or deontological ethic, however, they do not show that all individual uses of these techniques are immoral, much less that public policy should restrict or discourage their use.

As later chapters will show, these criticisms seldom meet the high standard necessary to limit procreative choice. Many of them are mere hypothetical or speculative possibilities. Others reflect moralisms concerning a "right" view of reproduction, which individuals in a pluralistic society hold or reject to varying degrees. In any event, without a clear showing of substantial harm to the tangible interests of others, speculation or mere moral objections alone should not override the moral right of infertile couples to use those techniques to form families. Given the primacy of procreative liberty, the use of these techniques should be accorded the same high protection granted to coital reproduction.

Legal Status of the Right to Reproduce

Because there have been few attempts by government to limit reproduction, there is little explicit law concerning the right to reproduce. However, judges in dicta often refer to such a right, and there seems little doubt that the right to procreate would be protected in most circumstances. Such statements generally assume a married couple that seeks to reproduce coitally.

The legal status of the right to reproduce involves the legal right to choose a willing sex or marital partner, to engage in sexual intercourse, to achieve conception and pregnancy, to treat infertility, and to carry pregnancy to term. While laws restricting marriage do affect procreation, there have been few attempts in the United States to restrict the desires of married couples to procreate. No license to become pregnant is needed, contraception is not mandatory, and no laws requiring married couples to be sterilized or to abort have existed. Past laws that required the sterilization of mentally handicapped persons are clearly in disfavor.

In the United States laws restricting coital reproduction by a married couple would have to withstand the strict scrutiny applied to interference with fundamental constitutional rights. Although no right to reproduce is explicitly mentioned in the Constitution, dicta in many cases suggest that such a right exists.[39]

The strongest precedent here is the case of *Skinner v. Oklahoma*, a 1942 case in which the Court struck down a state law that authorized thieves but not embezzlers to be sterilized without consent after a third conviction. Although relying on an equal protection rationale, the Court stressed the importance of marriage and procreation as among "the basic civil rights of man" and noted that "marriage and procreation are fundamental to the very existence and survival of the race."[40] Under this principle, persons cannot be selectively deprived of their right of procreation, and the state must justify any deprivation by showing a compelling state interest that could not be satisfied in alternative ways.

Many other Supreme Court cases contain statements that support the protected status of decisions to reproduce. In *Meyer v. Nebraska*, where the right of parents to have their children learn a foreign language was upheld, the Court stated that constitutional liberty includes "the right of an individual to marry, establish a home and bring up children."[41] In *Stanley v. Illinois*, the Court, in upholding an unmarried father's right to rear his child, stated that "rights to conceive and raise one's children have been deemed 'essential,' 'basic civil rights of man,' and 'rights far more precious than property rights.' "[42] *Cleveland Bd. of Education v. LaFleur* recognized a pregnant teacher's right to continue to teach in part because "freedom of personal choice in matters of marriage and family life is one of the liberties protected by the Due Process clause of the Fourteenth Amendment."[43] The most ringing endorsement of this right occurred in *Eisenstadt v. Baird* when the Court extended the right to obtain contraceptives to unmarried persons. Justice Brennan, in an opinion for the Court, stated:[44] "If the right of privacy means anything, it is the right of the individual, married or single, to be free of unwarranted governmental intrusion into matters so fundamentally affecting a person as the decision whether to bear or beget a child." Most recently, in the 1992 decision in *Casey v. Planned Parenthood*, Justices O'Connor, Kennedy, and Souter stated that "our law affords constitutional protection to personal decisions relating to marriage, procreation, contraception, family relationships, childrearing and education. [These] matters, involving the most intimate and personal choices a person may make in a lifetime, choices central to personal dignity and autonomy, are central to the liberty protected by the Fourteenth Amendment."[45]

Such statements suggest that a married couple's right to reproduce would be recognized even by conservative justices if a case restricting coital reproduction ever reached the Supreme Court. Coital reproduction has been traditionally recognized as one of the main functions of marriage and family.[46] The right of bodily integrity would also protect the right to procreate coitally to the extent that state interference with procreation mandated sterilization, contraception, or abortion.

As a consequence, married couples would have a fundamental constitutional right against state limits on coital reproduction, whether it takes the form of penalizing them for having more than a set number of children, requiring licenses to parent, or mandating sterilization, contraception, or abortion.[47] Restrictions on marital reproduction are theoretically possible only if the state can show great harm to others from the reproduction in question.

A situation that might justify such a limitation would be severe overpopulation, but such a restriction would have to be equitably distributed and structured to minimize coercion and unwanted bodily intrusion. Other situations involving harm to offspring or great costs to others can be envisaged, but it is unclear whether they would satisfy the high level of substantive justification necessary. For example, women on welfare who have more than a designated number of children could not be criminally punished for additional reproduction, much less forcibly sterilized or aborted, though they might not qualify for additional welfare payments.[48] Similarly, married couples with HIV could not be punished for having offspring.[49] A child infected with HIV who has no other way to be born disease-free has not been harmed, and the avoidance of medical costs is not a compelling justification for limiting reproduction.

One of the few court cases that has dealt directly with limitations on marital reproduction denied a married federal prison inmate the right to hand his wife a container of his sperm so that she might be artificially inseminated outside of prison and thus produce offspring of the marriage.[50] The federal appeals court's analysis of the competing interests in that case gave insufficient weight to the couple's reproductive interest and too much weight to the prison authorities' claims of administrative inconvenience.[51] Because the case arose in the special setting of a prison, it is not a strong precedent for limiting procreative choice in nonprison settings.

Unmarried persons may have strong interests in reproducing outside of marriage, and in many cases may be excellent child rearers. It is unclear, however, whether unmarried persons have the same constitutional rights to reproduce coitally that married persons do. Although the Court has recognized the right of unmarried persons to use birth control and terminate pregnancies, this is a right to avoid pregnancy and reproduction. It does not necessarily imply a right to engage in coitus in order to get pregnant. The Supreme Court has never recognized a right to engage in fornication, adultery, or incest, even though those actions could lead to procreation.[52] Because those laws have a pedigree and tradition as long as the practice of marital reproduction, the Court might be extremely reluctant to strike down fornication laws on the ground that they interfere with nonmarital procreation, much less recognize the right to engage in adulterous, polygamous, incestuous, or nonconsensual sex in order to procreate.

As a practical matter, however, the state's possible constitutional power to ban nonmarital forms of sexual intercourse gives it only a limited tool to restrict nonmarital reproduction. With over 30 percent of births in 1993 occurring out of wedlock, it is unrealistic to think that laws prohibiting nonmarital sex or penalizing unmarried reproduction would accomplish much.[53] Only a minority of states have such laws, and they are seldom enforced. Moreover, this power would not imply the right to require that unmarried persons be sterilized, use contraception, undergo involuntary abortion, or lose custody of illegitimate children.[54]

The main significance of denying unmarried persons a constitutional right to procreate would arise with state restrictions on access to infertility treatment and assisted conception. If an unmarried person's right to procreate is not constitutionally recognized, states could limit access to infertility treatments on the basis of marital status, sexual orientation, disability, or other factors that are not prohibited by state or federal antidiscrimination laws. Such a status could effectively bar some persons with valid interests in reproducing from access to noncoital means of reproduction.

The Legal Status of Noncoital Reproduction

The law has not yet dealt with legal claims of infertile persons to procreate, yet the principles that underlie a constitutional right to reproduce would seem to apply to the infertile as well. If so, they would have a negative constitutional right to use a wide variety of reproductive technologies to have offspring.[55]

If married (and possibly even single) persons have a presumptive right to reproduce coitally, what then about persons who cannot reproduce coitally? Coital infertility is no indication of a couple's adequacy as child rearers. Their desire to have a family—to beget, bear, and rear offspring—is as strong as in fertile couples. Because the values and interests that undergird the right of coital reproduction clearly exist with the coitally infertile, their actions to form a family also deserve respect. If so, the same standard of scrutiny applied to state action that restricts coital reproduction should apply to state restrictions on noncoital means of treating infertility.

Yet some people have challenged this notion, arguing that there is no legal right to reproduce if one lacks the physical ability to do so. But consider the analogous effect of blindness on the First Amendment right to read books. Surely a blind person has the same right to acquire information from books that a sighted person has. The inability to read visually would not bar the person from using braille, recordings, or a sighted reader to acquire the information contained in the book. Because receipt of the book's information is protected by the First Amendment, the means by which the information is received does not itself determine the presence or absence of First Amendment rights.

Similarly, if bearing, begetting, or parenting children is protected as part of personal privacy or liberty, those experiences should be protected whether they are achieved coitally or noncoitally. In either case they satisfy the basic biologic, social, and psychological drive to have a biologically related family. Although full genetic reproduction might not exist in each case, the interest of the couple in rearing children who are biologically related to one or both rearing partners is so close to the coital model that it should be treated equivalently. Noncoital reproduction should thus be constitutionally protected to the same extent as is coital reproduction, with the state having the burden of showing severe harm if the practice is unrestricted.

This conclusion is clearest with noncoital techniques that employ the couple's egg and sperm, as occurs with IVF or artificial insemination with husband sperm. Religious or moral objections to the separation of sex and reproduction should not override the use of these techniques for forming a family. However, because the only case dealing with artificial insemination with husband sperm arose in a prison setting, a direct precedent for the right to use these techniques has not yet been established.[56]

Similar protection should extend to the use of gamete donation to overcome gametic infertility in one member of the couple, as occurs in sperm and egg donation. Gamete donation permits the married couple to raise offspring biologically related to one or both parents (as in the case of egg donation). Again, moral objections to the noncoital nature per se of the conception or to the involvement of a third party without further indication of harm should not suffice to ban such procedures.

Use of a surrogate should also be presumptively protected, since it enables an infertile couple to have and rear the genetic offspring of both husband and wife in the case of gestational surrogacy, and of the husband in the case of full surrogacy. Indeed, recognizing the couple's right to use a surrogate is necessary to avoid discrimination against infertile wives. If an infertile male can parent his wife's child through the use of donor sperm, an infertile woman should be free to parent her husband's child through use of a surrogate. This is all the clearer if the surrogate is carrying the embryo of the couple.[57]

Of course, finding that the interests that underlie coital reproduction are present in noncoital and collaborative reproduction does not eliminate the harms or ill effects that some persons fear. Presumptive protection of these techniques, however, shifts the burden to those who would restrict them to establish the compelling harm that would outweigh the couple's reproductive liberty. As later chapters will show, it is difficult to show that the alleged harms of noncoital reproduction are sufficient to justify overriding procreative liberty.

Similar issues arise with legal regulation of technologies that alter the temporal sequence of reproduction, that affect the genetic makeup of offspring, and that allow tissue or embryos to be produced for research or transplant. In resolving these legal disputes, the constitutional primacy of procreative liberty and the need for strict scrutiny of competing state interests should be recognized.

RESOLVING DISPUTES OVER PROCREATIVE LIBERTY

As this brief survey shows, new reproductive technologies will generate ethical and legal disputes about the meaning and scope of procreative liberty. Because procreative liberty has never been fully elaborated, the importance of procreative choice in many novel settings will be a question of first impression. The ultimate decision reached will reflect the value assigned to the procreative interest at stake in light of the effects causing concern. In an important sense, the meaning of procreative liberty will be created or constituted for society in the process of resolving such disputes.

If procreative liberty is taken seriously, a strong presumption in favor of using technologies that centrally implicate reproductive interests should be recognized. Although procreative rights are not absolute, those who would limit procreative choice should have the burden of establishing substantial harm. This is the standard used in ethical and legal analyses of restrictions on traditional reproductive decisions. Because the same procreative goals are involved, the same standard of scrutiny should be used for assessing moral or governmental restrictions on novel reproductive techniques.

In arbitrating these disputes, one has to come to terms with the importance of procreative interests relative to other concerns. The precise procreative interest at stake must be identified and weighed against the core values of reproduction. As noted, this will raise novel and unique questions when the technology deviates from the model of two-person coital reproduction, or otherwise disaggregates or alters ordinary reproductive practices. However, if an important reproductive interest exists, then use of the technology should be presumptively permitted. Only substantial harm to tangible interests of others should then justify restriction.

In determining whether such harm exists, it will be necessary to distinguish between harms to individuals and harms to personal conceptions of morality, right order, or offense, discounted by their probability of occurrence. As previously noted, many objections to reproductive technology rest on differing views of what "proper" or "right" reproduction is aside from tangible effects on others. For example, concerns about the decomposition of parenthood through the use of donors and surrogates, about the temporal alteration of conception, gestation and birth, about the alienation or commercialization of gestational capacity, and about selection and control of offspring characteristics do not directly affect persons so much as they affect notions of right behavior. Disputes over early abortion and discard or manipulation of IVF-created embryos also exemplify this distinction, if we grant that the embryo/previable fetus is not a person or entity with rights in itself.

At issue in these cases is the symbolic or constitutive meaning of actions regarding prenatal life, family, maternal gestation, and respect for persons over which people in a secular, pluralistic society often differ. A majoritarian view of "right" reproduction or "right" valuation of prenatal life, family, or the role of women should not suffice to restrict actions based on differing individual views of such preeminently personal issues. At a certain point, however, a practice such as cloning, enhancement, or intentional diminishment of offspring may be so far removed from even pluralistic notions of reproductive meaning that they leave the realm of protected reproductive choice.[58] People may differ over where that point is, but it will not easily exclude most reproductive technologies of current interest.

To take procreative liberty seriously, then, is to allow it to have presumptive priority in an individual's life. This will give persons directly involved the final say about use of a particular technology, unless tangible harm to the interests of others can be shown. Of course, people may differ over whether an important procreative interest is at stake or over how serious the harm posed from use of the reproductive technology is. Such a focused debate, however, is legitimate and ultimately essential in developing ethical standards and public policy for use of new reproductive technologies.

THE LIMITS OF PROCREATIVE LIBERTY

The emphasis on procreative liberty that informs this book provides a useful but by no means complete or final perspective on the technologies in question. Theological, social, psychological, economic, and feminist perspectives would emphasize different aspects of reproductive technology, and might be much less sanguine about potential benefits and risks. Such perspectives might also offer better guidance in how to use these technologies to protect offspring, respect women, and maintain other important values.

A strong rights perspective has other limitations as well. Recognition of procreative liberty, whether in traditional or in new technological settings, does not guarantee that people will achieve their reproductive goals, much less that they will be happy with what they do achieve. Nature may be recalcitrant to the latest technology. Individuals may lack the will, the perseverance, or the resources to use effective technologies. Even if they do succeed, the results may be less satisfying than envisaged. In addition, many individual instances of procreative choice may cumulate into larger social changes that from our current vantage point seem highly undesirable. But these are the hazards and limitations of any scheme of individual rights.

Recognition of procreative liberty will protect the right of persons to use technology in pursuing their reproductive goals, but it will not eliminate the ambivalence that such technologies engender. Societal ambivalence about reproductive technology is recapitulated at the individual level, as individuals and couples struggle with whether to use the technologies in question. Thus recognition of procreative liberty will not eliminate the dilemmas of personal choice and responsibility that reproductive choice entails. The freedom to act does not mean that we will act wisely, yet denying that freedom may be even more unwise, for it denies individuals' respect in the most fundamental choices of their lives.

ABORTION AND CONTRACEPTION

CHAPTER 3

Abortion, Contragestion, and the Resuscitation of *Roe v. Wade*

THE FORTUNES of adversaries in the abortion debate have waxed and waned with political and legal change. In 1992 the election of President Bill Clinton and the Supreme Court's reaffirmation of abortion rights in *Planned Parenthood v. Casey* placed the pro-choice position in ascendancy.[1] The goal of prohibiting abortion is no longer on the public agenda.

Casey, however, modified *Roe v. Wade*'s rigid protection of abortion rights by accepting an undue burden test for governmental regulation. This test allows states considerable elbow room to discourage abortion through waiting periods, informed consent, and other regulatory requirements. The result is a modified pro-choice position that is likely to dominate ethical, legal, and popular thinking about abortion for the foreseeable future.

An important influence in the current situation is the increasing attention being paid to nuances of prenatal biology. The spread of in vitro fertilization has helped to focus attention on the earliest stages of human life. New contragestive drugs prevent fertilized eggs from implanting or interrupt implantation shortly after it occurs. As these techniques become routine, abortions will increasingly occur at the embryonic or prefetal stage of development. This will reinforce the modified pro-choice position and may help defuse the abortion controversy.

These developments will not cause the fervent pro-life minority that is willing to picket, protest, and pummel for pro-life causes to fold up their tents. However, with the loss of the White House, these groups have lost their main channel to legal change and their power is clearly in decline.[2] Others leery of abortion will be less energized to fight a policy that allows abortion while actively seeking to discourage it, particularly as advances in technology push pregnancy terminations to the earliest possible time. Law and technology together thus have the potential to dampen the abortion wars that have racked the country for the last 20 years. They will also influence how other technologies for avoiding reproduction are received.[3]

After describing the modified pro-choice position, this chapter will first consider the morality of early abortion. It will then describe the modified pro-choice legal situation, which is likely to remain fixed for the foreseeable future. Finally, it will address the potential role of contragestive technology in modulating the abortion debate, and the larger symbolic meanings that animate the abortion controversy.

THE MIDDLE GROUND: DISCOURAGE BUT
PERMIT ABORTIONS

The dominant emerging consensus about the moral and legal status of abortion lies between the two extremes of total pro-choice and absolute right to life, though it is much closer to the pro-choice position than its opposite. To paraphrase President Clinton, abortion should be safe, legal, and rare.

This middle position may be characterized as one in which abortion at early stages of pregnancy is generally viewed in most circumstances to be an ethically and legally acceptable act, but an act that should be discouraged or avoided whenever possible. As pregnancy progresses, abortion becomes more morally questionable, and greater efforts to discourage it through informed-consent policies and waiting periods are justified. At or near viability, abortions can be prohibited altogether, except when necessary to protect the life or health of the mother. No limits on the reasons for abortion can be imposed prior to viability, nor can third parties be given veto power over the woman's choice. However, public funding is not required, and parents can be notified or asked to consent to a minor's abortion as long as an alternative for minors unwilling to inform parents is provided.

Although this position is very close to the law's pro-choice position that has been in force since 1973, it does leave room for discouragement of abortion—the position that the vast majority seem to accept. For example, Congress and most states have chosen not to fund abortions for indigents. In addition, *Casey* recognizes the state's role as an educator and persuader, though not a coercer. It permits state efforts to inform women of facts of fetal status and adoption alternatives and to require reasonable waiting periods to contemplate their decision.

There is also ample room to prevent abortion through sex education and provision of contraception, though these means are controversial when directed at minors. A society committed to reducing the incidence of abortion could make sex education and provision of contraceptives a hallmark of public policy, as well as make child-care support available for pregnant women who feel they have no alternative to abortion. In addition, public policy efforts could be directed at having abortions occur at the earliest possible time, when they are least ethically problematic. To do so, both the morning-after pill and contragestives such as RU486 should be made available. As these actions occur, they will further entrench the middle position.

A public policy that permits abortion but tries to minimize its incidence most accurately reflects present ethical, legal, and public thinking. The ethical and legal bases for this statement are discussed in greater depth below. But there is ample evidence that it also reflects public opinion. Polls have consistently shown that a majority of Americans oppose abortion on demand, but are not willing to make it a crime.[4] Furthermore, a clear majority favors abortion to protect the life and health of the mother, in cases of rape or incest, and to prevent handicapped births.[5] As law, social practice, and new technology encourage earlier abortion, support for this position is likely to grow, for it has the greatest chance of minimizing abortion while permitting women this option.

However, the dominant middle position has two major drawbacks. One is that it will not immediately end the polarization and conflict that have swirled around abortion. Right-to-life groups have lost the battle to criminalize abortion, but they will not "go gently into that good night." They are likely to remain a powerful legislative force at both the state and federal levels. They will be successful in some states in getting informed consent, waiting periods, and parental-notice provisions passed that effectively deny abortion to younger and poorer women. They may also succeed in blocking the federal Freedom of Choice Act that would codify *Roe v. Wade* and in excluding abortion from any national health insurance plan. Their more militant wing is likely to continue intrusive picketing, vandalism, violence, and even murder against abortion providers for some time.[6] Still, informed consent, waiting periods, parental notice, and policies to prevent abortion are a significant step toward the middle. The result begins to look like the compromise position that some scholars claim has prevented extreme polarization on abortion in Europe.[7]

The second drawback of the emerging middle position is endemic to the classic liberal position on rights, which places a premium on education and means. Those who have the means and knowledge to exercise their rights are well protected. Those who lack the means have the right in name only. Persons too young, poor, or uneducated to use contraceptives or get access to early abortion will end up with less reproductive choice than those with wealth, power, and knowledge. Yet they are the group that will be most affected by informed consent, waiting periods, and other state efforts to discourage abortion. They are also more likely to seek later abortions.

To prevent such distributive inequities, public policy should focus on sex education, including information about contraception and early abortion, and fund or provide contraceptive and abortion services. With the legal right to abortion no longer in question, controversy over assuring all women effective access to this right is likely to continue.

ETHICAL JUSTIFICATIONS

Abortion has been an intractable issue because of the clash of moral absolutes it presents.[8] On one side are pregnant women who want to be free of the burdens of unwanted pregnancy. To deny them the right to terminate pregnancy effectively denies them the right to avoid reproduction, because birth control may be unavailable or ineffective. On the other hand, abortion destroys an embryo or fetus, and thus displays a willingness to take human life. How is such a fierce conflict to be resolved?

Morally, it seems wrong to deny women control over this most important decision, yet it does not follow that they should be able to abort at all stages of pregnancy. No one can cause a newborn's death to avoid the burdens of child rearing or the pain of relinquishing an infant for adoption. If the fetus is very close to a newborn in neurological and cognitive development, abortion should also be limited. At earlier stages, there are also ethical and symbolic considerations that counsel discouragement, even if they do not justify prohibition. It is clearly preferable to control fertility with contraceptives and abstinence rather than with abortion. If contraceptives fail or are unavailable and abstinence is not possible, then abortion should occur at the earliest possible time. Finally, asking women who abort to consider carefully their position for a set period before the abortion may also be defensible.[9]

A position that opposes all abortion is hard to justify, except for persons who hold extreme right-to-life views. Although abortion shows a disregard for prenatal human life, it is difficult to equate abortion with murder, which traditionally has been defined as the killing of a live-born person separate from the mother, a category that never covered fetuses.[10] Calling all abortion "murder" overlooks the very different biologic stages of embryonic and fetal development, and the moral distinctions that rest on them. A moral position that values all postconception, prenatal stages equally will not appeal to the widely shared, commonsense moral perception that human potential at early stages of gestation is not always an overriding value.

For these reasons, the modified pro-choice position that recognizes a moral and legal right to early abortion but seeks to discourage or prevent abortion has much greater appeal. It does not deny the symbolic meanings that attend the destruction of prenatal life, even though it permits women to abort up until the point of viability. At the same time, it allows room for actions to discourage abortion through education, persuasion, and other services even though a woman's final choice over such a fundamental matter must be respected.

But can this middle position be morally justified? At issue is the priority of bodily integrity and autonomy over prenatal life, of avoidance of gestational and reproductive burdens versus fetal status and respect for human life. A more extended discussion of these issues follows.

Abortion and Procreative Liberty

The moral argument for the modified pro-choice position begins with a recognition of the importance of abortion for the freedom to avoid reproduction. While abstinence and contraception are an essential bulwark of this liberty, many women do not have access to effective contraception, and abstinence may not be a realistic option.[11] Even with assiduous contraceptive use, unwanted pregnancies will occur. Control over pregnancy and parenthood is thus intimately tied to continued access to abortion.

If women lack the liberty to end unwanted pregnancy, they will undergo major physical, social, and pyschological burdens that deprive them of control of the physical and social self in essential ways. Most immediately, the burden is felt in physical terms, as their bodies are taken over by pregnancy. But pregnancy carried to term also entails responsibility for offspring. Even if the child is relinquished for adoption, there will be powerful feelings of attachment, responsibility, and guilt that will, in many cases, last a lifetime. Men whose children are reared by others may also feel responsibility and guilt, even if they avoid financial or other rearing responsibility for their offspring.

Abortion, as well as other issues of avoidance of reproduction, is about escaping those burdens.[12] Any account of individual autonomy and respect for persons must recognize the prima facie liberty interest of women in being free of the burdens of unwanted reproduction. To deny presumptive right status to this interest is to deny that a woman has the fundamental right to control what is done to her body and her life. Denying women the presumptive right to end pregnancy in effect commandeers or "takes" their bodies, treating them as public property or resources to advance other interests. It is not surprising that the language of involuntary servitude and conscription has come increasingly to characterize the pro-choice position.[13]

But presumptive rights are not absolute rights. Abortion presents the question of whether the presumptive right to avoid reproduction through abstinence and contraception remains once a woman has sex and gets pregnant. Her interest in avoiding reproduction is now no longer an abstraction, but an acute reality directly impinging on her. The question of whether she retains the right to avoid reproduction after conception and pregnancy is really a question of whether competing interests in protecting prenatal life justify imposing the heavy burdens of unwanted pregnancy and reproduction upon her.

In assessing this question, we must remember that no right is absolute and that even fundamental moral or constitutional rights have limits when substantial, unjustified harm to others can be shown. Thus a person's keen interest in avoiding the social burdens of reproduction does not justify infanticide nor assault on a pregnant woman to prevent her from giving birth. The moral question raised by abortion is whether protection of fertilized eggs, embryos, and fetuses is close enough to the protection of persons after birth for abortion to be justifiably limited.

In addressing this question, an essential point is that a high standard of justification should be met to warrant overriding the woman's presumptive right to end pregnancy. Protecting the life or health of others would ordinarily satisfy that standard. However, moral objections or symbolic commitments alone, over which individuals in a pluralistic society usually make their own choice, will not. The ethical argument for or against abortion will thus turn on whether interests affected by abortion meet this high standard of justification.

Abortion and Fetal Status

The most commonly articulated basis for opposition to abortion rests on views of the moral status of the fetus. This argument is made in both a strong and a weak form. The strong form takes the position that fertilized eggs, embryos, and fetuses are already persons with rights and interests to be protected. The weak form of the argument asserts not that the fetus is already a person, but that its clear potential to become one requires that actions that would harm or destroy it be avoided.

THE STRONG FORM: FETUS AS PERSON

Some persons opposed to abortion take the strong view that fertilization and subsequent stages of prenatal development involve a new person. To them, fertilization is the crucial event, because it produces a genetically unique, alive, human entity—an "unborn child"—that has all the rights and interests of born children. Abortion is therefore regarded as the murder or destruction of an "innocent human life" and should be prohibited.

A response to the strong claim can be made both on biologic and on moral grounds.[14] In biologic terms, a fertilized egg, embryo, or fetus cannot be a person or even a moral subject with interests and rights because it is too undeveloped biologically. In the earliest stages, it lacks differentiated organs and a nervous system.[15] Even when those are developed, they still are far short of the cognitive ability to reason or even to feel pain and sensation that make a living entity a moral subject in its own right. Not until sentience is reached, roughly at viability in the twenty-fourth to twenty-sixth weeks of pregnancy, does the fetus develop interests in its own right. Viability does not, however, mark personhood in the moral sense, because the viable fetus still lacks the ability to reason or make choices, though it might be a moral subject because it is sentient. The strong view's claim of personhood thus appears to mistake potential for actual personhood.[16]

This argument will not, of course, persuade those who view the fertilized egg as a person that they are mistaken. It will, however, appeal to persons who think that a certain degree of biological development or maturity is essential before fetuses are owed respect in their own right. It also explains the appeal of a cutoff line for abortion at viability.

The strong version also mistakenly assumes that even if the embryo or fetus were clearly a person, a woman would always be morally obligated to allow it to occupy her body for nine months. As the philosopher Judith Jarvis Thomson has shown in a classic article, acceptance of fetal personhood does not itself determine that the fetus has the right to occupy a woman's body.[17] Since it is the woman's body, giving the embryo/fetus-person a right to occupy it would have to depend on some premise other than its personhood alone. Thomson shows that in many cases, such as rape and sexual intercourse with contraception, a persuasive moral claim that the fetus has the right to use the body of another cannot be made. So even if the fetus were a person, it would not follow that abortion—expelling the fetus—would be wrong in all cases.

At the very least, viewing the fetus as person should allow the woman who is not morally responsible for its attachment to be free to unhook the fetus, in order to relieve her of further bodily burdens.[18] It would not necessarily give her the right to cause its death in unhooking, if safe unhooking were otherwise possible, nor in causing its death once the fetus were expelled. Her morally protectable interest is in becoming free of bodily burdens and not in avoiding reproduction altogether.

The Thomson analysis is extremely useful for focusing attention on the competing interests at stake, and on the all-important question of under what circumstances one person has a moral obligation to provide his or her body or its parts to another. Although the analysis responds directly to the claim that the fetus is a person, it is also relevant when persons argue that abortion is inherently disrespectful of human life.

THE WEAK FORM: THE DUTY TO RESPECT POTENTIAL PERSONS

In the weaker version, the claim is not that the fertilized egg, embryo, or fetus is already a person or moral subject, but that it is genetically unique and will, if no interruption occurs, become one at birth. Because it is human, genetically unique, and has the potential to become a person, it should be protected out of respect for human life generally. Thus abortion is immoral and should be prohibited because it demonstrates a disregard for a human life that soon will be a person.

One may recognize the potentiality of the fetus, however, without also concluding that abortion is always wrong and should be prohibited. The essence of this claim is that we ought to respect embryos and fetuses, not because they are entities that in themselves have moral claims on us, but because they have the potential to develop into persons, and thus are an important setting in which to demonstrate our respect for human life generally.[19] Even if abortion is not the equivalent of murder, abortion still denotes a devaluation of the sanctity of human life because it ranks avoidance of the burdens of pregnancy over commitment to potential persons.

But acceptance of this view does not necessarily lead to the conclusion that abortion is inherently immoral or always should be prohibited. Rather, it emphasizes the symbolic dimensions of abortion—abortion is wrong because it symbolizes disrespect for human life. But if the harm of abortion is a symbolic loss of respect for human life and not a substantive violation of fetal rights, then the costs and benefits of this symbolic loss, relative to other values, such as the woman's interest in avoiding unwanted pregnancy, must be compared. Given the great impact of unwanted pregnancy, reasonable persons might find that the benefits to the woman of abortion far outweigh its symbolic costs, particularly at early stages of pregnancy. In any event, given that people may reasonably differ over the existence and extent of those costs, should not the pregnant woman's weighing of the competing interests be presumptively respected?

At the very least, the weak version should lead to closer distinctions about the circumstances of the abortion, including the stage of pregnancy and why abortion is being sought. For example, an early abortion should be symbolically more acceptable than a later one, because the loss of an early embryo or fetus shows less disrespect for life than an abortion of a fully developed or viable fetus. Also, a woman's circumstances and reasons for abortion might also be relevant to an assessment of symbolic effects. For example, a second-trimester abortion to avoid female offspring would be viewed differently than an early abortion for a fourteen-year-old girl, a woman with three children under five whose birth control failed, or a woman who is simply unwilling to parent a child. A fuller discussion of acceptable or unacceptable reasons for abortion is needed to analyze these differences. Even if one's moral evaluation of her judgment will vary, it is still reasonable to conclude that the final decision in most circumstances should be left to the woman directly affected.

In any event, the weak version of the anti-abortion argument, in granting that the embryo or fetus has no rights in itself but is a powerful symbol, allows more nuanced moral judgments about the propriety of abortion. Even if abortion should be avoided whenever possible, there will be many circumstances in which avoiding the burdens of unwanted pregnancy will still be morally justified. When pushed to the limit, such a view supports privileging the pregnant woman's views of when an unwanted pregnancy may be terminated.

THE IMPORTANCE OF VIABILITY

The intermediate position of discouragement but not prohibition of abortion has a limit at viability. The viability line recognizes the biological reality of progressive fetal development: that at some point before birth the fetus is sufficiently developed so that abortion becomes morally unacceptable. Viability, which is defined as the ability to survive outside the uterus, is generally put at twenty-four to twenty-six weeks. At this point a large percentage of aggressively treated premature infants survive, although they often have handicaps.

While physicians may debate when exactly viability is reached, it is important to be clear about why this line should count. In *Roe v. Wade*, the Supreme Court gave a definition of viability ("potentially able to live outside the mother's womb, albeit with artificial aid"), but omitted the syllogism that explained why external survival should count as grounds for overriding the woman's interests in aborting.[20] An explanation often given is that at viability a viable fetus so strongly resembles a newborn infant that the two should be treated similarly. But this account overlooks the great differences in physical development that remain, and fails to specify why or what degree of resemblance is sufficient to make resemblance a determinative moral factor.

A more cogent explanation is that at or around viability the fetus acquires the neurologic capacity for sentience, and thus has interests in its own right. If so, at viability the concern is no longer merely symbolic, but the concern is to protect a subject with interests from harm. If technology pushes viability back to earlier presentient stages, it will cease to have this moral significance, because survivability will no longer correlate with sentience. Note, however, that having interests is not the same as achieving personhood.[21] Moral duties can be owed to sentient beings, such as animals, that are not persons.

One might also understand the viability line in symbolic terms. At viability the symbolic costs of destroying a potential person simply become too great. Because a viable fetus that can be valued for itself and not merely its potential now exists, destroying it has much greater symbolic costs than abortion earlier in pregnancy. In addition, abortion ordinarily could have occurred at an earlier, less symbolically charged stage of pregnancy. Unless there is a compelling reason for late termination, the gain to the woman at this late stage would appear to be outweighed by the symbolic cost of aborting such a well-developed entity.

Clarity about why viability is a limit is essential to avoid the contradictions that arise from an emphasis on survivability alone. Although abortion is usually associated with the death of the fetus or embryo, this is not always the case. While some abortion techniques (aspiration or curettage) dismember and thus directly kill the fetus, other techniques (prostaglandin induction) cause the fetus to be expelled from the uterus. If expulsion occurs at viability, the fetus could survive, thus enabling the woman's interest in avoiding gestation to be met without also causing fetal demise.

The Supreme Court's emphasis on survivability rather than sentience leads to a contradiction. If ability to survive is key, then termination of pregnancy without causing fetal death should be permitted rather than prohibited at viability, because fetuses could then survive and a woman would be freed of further gestation. Similarly, previable abortions should then be postponed until viability, to assure fetal survival.[22] Yet these conclusions are the exact opposite of the Court's holding in *Roe*.

This contradiction can be avoided by making the fetus's interests in its own right rather than survivability key. Once the fetus becomes a subject in its own right, its interests are to avoid pain and to continue to grow and to be delivered as healthy as possible. Expelling the fetus nonlethally at viability will produce a premature newborn who is much worse off than if the pregnancy were not aborted. The child then faces a long, costly stay in a neonatal intensive care unit and the possibility of severe physical and mental deficits.[23] If it has interests at viability, its interests are to be brought into the world as healthy as possible. Termination at viability without demise is preferable only if demise is the only other alternative.

From the woman's perspective, abortion at viability does relieve her of further gestation, but she will remain responsible for the premature newborn's well-being until she terminates legal custody, and may feel guilt and concern at having caused her surviving son or daughter to survive with handicaps due to premature birth. Her interest in not procreating will not have been satisfied, except to the extent that she has avoided several weeks of gestation.

The technical ability to separate gestation and fetal survival is a solution to the abortion problem only in cases where one thinks that the woman has a strong interest in a late-term abortion. Lack of access or diagnostic uncertainty about the woman's or fetus's health may occasionally cause the need for a postviability abortion. One could minimize fetal harm and symbolic costs while still permitting abortions at this stage by requiring that they be done with prostaglandins or other methods that maximize the chance of fetal survival. Such a solution, however, is hardly ideal, and will affect only a small number of abortions.

SPECIAL RESPECT FOR PRENATAL LIFE AS AN
INTERMEDIATE POSITION

This analysis of fetal interests responds to the deeply felt sense that biological status is morally relevant. Persons who oppose this view must take either the strong view that embryos and fetuses are persons since fertilization, or the weak view of the symbolic importance of protecting prenatal life. Yet both views seem inadequate to justify depriving a woman of choice over an unwanted pregnancy prior to viability. The strong view must overcome the biological reality that the ordinary attributes of persons are missing in fertilized eggs, embryos, and fetuses.[24] The weak view must show why the symbolic meanings of early abortion should take priority over the reasonable views of the pregnant woman and others of the greater importance of ending pregnancy.

Whatever one's ultimate assessment of these arguments, it is important to recognize that some common ground for respecting prenatal life remains. Although people may differ over whether the embryo/fetus is a person or whether abortion should be permitted, they may still accord prenatal life special respect because it is genetically unique, living, human tissue that, as pregnancy progresses, increases in capacity and eventually becomes a newborn infant.[25]

Treating the embryo/fetus with special respect does not depend on metaphysical assumption or religious belief, though it does depend on openness to the meanings that prenatal life stimulates. Precisely because the embryo/fetus is genetically unique and has the potential to become more, it operates as a powerful symbol of the unique gift of human existence.[26] Because it stimulates consciousness of the human community more directly and efficiently than other human tissue, it deserves special consideration even if it is not itself a moral subject or rights-holder. The flag, the Torah, certain works of art, national monuments, religious relics, and human remains are examples of other objects that are revered and respected because of their symbolic import, even though they are not themselves moral subjects or rights-bearers.[27]

However, respecting the embryo and fetus as a symbol or reminder of our membership in the human community should remain a matter of choice, not moral duty. Valuing previable stages of human life is constitutive but not morally obligatory.[28] While other objects or entities may also serve this function, the embryo/fetus serves it especially well because of its role in the series of events that lead to the birth of a child. Yet because of its rudimentary development, especially at earlier stages, it is less constitutive of human community than are viable fetuses or recently dead cadavers.

A symbolic view of the embryo/fetus, however, does not require that everyone find the same symbolic meaning in it, or that everyone act according to the meanings that others find. Those who choose to invest the embryo/fetus with special meanings define themselves and their moral commitments in so doing, just as members of a national or religious community constitute themselves by respect for the American flag, a Torah, or a crucifix. Divergent views, however, should be tolerated, for no well-established tradition so invests the embryo/fetus with a clear meaning that one would question the character of a person who denied that the embryo/fetus itself had rights, or who thought that other human interests might take priority.[29]

This view of the symbolic significance of embryos and fetuses supports the modified pro-choice position. Although previable fetuses are not sufficiently developed to have rights or interests in themselves, they are a vehicle for symbolic meanings about respect for human life. Respecting and preserving that symbolic meaning, however, is morally optional and not required before viability. Individuals may choose to give the utmost respect to prenatal life, but they violate no moral duty to fetuses or the community if they rank a woman's control over pregnancy higher. In a pluralistic society, those with differing views are not morally justified in controlling the actions of others on the basis of deeply personal meanings that many persons do not share.

If one accepts this view, the best course of action would be to prevent the need for abortion through education, contraception, and support for parenting. If abortion must occur, it is preferable that it occur as early as possible, with drugs that prevent or interrupt implantation. To mark the symbolic importance of the decision, it should also be permissible to have women carefully consider the implications of their decision before acting. In the end, however, the pregnant woman should be allowed to decide whether she wishes to demonstrate her symbolic respect for human life by continuing the pregnancy.

A similar analysis will apply to many of the issues that arise with new reproductive technologies involving fertilized eggs, embryos, and fetuses. Technologies that create, manipulate, and destroy early embryos should be assessed in terms of their impact on reproductive interests and the symbolic meanings that the actions in question convey. Similarly, techniques to create embryos and fetuses in order to obtain tissue for research or transplant may impose symbolic costs in the pursuit of reproductive or other goals. In each instance, the conflict will be resolved by how one weighs and evaluates the reproductive interests at stake versus symbolic interests in respect for prenatal life.

LEGAL ISSUES

Debates about the legal status of abortion view the same issues through a constitutional lens. *Roe v. Wade*, decided on 22 January 1973, was a ringing endorsement of procreative liberty.[30] By recognizing the right to terminate a pregnancy up until viability, the Court gave constitutional status to a pregnant woman's choice to abort. This decision effectively invalidated all state abortion laws, and narrowly circumscribed state power to regulate abortion.

The constitutional outcome in *Roe* rested on two premises. Both premises rested on the assumption that embryos and fetuses are not persons within the Fourteenth Amendment, thus there is no constitutional obligation to accord them rights. Any respect or protection accorded them is a matter of state discretion, subject to other constitutional constraints. Interestingly, none of the dissenting justices in *Roe* or *Casey* disputed this point.[31]

The two premises of the decision tracked the ethical analysis just addressed. One premise was that the woman's interest in terminating an unwanted pregnancy is a fundamental right, which can be infringed only upon a showing of a compelling state interest. The second premise was that the state's optional decision to protect fetuses by banning abortion does not constitute a compelling state interest prior to viability.

While critics of *Roe* have attacked both premises, a cogent defense of each exists. Given *Griswold v. Connecticut*'s recognition of a fundamental right of married persons who have sex to avoid reproduction by contraception, it is an incremental step to say that the same fundamental right presumptively exists when the woman is already pregnant.[32] To deny *Griswold*, however, is to deny the whole tradition of unenumerated right, substantive due process lawmaking that persists and endures in constitutional adjudication. Despite perennial claims that substantive due process has no constitutional foundation, the Supreme Court has never rejected it. Given a well-established tradition of identifying unenumerated constitutional rights, the presumptive right to avoid reproduction, like the right to reproduce, is a strong contender for recognition. If a due process and liberty grounding for the right to abort is rejected, textual support might be found in the Thirteenth Amendment's ban on forced labor and involuntary servitude.[33]

The other premise in *Roe* concerns what counts as a compelling state interest. Here the Court applied the well-established principle that a moral purpose or objection alone could not trump a fundamental right. Because the moral status of previable embryos and fetuses is itself morally contested, with no consensus among people or religious groups, it would be arbitrary to allow what is ordinarily left to pluralistic decision making to overcome such a right.[34] A state is free to value the fetus as it wishes, as long as it does not interfere with a woman's right to value the fetus as she wants and terminate pregnancy. At viability, however, the fetus's advanced development lends itself to a more objective valuation of its interests, and the woman's interest in ending pregnancy can be limited.[35]

Opponents of *Roe* have attacked both premises, and criticized the Court for removing an issue from legislative discretion on the basis of an unenumerated right not firmly grounded in precedent or tradition.[36] As these criticisms converged with the Reagan-Bush administration's appointment of several conservative justices to the Supreme Court, the continued survival of *Roe* and the basic right to abortion appeared to be in serious doubt.

The Expected Demise of Roe v. Wade

In June 1992, it was widely expected that the Supreme Court would soon reverse *Roe v. Wade* and give states the power to restrict abortion. A majority in the 1989 case of *Webster v. Reproductive Services* was ready to scrap the trimester structure of *Roe*.[37] The replacement of Justices Marshall and Brennan, staunch defenders of *Roe*, with Justices Souter and Thomas suggested that *Roe* would soon be overruled. The case of *Planned Parenthood v. Casey* then before the Supreme Court was expected to signal *Roe*'s imminent demise, with the coup de grace expected in cases from Guam, Louisiana, or Utah that directly restricted early abortions.

A reversal of *Roe v. Wade* would have substantially diminished procreative liberty. For the first time since 1973 states would have been permitted to prohibit or greatly restrict a pregnant woman's access to abortion, a power which ten to twenty states would undoubtedly have exercised. Although the precise scope of state power would have depended on the grounds of the reversal, it is likely that the Court would have given states the power to restrict abortion as much as the legislature in a particular jurisdiction wished, including the power to ban postcoital methods of birth control and contragestive agents such as RU486. The only uncertainty concerned whether a state would have been obligated to grant exceptions for the life or health of the mother, rape and incest, or permit exceptions for fetal deformity.

Such a broad power over abortion was likely because a reversal of *Roe* would rest on the Court's rejecting either or both major premises that underlie Roe's finding of a right to abortion. With the legal status of the fetus under the Fourteenth Amendment not itself directly challenged, it was expected that the Court would deny that terminating unwanted pregnancy is a fundamental right that demands anything more than a rational basis for restrictive state action.[38]

Even if the Court retained some protected status for choices to abort, it would most likely find that the state's interest in prenatal life is legitimate and compelling at all stages of pregnancy. Indeed, it would not have been surprising if a Court intent on reversing *Roe* had combined both approaches, finding that avoiding unwanted pregnancy is a protected liberty interest but not a fundamental right, but that the state's interest in protecting prenatal life suffices to override that liberty at all stages of pregnancy.

Whatever the precise approach taken, states would then be free to ban, regulate, or permit abortion according to how the state chose to balance procreative liberty and prenatal human life. Access to abortion would then depend on where one lived and one's ability to go elsewhere. Young, poor, and minority women would have been hit especially hard. They—and many others—might be prevented from having abortions, or be forced to have them much later than they otherwise would. Self-administered and illegal abortions would increase to some unknown extent, with some women being injured or even dying. Of course, increased attention to birth control and better support for adoption would offset some of these effects. Overall, however, there would appear to be a substantial net loss of procreative liberty.

If *Roe* had been reversed, it is also likely that states could have banned postcoital contraception and contragestive agents such as RU486. If the reversal of *Roe* were based on a finding that no fundamental right is involved in the abortion decision, protecting fertilized eggs and early embryos would be a rational basis for state restriction. Alternatively, if a fundamental right or protected liberty interest in abortion remained but the Court found that the state's interest in protecting prenatal life at all stages of pregnancy is sufficient to override the liberty interest in abortion, any state action to protect fertilized eggs would also have been constititutional. Under either rationale, the state would have the power to ban contragestive drugs and postcoital methods of birth control.[39]

A reversal of *Roe* would thus have limited the continued vitality of *Griswold* to prefertilization methods of birth control. Postcoital methods, such as the intrauterine device, low-dose birth control pills, and the morning-after pill, which operate by preventing implantation of fertilized eggs, could be banned under the state's power to protect all stages of postfertilized human life. Given the right-to-life premise that a new person exists from the time of fertilization, it would not be surprising if some states had banned postcoital contraceptives as well. Indeed, for persons holding this view a failure to protect preimplantation embryos would be arbitrary, because the developmental differences immediately after implantation are not great enough to justify different moral or legal treatment of embryos just before implantation.[40]

Casey *and the Modified Middle Position*

By a 5–4 vote in June 1992, the Supreme Court in *Planned Parenthood v. Casey* reaffirmed the basic principle of *Roe v. Wade* that a woman has a right to terminate pregnancy up until viability and thereafter when necessary to protect her life or health.[41] However, the Court modified the trimester structure of *Roe*. It adopted an undue burden test that allows states to inform pregnant women about abortion alternatives and the fetus's anatomical status and to require that they wait 24 hours after receving this information before having an abortion.

The Pennsylvania law at issue in *Casey* did not directly challenge the right to early abortion, though it restricted it with informed consent, waiting periods, and husband and parental-notification requirements. While most of Pennsylvania's restrictions would have been found unconstitutional under the trimester structure of *Roe*, statements in *Webster* strongly suggested that a majority of the Court would uphold these provisions. Many persons also expected Justices Souter and Thomas as well as Justices Kennedy and O'Connor to signal their disapproval of the essence of *Roe*, which would require a later case for direct reversal.

However, with the emergence of a solid three-vote center of Justices O'Connor, Kennedy, and Souter, the Court surprised almost everyone, and left pro-life forces reeling.[42] The Court accomplished this startling result by reaffirming its authority to define fundamental unenumerated rights through "reasoned judgment" in interpreting the liberty clause of the Fourteenth Amendment. Recognizing that basic rights of "liberty" are not confined to those rights mentioned in the Bill of Rights, nor those specifically recognized by past traditions, it drew upon past cases recognizing rights to bodily integrity and "a person's most basic decisions about family and parenthood."[43] If past decisions protect personal decisions "relating to marriage, procreation, contraception, family relationships, childrearing and education," then a woman must also have a basic right to terminate pregnancy, because it is so closely tied to, indeed, is a central aspect of that protected sphere of decision making.[44]

Having reaffirmed the basic liberty right to terminate pregnancy established in *Roe*, the Court also reaffirmed that the state's otherwise "important and legitimate interest in potential life" did not outweigh this right until viability at roughly the twenty-fourth week of pregnancy.[45] As in *Roe*, it merely restated the meaning of viability to justify this conclusion—"a realistic possibility of maintaining and nourishing a life outside the womb."[46] However, the Court indirectly addressed the issue of fetal status in explaining why personal liberty must include the decision to abort. Prior to viability, one's assessment of the priority to be granted fetal status was a matter of "the right to define one's own concept of existence, of meaning of the universe, and of the mystery of human life. . . . The destiny of the woman must be shaped to a large extent on her own conception of her spiritual imperatives and her place in society."[47]

The *Casey* Court did, however, modify the strong pro-choice slant of *Roe* by rejecting *Roe*'s trimester framework for measuring abortion regulations. The trimester framework did not sufficiently recognize the state's legitimate interests in potential life and maternal health which even *Roe* admitted existed throughout pregnancy. Accordingly, it found that state laws that aim to ensure that the abortion decision is "thoughtful and informed" are valid if they do not impose an "undue burden" or "substantial obstacle" on access to abortion.[48] On this standard, state regulations that serve legitimate state concerns in how abortions are provided but which do not substantially limit access to abortion do not create an "undue burden" and are acceptable. As long as the core interest in terminating an unwanted pregnancy is protected, ancillary restrictions that only marginally increase the costs or burdens of abortion are not "undue" and are therefore permissible.

The undue-burden test allows some restrictions that could not be justified under the strict scrutiny standard of *Roe*. It may be that this test, as pro-choice activists strongly argue, poses a major threat to procreative choice because of its potential to be interpreted as a very loose constraint on restrictive abortion policies. By definition, however, the restrictions permitted under the test cannot be "substantial" or "unduly" burdensome, or they will be struck down. The effect of state restrictions on access to abortion will thus depend ultimately on how courts view the burdens created by particular regulations. If they are faithful to *Roe* and *Casey*'s recognition of a fundamental right to abortion, the test will not permit states to limit greatly a woman's access to abortion.

In *Casey* itself the Supreme Court found that physician disclosure and 24-hour waiting period provisions, which had previously been struck down under *Roe*'s strict-scrutiny approach, did not create a substantial barrier to abortion and thus were upheld.[49] It viewed these provisions as merely assuring that women contemplating abortion were aware of "philosophic and social arguments" in favor of continuing pregnancy and of the "procedures and institutions" concerning alternatives such as adoption and child support if the woman chose to raise the child herself.[50] The record contained no evidence that a 24-hour waiting period would so increase the burdens and costs of travel to clinics that it constituted an "undue burden" on the right to have an abortion. However, the Court left open the possibility that actual experience might show otherwise, in which case a challenge to those provisions could later be entertained. At the same time, the Court struck down a spousal notification provision, because of much clearer evidence that informing abusive and controlling spouses of a desire to terminate pregnancy would effectively prevent many women from obtaining abortions.

The Impact of Casey

Where then does *Casey* leave abortion law and other issues of procreative liberty? As long as Justices Blackmun, Stevens, O'Connor, Kennedy, and Souter stay on the Court, the right to abortion recognized in *Roe* will remain viable. If any of them retire, a pro-choice president is likely to appoint replacements who will protect the basic right to abortion, as President Clinton has done in his appointment of Ruth Bader Ginsburg to replace Justice Byron White, a dissenter in *Roe* and *Casey*. Congressional passage of the Freedom of Choice Act, which is designed to codify the essential holding of *Roe v. Wade*, will also protect the right to abortion.

Casey's resuscitation of *Roe v. Wade*, however, does alter the landscape of abortion legislation in some significant ways. The undue-burden test will permit states to impose informed consent and waiting-period requirements along the lines of the Pennsylvania law upheld in *Casey*. An important question will be whether states may increase the waiting period beyond 24 hours, as many European countries do. The validity of longer waiting periods will turn on whether such a period of reflection actually aids an informed decision or is merely obstructionist, and whether a record of substantial obstacle to obtaining an abortion can be established.[51] Bitter battles are likely to continue in legislatures and courts as these issues are thrashed out, with perhaps ten to twenty states passing such regulations. The outcome of these battles will determine the extent to which the modified pro-choice position, which is now constitutionally permissible, will define the legal landscape in which abortion occurs.

Many persons will find the *Casey* system of access to abortion with some regulation a desirable compromise. Professor Mary Ann Glendon and others have pointed out that the American system of very liberal abortion rights is unnecessarily politicized because constitutionalizing the issue has removed almost all ability for compromise by either side.[52] *Casey* will open the door to more compromises in procedures for obtaining abortion and could bring the United States much closer to the European system for obtaining abortion, at least in those states that enact counseling requirements and waiting periods.

As long as *Roe-Casey* survives, however, important differences from the European model will remain, with continued politicization likely. Abortions later than the first trimester will still be possible, which is less often the case in Europe.[53] Nor will there be a requirement that a woman show that abortion is necessary to prevent severe distress, as German law requires.[54] Under *Roe-Casey* no check on her reasons is permitted—her desire to end pregnancy for any reason is enough. Finally, consent and waiting periods will have a much greater chance of preventing women from having abortions in America than in Europe. The paucity of abortion providers and the need to travel long distances to obtain an abortion is less of a problem in Europe than it is in many American states.

Finally, it should be noted that *Casey*'s revival of *Roe* will not necessarily change the status of other technologies affecting embryos and fetuses. *Roe*, for example, does not control disposition of embryos outside the body, because no pregnancy is involved.[55] Nor would a reversal of *Roe* have prevented selective reduction of multifetal pregnancies when they posed a serious risk to the mother's life or health.[56] However, *Roe-Casey* does prohibit any inquiry into motives or reasons for abortion, and thus probably protects conceptions and abortions designed to produce embryos or fetal tissue for research or transplant, and even abortion on gender grounds.[57]

RU486 AND CONTRAGESTION

The modified pro-choice position will receive even more support once contragestive agents such as RU486 are available in the United States. These agents prevent or interrupt implantation soon after it has occurred. Thus they act both as postcoital birth control when they prevent implantation from occurring and as abortifacients when they induce miscarriage.

Because they operate so soon after conception, often before pregnancy itself has begun, they have the potential to defuse some of the heat of the abortion controversy by greatly increasing the number of terminations that occur at or shortly after implantation. While low-dose birth control pills, intrauterine devices, and the morning-after pill are contragestives, the most controversial contragestive drug is RU486, an antiprogesterone agent. RU486 occupies the progesterone receptor sites in the cells of the endometrium, thus depriving the uterus of the progesterone it needs to maintain pregnancy. As a result, the developing embryo will not attach to the walls of the uterus. If already attached, it will in effect unhook, and be shed.[58]

RU486 is now used for about a third of the abortions performed in France. It has been approved for use in Great Britain and the Netherlands, and is currently being tested in Sweden and China. Because of right-to-life opposition, however, Roussel Uclaf, the French company that holds the patent, and its German parent, A. G. Hoechst, had not sought FDA approval in the United States nor licensed another drug company to do so. The election of President Bill Clinton has now overcome their reluctance to seek testing and marketing approval in the United States. Americans' access to RU486 and other antiprogesterone agents is likely to occur in the next three to five years.

The Advantages of Contragestion

Contragestives operate medically, and are safer and cheaper than surgical abortion. They are also morally and symbolically preferable to later abortions, because they prevent or interrupt pregnancy at the very earliest stages of embryonic development. In their contraceptive mode, they prevent implantation of a blastocyst, a stage at which no differentiated organs or neurological structures have developed.[59] Only persons holding strict right-to-life views would hold that there is a moral duty to have all fertilized eggs and blastocysts implant in the uterus.

As abortifacients, contragestives interrupt implantation at the embryo stage before a fetus has developed. The postimplantation embryo is still so rudimentary in development that it can reasonably be viewed as lacking interests in its own right, and thus is not the subject of a moral duty to assure its continued survival.

Because contragestives operate so early, before or shortly after pregnancy has been established, their use should be preferable to later abortions performed on more developed fetuses. Preventing a fertilized egg from implanting or interrupting implantation shortly after an embryo has developed is less morally or symbolically problematic than surgically destroying a much more developed fetus. Indeed, if most pregnancy terminations occurred at or shortly after implantation, much of the moral heat of the abortion controversy would no doubt lessen. Making RU486 available in the United States will be a significant step toward resolution of this wrenching social issue.

Pro-Life Opposition to Contragestion

Contragestion may appeal to persons who view prenatal moral status as an evolutionary process dependent on biological development, but it will have little appeal for persons who view any destruction of a fertilized egg as murder. For those persons, it matters not a whit that abortion would occur before a fetus had developed, much less a fetus with a sentient nervous system. They view all stages of human life as of equivalent value and equally deserving protection. Whether characterized as birth control or abortifacient, contragestives destroy or prevent embryonic "persons" from continued life.

As a nonsurgical, office-based procedure, contragestion also hides the moral wrong they perceive in termination of pregnancy. Women who use contragestion may mistakenly think that they are not destroying an innocent human life because they are taking a pill that ends or prevents implantation. In addition, many more physicians will prescribe contragestives than perform surgical abortions, thus relieving the problems of access to abortion that exist in many areas. They also enable women to evade the public scrutiny of going to an abortion clinic—Operation Rescue cannot realistically picket the office of every doctor who prescribes RU486. RU486 will thus help institutionalize the willingness to destroy innocent human life.

As a result, right-to-life groups in the United States and Europe have vigorously fought to prevent the introduction of RU486 into medical practice. Their demonstrations and threats of boycott would have led Roussel Uclaf to withdraw RU486 from marketing in France if the French Ministry of Health had not intervened.[60] This experience has led Roussel Uclaf and its parent company, A. G. Hoechst, to move cautiously in other countries and deterred them until recently from seeking marketing approval in the United States, where pro-life groups have threatened boycotts of their other products.

Despite their waning political influence, right-to-life groups are likely to continue vehement opposition to the introduction of RU486. If RU486 becomes widely available, little steam will remain in the right-to-life movement. It will be much harder to mobilize opposition to contragestive pills that operate around the blurry time when pregnancy has not yet occurred or has just started. Because RU486 seriously undermines the right-to-life movement, it has fought tooth and nail to keep it out, even though the effect is to make abortions occur later than is necessary.

With *Roe* reaffirmed in *Casey* and a pro-choice president in office, Roussel Uclaf and A. G. Hoechst have now found that enough consensus about the acceptability of abortion exists in the United States to satisfy its self-imposed conditions for release of the drug for testing and marketing. (A reversal of *Roe* would have kept the drug out of the United States for many years.) Requests by public officials, by public health and women's groups, and by President Clinton himself were instrumental in persuading Roussel Uclaf and A. G. Hoechst to release RU486 for testing in the United States.[61] Ultimately, a combination of politics and profits will determine the availability of RU486 and other contragestive agents.

If pro-life groups had succeeded in keeping contragestive drugs permanently off the market, an important opportunity for compromise or modulation of the abortion controversy would have been lost. If abortions occur, it is far preferable that they occur earlier and medically rather than later and surgically. RU486 thus provides an opportunity for compromise and consensus based on abortions occurring at the earliest stages of prenatal development.

ABORTION REGULATION AND THE CONTROL OF WOMEN

The manifest message of anti-choice legislation is the importance of protecting "innocent human life." Yet the extremes to which the anti-choice forces go in their denial of biologic distinctions, their inconsistencies in granting exceptions for health, rape, and fetal deformity, and their utter disregard of the impact of unwanted pregnancy on women's lives suggest that a latent agenda animates their fervent efforts. This agenda appears to be the control of women—punishing them for their sexuality and keeping them in certain reproductive and family roles.

The existence of this latent agenda reveals itself in the extremes and inconsistencies of the anti-choice program. The pro-life position that even fertilized eggs and blastocysts—microscopic entities consisting of undifferentiated cells without a nervous system—must be protected ignores the physical and social burdens that such protection imposes on women. Strict right-to-lifers recognize no exceptions, while others pick and choose among the fetuses and embryos to be protected, with some allowing abortion in pregnancies due to rape and others when there is severe fetal deformity.

The willingness to burden women is also evident in Judith Thomson's perceptive analysis of the moral rights and duties in abortion. As she has shown, the fact of fetal personhood merely raises the issue of when and whether women may be required to be Splendid Samaritans and lend their body to the fetus; it does not automatically require that conclusion. The alacrity, however, with which pro-life groups assume that women have a moral duty to lend their bodies to serve fetal needs—far beyond any other duties to rescue recognized in law—betrays an underlying attitude that a woman's role is to sacrifice her own interests and reproduce. Yet those same groups do not urge that laws be enacted to require that people generally rescue others, much less require that mothers and fathers donate their tissue or organs to enable others to survive.[62] They also are not strong supporters of the social programs that would prevent the need for abortion or which would make childbirth an attractive alternative for women who are pregnant. The pro-choice quip that anti-abortion groups respect the right to life only from fertilization to childbirth is not mere hyperbole.

The latent agenda point has been best articulated by Kristin Luker in her important study of the politics of abortion.[63] Luker's theory is that abortion is really a symbolic battleground for what appropriate female social roles are. The pro-life forces tend to be dominated by women who are less educated, have fewer careers, and primarily raise children in conventional marriages. The pro-choice activists are better educated, and careerist, and do not identify womanhood with reproduction.

Luker theorizes that the pro-life forces see birth control and abortion as an attack on or devaluation of their life-style, for it calls into question the importance of the childbearing and rearing that is their main enterprise. They are fighting to the core to preserve the association between being a woman and being a reproducer versus the careerism of the opposing view. Male activists may also share these traditional views of a woman's role.

The pro-choice forces, on the other hand, see meaning in work and career rather than primarily in defining themselves as mothers who raise children. Their struggle has been for recognition of a woman's right to work and to be free of the demands of childbearing. For them, the ability to control the timing and fact of pregnancy through birth control and abortion is central to work and career. Even if they never have abortions themselves, the right to do so is an important symbol of their freedom that must be preserved.

Closely allied to this view of the reproductive role of women is a view of sex as designed for reproduction and marriage. Although married women have abortions, abortion is commonly seen by opponents as a form of birth control that enables alienated, uncommitted sex to occur. For them, a policy of "abortion on demand" denigrates the importance of sex and marriage and demeans human life. Strict limits on abortion are thus needed to prevent sex from being trivialized or abused. However, as with differing views of prenatal status, these views are too idiosyncratic and personal to be imposed on others who have a different view of the meanings that attend sex and reproduction.

Given these competing symbolic agendas, it is no surprise that the abortion debate has been so recalcitrant to resolution, and is likely to continue even as new abortion technologies become available. Only when women are no longer so totally identified with procreation and motherhood will there be full acceptance of their right to terminate pregnancy.

CONCLUSION

The ascendancy of the modified pro-choice position will not immediately quiet the clamor over abortion, nor dispel the ambivalence that many people continue to have about the destruction of prenatal life. However, by providing a stable legal framework, it may help move the social debate from prohibition to methods of prevention, even as abortion remains available.

If so, technologies that prevent or end pregnancy shortly after implantation offer many advantages over later surgical abortion. Not only are they safer and less intrusive, but they operate at a very early stage of embryonic development. Together with increased access to birth control, they present an important opportunity to expand procreative choice while deescalating the abortion controversy. While they should not be the central part of a preventive strategy, they have an important role to play when abortions do occur.

In the final analysis, however, the battle over abortion, like the battle over other reproductive technologies, may be more dependent on emotion than on reason. Although usually viewed as a conflict between prenatal human life and the burdens of unwanted pregnancy, the rigid resistance of pro-life opponents to distinctions based on biological development and impact on women suggests that deeper forces are at work. At the most basic level, the conflict goes beyond views of prenatal status to highly charged views about life, death, sexuality, and women's reproductive and social roles. These views will continue to influence the abortion debate and other technologies affecting prenatal life.

CHAPTER 4

Norplant, Forced Contraception, and Irresponsible Reproduction

NORPLANT offers safe and effective contraception for up to five years, thus increasing options for women seeking to control their fertility. Yet shortly after FDA approval in 1990, proposals surfaced to have Norplant implanted in child abusers, welfare mothers, and teenagers. Because the contraceptive effect of Norplant is reversible at any time, it appeared to offer an acceptable technological solution for harmful or irresponsible reproduction.

However, the notion of state intervention to limit reproduction is anathema to many people. If procreation is a basic right, then people must be allowed to reproduce as they wish and the consequences tolerated, just as the consequences of free speech or the due-process rights of criminals must be tolerated. Still, the possibility of temporary interference with irresponsible reproduction is an attractive option. At the very least, this technology forces us to address issues of reproductive responsibility that have long been ignored. This chapter discusses irresponsible reproduction and the social policies that may be adopted to discourage it.[1]

THE NORPLANT SYSTEM

On 10 December 1990, the Food and Drug Administration approved Norplant for use in the United States.[2] The Norplant system of contraception consists of six flexible silastic matchstick-sized capsules that contain levonorgestrel, a synthetic progestin widely used in oral contraceptives. The capsules are inserted under the skin of the upper arm in a 10 to 15 minute procedure done with local anesthesia. Women can feel the implant under the skin, but it is not ordinarily visible.

Once implanted, the levonorgestrel slowly diffuses through the walls of the capsules into the bloodstream.[3] Norplant achieves contraception by suppressing ovulation, like contraceptive pills, and by thickening a woman's cervical mucus to impede passage of sperm into the uterus. The chance of becoming pregnant with Norplant averages less than 5 percent per year over five years, making the Norplant system the most effective

contraceptive available, except for permanent sterilization. Since it is es-
trogen-free, it can be used safely in women who are hypertensive or dia-
betic, who have migraine headaches, or who are over forty years old and
smoke.

Norplant is also very convenient for users. Once implanted, nothing
further need be done—a distinct advantage over barrier methods and the
pill. The most common side effect is a disruption of menstrual patterns,
with some women experiencing amenorrhea and others irregular bleeding. Some users also experience headaches, weight change, and acne. Current studies show, however, that when the chance of these effects is explained, 94 percent of women are satisfied with the implants, with 71
percent stating that they would use this method again.[4]

A major advantage is that Norplant's contraceptive effect is reversible
at any time.[5] When the woman wishes to regain fertility, the capsules are
removed under local anesthesia through a small incision in the skin.
Within a week of removal, the level of levonorgestrel is almost undetect-
able in the bloodstream, and normal ovulation is soon restored.

The current cost of Norplant is $365, with an additional charge of
$150 to $650 for the insertion, counseling, and checkups. A $150 to
$300 fee for removal may also be charged. While the $365 price com-
pares favorably with the cost of five years of oral contraceptives, that
comparison does not take surgical fees for implantation and removal into
account. Also, if removal occurs before five years, the cost advantage is
lost. For women who tolerate the relatively minor side effects and who
can afford it, it will be preferable to the inconvenience of taking an oral
contraceptive or using barrier methods. However, it provides no protection against sexually transmitted disease.

ACCESS TO NORPLANT

A major problem with Norplant is making the system available to women
who cannot pay the relatively high, up-front cost. Wyeth-Ayerst, the dis-
tributor of the system, is charging both public and private providers $365
for the silastic tubes. While Medicaid will cover this fee for the medically
indigent, low Medicaid reimbursement rates for insertion may deter some
doctors from providing it. Also, there are millions of women who are not
poor enough to qualify for Medicaid nor rich enough to pay the full up-
front cost of the device, which health insurance usually does not cover.[6]
Private agencies such as Planned Parenthood will fill some of that gap, but
many women who want the device may not be able to afford it. If women
are to be guaranteed control over their fertility through contraception,

long-acting contraceptives such as Norplant should be made available to all women who desire it.[7]

A related question concerns access by teenagers who are at risk of pregnancy. The issues are no different than those that arise with other contraceptives for teenagers. If parents approve and are willing to pay the cost, access is not a problem. In other cases, lack of information, the need for parental consent, and money will be a substantial barrier to teenage access. In addition, public programs to provide teenagers with Norplant will have to overcome perceptions that provision of contraceptives encourages sexual activity or is otherwise coercive.

NORPLANT CONTROVERSIES

As a voluntary method of contraception that has met regulatory standards of safety and efficacy, Norplant presents no major ethical or legal issues, beyond making it available to all women who want it and assuring that women are informed of its side effects. Voluntary use by adolescents raises issues of parental consent and impact on nonmarital sexual activity, but these issues arise with any contraceptive use by minors.

Norplant has become controversial, however, because of attempts by judges, legislators, and others to require that certain women use Norplant to avoid reproduction that is alleged to be irresponsible or harmful to children and society. Within a month of FDA approval, for example, a trial judge in California offered to release from prison a woman convicted of child abuse, if she would consent to use of Norplant. Other judges have offered similar deals to women, and legislation authorizing involuntary insertion of Norplant in alchoholics and drug addicts who have given birth to children has been introduced.[8]

Legislators have also been quick to offer Norplant to women on welfare. In 1991, a Kansas legislator introduced a bill that would pay $500 to any mother on welfare who had Norplant implanted, and $50 a year to maintain it. David Duke introduced a similar bill in Louisiana, with a $100 reward. A 1990 editorial in the *The Philadelphia Inquirer* proposed making use of Norplant a condition of receiving welfare as a way to reduce the size of the "underclass."[9] In January 1993, the governor of Maryland proposed that use of Norplant be made mandatory in certain cases.[10]

Mental health professionals have considered use of Norplant with retarded and mentally ill women who are at risk of sexual exploitation in residential facilities. Others have proposed that Norplant be required or offered to women who are HIV-infected, and to women who are at risk for offspring with severe genetic disease. Still others would provide Norplant to teenagers at school clinics.[11] Proposals to have Norplant inserted in all girls at puberty have also surfaced.[12]

Reactions to such proposals have varied from enthusiastic approval to horror and outrage. Approval comes from those persons who believe that certain kinds of reproduction are irresponsible, and that the state may take steps to prevent irresponsibile reproduction with an easily reversible device such as Norplant. Others see proposals to offer, entice, or compel women to use Norplant as a violation of basic human rights—a racist or elitist response to problems that should be resolved by other means. They also oppose such an approach, because women vary in their tolerance of Norplant's irregular bleeding and other side effects.

Whatever one's views about these proposals, it is clear that Norplant has succeeded in reintroducing a discourse of reproductive responsibility into public life. Because Norplant is easily inserted and fully reversible, it appears to be much less intrusive of personal rights and dignity than is compulsory sterilization, which is now widely opposed. Moreover, many of the proposals are not directly coercive, but merely provide incentives for target groups to use Norplant. The result is a long overdue discussion of reproductive responsibility and the state's role in promoting such responsibility.

REPRODUCTIVE RESPONSIBILITY

Chapter 2 presented the case for recognition of both a moral and legal right to reproduce. Arguing that reproduction is important to individuals because of the personal and social meanings that surround it, the chapter concluded that decisions to reproduce should be viewed as presumptive rights that are subject to limitation only upon the showing of substantial harm to the interests of others. The development of Norplant now requires us to address what kinds of harm would constitute a sufficient basis for limitation of that right.

Any discussion of reproductive responsibility and governmental action to limit reproduction is a touchy subject, however.[13] The history of attempts to limit "irresponsible reproduction" is replete with abuse and discrimination. From 1920 to 1960 more than 60,000 "mental defectives" were forcibly sterilized on eugenics grounds, even though the risk of transmission of genetic disease was low and diagnostic errors of mental deficiency abounded.[14] Poor and minority women have also been sterilized without consent under both public and private programs well into the 1970s.[15] As a result, there is an extreme reluctance to even discuss the idea of irresponsible reproduction, much less propose public policies, for fear that it will be viewed as racist or lead to coercive state policies that will replicate earlier abuses.

Nevertheless, it is essential that conversations about reproductive responsibility take place. Reproduction always has moral significance because it leads to the birth of another person, whose needs for love, nurturing, and resources have to be met. Clearly, one can act responsibly or irresponsibly in reproducing, because of the impact that one's actions will have on offspring and others, including existing children. A dialogue about the circumstances that make reproduction desirable or undesirable, advised or ill-advised, responsible or irresponsible is needed to help us determine the parameters of morally and socially acceptable conduct, and to guide or limit governmental action that affects reproductive choice.

Any judgment about the reproductive responsibility of individuals must pay attention to four issues: the importance of the reproduction in question to the person(s) reproducing; the ease or difficulty with which they could avoid that reproduction; the burdens that reproduction will cause resulting offspring; and the burdens or costs imposed on society and others.[16] Clarifying these parameters is necessary before they are applied to individual cases and questions of public policy are addressed.

Reproductive Interest

Reproduction is often said to be irresponsible because of the costs imposed on others. Implicit in such a judgment is the assumption that the person reproducing has little or no reproductive interest to justify those costs. What counts as a reproductive interest? What distinctions can be made on this score?

An important issue here will be whether the persons will be involved in rearing resulting offspring. Although reproduction may occur without rearing, one reason why reproduction is highly valued is because of the rearing and family experiences it makes possible. A person who reproduces but has no contact with offspring may have a lesser interest in reproduction than a person who reproduces with the intent to rear children. Whether the reproduction of either is undesirable will depend on the costs imposed on offspring and society. However, in balancing those costs against the value of the reproductive experience, the capacity and likelihood of rearing is a relevant factor.

On this parameter a man who fathers many children with different women but who has no contact with any of them and provides no support is more easily open to a charge of irresponsibility. At the opposite extreme would be the cases where the person reproducing is seeking to nurture and rear her offspring. HIV women, welfare mothers, and unmarried teenagers may fit this category. Although their reproduction may be undesirable because of consequences for offspring and the welfare system, they have substantial reproductive interests at stake when they will also rear their offspring. Because reproduction with rearing is presumptively protected, a correspondingly high level of harm will have to be shown to justify overriding their procreative freedom.

Other cases will fall in between these two extremes with many variations among them. Some persons may have minimal contact with offspring, rear intermittently, or require the assistance of other rearers. Some may rear fully but die while offspring are still young. Also relevant in assessing the value of the reproductive interest at stake will be whether the person has previously reproduced, or will be able to reproduce in the future if a present opportunity is denied.

The key question in each case will be the value to the person and others of the precise reproductive experience that is occurring. Answering this question, however, will pose many problems beyond merely determining whether genetic reproduction *tout court* should be valued as much as genetic reproduction cum rearing. If the question is pushed, questions of the worth of the experience to the person will have to be faced, and distinctions must be drawn based on previous and likely future reproductive experiences, expected life span, the amount of rearing, and the like. Because of these complications, it may not be possible as a practical matter in most cases to go beyond whether the persons reproducing will be aware that they have reproduced and whether they will have some rearing role or contact with offspring.

Burdens of Avoiding Reproduction

Judgments of irresponsible reproduction will also have to factor in the ease or burdens of alternatives open to the person to avoid reproduction. Even if reproduction imposes high costs on others and the person has only a minimal reproductive interest at stake, a charge of irresponsibility will fit only if the person has reasonable alternatives to reproduction. A person who could have been abstinent, used birth control, or terminated pregnancy would be acting irresponsibly if their failure to do so imposes high costs on others, particularly if they have no intention or ability to rear resulting offspring. On the other hand, if they have been raped, cannot reasonably remain abstinent, or birth control or abortion is dangerous, not available, or morally repugnant, then their responsibility is less.

The hard cases here will arise over whether alternatives to reproduction are reasonably available. For example, should a conscientious belief about the immorality of birth control or abortion justify actions that produce little or no significant reproductive experience and impose high costs on others? Must a woman insist that she or her partner use contraception? The lack of moral accountability for undesirable reproduction does not lessen the costs which that reproduction imposes on others, nor does it increase the signficance of marginal reproductive interests. Of course, questions of the burdens of avoidance do not determine whether the reproductive outcome is desirable or advised, but merely whether a person can be held responsible for undesirable outcomes. It also does not prevent society from acting to prevent the reproduction in question.

Impact on Offspring

Reproduction is said to be irresponsible when it is reasonably foreseeable that the parents will be unable to produce healthy offspring or will otherwise rear them in circumstances that deny them a minimum level of care, nurture, and protection. Parents who abuse their children by prenatal or postnatal conduct, rear them in disadvantageous circumstances, or pass on genetic or infectious disease would appear to fit this category.[17] The consequences for offspring, when coupled with an unwillingness or inability to rear and reasonable alternatives to reproduction, would arguably make this reproduction irresponsible.

There is, however, a major problem with finding harm to offspring in these circumstances, and hence with claiming that the reproduction is irresponsible. The problem is that in many cases of concern the alleged harm to offspring occurs from birth itself. Either the harm is congenital and unavoidable if birth is to occur, or the harm is avoidable after birth occurs, but the parents will not refrain from the harmful action. Preventing harm would mean preventing the birth of the child whose interests one is trying to protect. Yet a child's interests are hardly protected by preventing the child's existence. If the child has no way to be born or raised free of that harm, a person is not injuring the child by enabling her to be born in the circumstances of concern. The overwhelming majority of courts faced with this question in wrongful-life cases brought on behalf of the child have reached the same conclusion.[18]

Of course, this objection would not hold if the harmful conditions are such that the very existence of the child is a wrong to it. Such a case would arise where from the perspective of the child, viewed solely in light of his interests as he is then situated, any life at all with the conditions of his birth would be so harmful to him that from his perspective he would prefer not to live. In such a case existence itself is a wrong. In theory cases of wrongful life could exist, but it is doubtful whether most of the cases of concern fit that extreme rubric. For example, children born with genetic handicap or HIV might have years of life that are a good for them, as would children born in illegitimacy, poverty, or to abusive parents, even though it is less good a life than they deserve. In fact, if true cases of wrongful life did arise, one's duty would be to act immediately to prevent continued existence in order to minimize the harm. Protecting offspring by preventing their birth thus prevents the birth of offspring whose life is a net benefit to them, and is not always necessary to protect them in cases where their life is truly wrongful.[19]

This point about wrongful life is key to any claim that reproduction is irresponsible because it harms offspring by bringing them into the world in a diseased, handicapped, or disadvantaged condition. If offspring are not injured because there is no alternative way for them to be born absent the condition of concern, then reproduction is not irresponsible because of the effect on offspring who are born less whole than is desirable. This is true both in cases in which the harms are congenitally unavoidable because of genetic or infectious disease, and cases in which the harm is avoidable after birth but parents will nevertheless not avoid injuring their offspring. If there is no injury to offspring from their birth alone, then reproduction is not irresponsible solely because children are born in undesirable circumstances.

Yet one may still morally condemn giving birth to offspring in such circumstances. Derek Parfit captures this point well in his example of a woman who is told by her physician that if she gets pregnant while on a certain medication she will give birth to a child with a mild deformity, such as a withered arm, but if she waits a month, she can conceive a perfectly normal child.[20] If the woman refuses to wait and has the child with the withered arm, she has not harmed that child, because there is no way that this *particular* child could have been born normal. Still, many would say that she has acted wrongly because she has gratuitously chosen to bring a suffering child into the world when a brief wait would have enabled her to have a normal, though different, child. Now one could argue that her action is morally justified by the net good provided the child born with the withered arm. However, if one concludes that her actions are wrong, it is not because she has harmed the child born with the withered arm, but because she has violated a norm against offending persons who are troubled by gratuitous suffering.[21]

Burdens on Society

A main ground for charging that reproduction is irresponsible is the costs or burdens imposed on others. These burdens may take a financial or nonfinancial form. A common kind of nonfinancial burden is the sense of outrage or offense felt when someone gratuitously has children who are born with disease or disadvantages, as in Parfit's example of the withered arm. Even though bringing children into the world who have no other practical way to be born healthy does not in itself injure them, it does injure the sensibilities of those persons offended by the action, particularly when the person reproducing could have easily avoided that outcome. In this case, the person reproducing is harming only those whose sensibilities are affected by this experience.

But there is a problem in using this notion of offense to condemn those who bring unavoidably handicapped children into the world. The sense of offense is grounded in the undesirability of handicapped or disadvantaged children, and is inescapably a judgment about their worth. A claim of irresponsibility that rests on the undesirability of handicapped persons will not be a strong basis for moral condemnation or public action to prevent such births, particularly if those reproducing plan to rear or have other strong reproductive interests in the birth in question, and cannot reproduce without risking the handicapped birth.

The most significant burdens on others thus turn out to be the rearing burdens and financial costs that reproduction will impose on others and on the public treasury in welfare payments, medical costs, educational costs, child-abuse monitoring, social workers, and so on. Unspecified costs such as the costs of crime and social disintegration that such reproduction helps cause could also be included here.

Now this category of costs is significant only if it significantly exceeds the costs which *any* birth imposes on society. It may be that any additional child makes demands on societal resources, and incurs public subsidies to some extent. It may also be that only some children subsidized in this way repay those costs over their lifetime through their own contributions. Only where the costs imposed or the subsidies demanded exceed a reasonable level might one be said to be harming others by their reproduction.

It is difficult to say which cases fall into that category and thus may be deemed irresponsible. Persons who reproduce knowing that they will depend on the welfare system or the charity of others to support their children will be imposing costs on others. The question is, however, whether those costs are beyond what we reasonably expect children to cost, or which we are willing to pay to enable persons to have offspring. If the costs do exceed that ceiling, there may be grounds for charging them with irresponsible reproduction because their reproduction requires others to pay more than can be reasonably expected to enable reproduction to occur.

The size of the cost will be determinative when the reproductive interest at stake is small, as in cases where reproduction will not lead to rearing, and will be less important as the reproductive interest mounts. Of course, how great that reproductive interest must be, and how the interests compare in individual cases, will require close judgments. Such judgments will affect the validity of state efforts to minimize the costs by discouraging the reproduction.

Another important issue of burdensome and possibly irresponsible reproduction is reproduction in the face of overpopulation. When are additional births irresponsible because of the large number of existing persons? To answer this question, we must first decide how many people there ought to be, and then allocate future reproduction accordingly. Parfit has shown that a number based either on the highest possible average level of happiness in the community or the highest total amount of happiness in the community will be inadequate.[22] Questions of population raise complex issues that are beyond the scope of this book. Although reproduction may be irresponsible due to overpopulation, this is not the source of the concerns that have led to proposals to require use of Norplant to prevent allegedly irresponsible reproduction in the United States.

The Parameters Applied

With this account of factors relevant to judgments of undesirable or irresponsible reproduction, one can assess the reproductive decisions of particular individuals. The judgment in any given case will reflect a balancing of the reproductive interests at stake, the ease or burdens of avoiding reproduction, and the effects on others. A careful assessment of these factors will often be difficult because of factual uncertainties and normative imponderables about the weight to be assigned to each factor. Yet this is the task that anyone who fairly attempts to judge reproductive responsibility must undertake.

SOCIAL POLICY ISSUES

The question of social policy to discourage irresponsible or undesirable reproduction presents a different set of issues. Even if we agree that reproduction in certain cases is undesirable or irresponsible, the question remains what to do about it. Should reproduction always be left to the individuals involved, or are governmental actions to discourage or prevent irresponsible reproduction appropriate?

Excluding the government as an actor/participant in the dialogue about reproductive responsibility is not justified. The state has responsibilities to protect citizens and to facilitate exercise of their rights. Because reproduction so directly affects others, and the state is often called upon to pay the costs of reproduction, there is a legitimate role for the state to speak on these matters.

More controversial, however, are the steps that the state may take to implement its views of reproductive responsibility. These range from providing subsidies, information, education, and access to the use of positive incentives, penalties, and seizures. An important distinction is between governmental programs that support or encourage voluntary choice and those that are more coercive. Programs that inform, educate, assist, and subsidize will be more easily accepted than more coercive actions. However, voluntarism may have dangers, even in purportedly benign government programs. Information can be delivered in settings or in styles that might be perceived as threatening. The very fact that the government is involved constitutes a judgment about the undesirability of conduct and may offend some persons. Charges of genocide or discrimination may arise because a voluntary program appears targeted to a particular ethnic or minority group. In general, however, programs designed to inform women or to provide access to Norplant are desirable and acceptable. This is true even if only particular groups are targeted, such as welfare mothers, teenagers, women with AIDS, or those convicted of child abuse.

More controversial governmental actions involve programs that offer incentives or condition program benefits in return for certain reproductive choices. In general, incentive programs are designed to preserve autonomy, even though they attempt to influence how the autonomy in question is exercised. However, offering rewards to use Norplant or conditioning the receipt of welfare benefits on its use may be perceived as burdening or coercing individual choice, especially when the choice is presented to welfare mothers, teenagers, and other vulnerable groups. As the discussion below will show, however, the legality of such offers and conditions should be distinguished from their wisdom as social policy. If the incentive offer or condition does not deprive a person of what she or he is otherwise entitled to, it will usually be legally permissible. However, one can question whether irresponsible reproduction is so serious a problem that focusing on these groups is a sound answer to serious social problems.

More coercive measures, such as penalties for reproducing irresponsibly or refusing birth control, have a strong presumption against them. Prudential questions aside, there may be legal or constitutional barriers against such policies. The power of the state to coerce or force people not to reproduce turns on whether its actions violate a fundamental right, and if so, whether there is a compelling interest to justify it. If the state's action interferes with or limits coital reproduction by a married couple, it would ordinarily be found to infringe a fundamental right to procreate, and thus require strong justification.[23]

An unresolved question at this point is whether courts evaluating such a claim would assess the relative importance of the reproduction at issue to the individuals involved. If the parents would rear, mere offense at what they are doing or costs to the taxpayer probably would be insufficient to justify intruding on their right. However, if the parents would not rear, because of unfitness, past neglect, impecunity, or other factors, the courts in particular cases could find that the reproductive interest is so slight as to allow a lesser state interest to justify intrusion.[24] Of course, direct seizures to implant Norplant or to sterilize individuals would require a very strong justification because of the intrusion on bodily integrity alone.

Policies directed at reproduction by unmarried persons or minors might have a lesser constitutional hurdle to surmount. Because the Supreme Court has not held that persons have a right to reproduce outside marriage, a lesser justification may be needed to uphold such policies.[25] In that case, costs to the community might justify laws that could not be justified against married persons. However, unmarried persons would still have rights against bodily intrusion. Thus state policies that required physical burdens or sacrifice, such as forcible implants or sterilization would have to meet the compelling interest standard. In those cases saving money or preventing insults to community sensibility may not be sufficient, even if the legally protected reproductive interest is less than in the case of married persons.

It appears that coercive sanctions will be rarely available to states seeking to minimize or discourage irresponsible reproduction. In most instances, the harms sought to be averted are costs to the community or to a sense of offense, because children themselves, who have no way to be born without the disadvantage in question, would not be harmed. These kinds of concerns will not justify coerced intrusions on the body, much less on strong reproductive interests. However, they could justify limitations on lesser reproductive interests, such as genetic reproduction *tout court*, or when persons have no protected reproductive interest because of age and marital status. Other than the severely retarded, there may be no group that fits the criteria for coercive action. In the end, government policy will almost invariably have to rely on information, education, counseling, subsidies and incentives, so that the freedom of choice in matters of reproduction is protected.

FIVE PROBLEMATIC CASES

With the parameters of reproductive responsibility and the range of policy options as background, we are now ready to discuss five problematic situations for which Norplant has been urged. In each case, we must balance the benefits of the questionable reproduction to the person involved against the claims of irresponsibility. The availability of state policies to discourage undesirable reproduction will depend on the extent to which those policies which interfere with fundamental rights can be justified by harmful effects on offspring, taxpayers, and society. The discussion will show that in most instances the alleged irresponsibility will not support coercive policies, though it will permit voluntary measures that use education, information, subsidies, and incentives.

Contraception As a Condition of Probation

The question of compulsory use of Norplant has been most frequently raised in cases involving women convicted of child abuse or homicide of their children. In these cases, the sentencing judge is faced with a problem. Although a prison sentence is justified, the judge recognizes that the woman might be better rehabilitated in the community. However, she also knows that if the woman has more children, rehabilitation will be more difficult and that there is a real danger that abuse of a new child might occur. In these situations, some judges have offered women the option of probation on condition that they consent to Norplant or other contraception as an alternative to the prison sentence that would otherwise be imposed.[26]

The most widely publicized case of mandatory contraception, *People v. Johnson*, involved a twenty-seven-year-old woman sentenced to two to four years in prison for child abuse.[27] She had been convicted of severely beating two of her four children with a belt. Toward the end of her first year, the trial judge offered to release the woman on probation if she would agree to have Norplant implanted for three years of probation. The woman initially agreed. Later she sought to appeal this sentence on the ground that it was coerced, that it violated her fundamental right to procreate, and that it was medically contraindicated.

In a rehearing after the woman revoked her initial agreement to the sentence, the judge noted that she had shown herself incapable of caring for her children and stated: "It is in the defendant's best interest and certainly in any unconceived child's interest that she not have any more children until she is mentally and emotionally prepared to do so. The birth of additional children until after she has successfully completed the court-ordered mental health counseling and parenting classes dooms both her and any subsequent children to repeat this vicious cycle."[28] He further noted: "Although the right to procreate is substantial and constitutionally protected, it is not absolute and can be limited in a proper case. The compelling state interest in the protection of the children supersedes this particular individual's right to procreate and does not interfere with her right of sexual expression."[29]

In considering the validity of contraception as a condition of probation, an important preliminary issue is whether the judge's sentencing power includes the power to impose contraception as a condition of probation. If the law does not authorize such a sentence, then such conditions are invalid.[30] If such probation conditions have been authorized, the question then is whether the authorized sentence is unconstitutional.

Ordinarily a state requirement or coercive offer that a woman take Norplant would require a compelling justification, for it intrudes into her body and limits her reproduction. A convicted child abuser could still have an interest in reproducing. She may wish to have and rear more children, precisely because of guilt she feels for her past behavior. However, if she will lose custody of any child upon birth because of her past record as an abuser, her reproductive interest may be reduced. If custody will not automatically be removed, or if she will be permitted to have some limited contact with offspring, her reproductive interest increases in importance. Even if she has no rearing role, she may still get important satisfaction from having produced another child. Although the facts of individual cases will vary, convicted child abusers will often retain the reproductive interests that enjoy presumptive protected status.

If that is so, any coercive state efforts to prevent her from reproduction would have to meet the compelling interest test. In this case the asserted state interest—protection of future offspring who will be injured by future abuse—may not exist. If the woman retains custody of future children, she may have been rehabilitated and no longer be an abuser. Or social workers may more closely monitor her to prevent abuse from occurring.[31] Even if she does abuse future children, it is not clear that they will enjoy such a horrible life that they never should have been born at all, and thus are harmed by being born to an abusing mother.[32] In short, the need to protect future offspring does not appear to justify overriding her right to procreate, because the means of protection prevents the birth of the children whom one is trying to protect.

Nor could limitations on her reproduction be justified by the need to protect society and the community. Child abusers who reproduce will cost the community more money and services in monitoring, treatment, and other services. If children are born and later injured, many people will experience outrage at her repetitive conduct. More demand on scarce foster parent resources will occur, at a time when those resources are severely strained. Costly medical and psychological treatment may be needed for the child.[33] In addition, people may lose confidence in a system that permits a woman who has severely beaten or murdered her children to produce more children. But these costs would ordinarily not support coercive sanctions that limit exercise of a fundamental right, and probably will not support coercive sanctions for failure to use Norplant.

However, the woman in question is a convicted child abuser and could be sent to prison. A condition of imprisonment is that men and women are ordinarily prevented from reproducing—from begetting and bearing children while in prison.[34] They have no constitutional right to conjugal visits, and no right to hand their sperm out for artificial insemination.[35] Since prisoners are ordinarily deprived of procreation during the term of imprisonment, could not the state place a person subject to imprisonment on probation with contraception, on the ground that the greater power to imprison implies the lesser power to impose contraception?

If the greater power to imprison does not imply the lesser power to impose contraception, then interfering in reproduction in this way will be a punishment that must satisfy Eighth Amendment standards against cruel and unusual punishment.[36] This provision bars punishments that are excessive or barbarous.[37] Because temporary loss of reproduction via Norplant does not appear to be excessive for the crime of abusing children, the question will turn on whether imposition of Norplant is inherently cruel or barbarous. Here the method is a choice—probation with Norplant or prison—that is akin to the choices presented defendants deciding whether to plead guilty, but one that focuses on their body and its functions. It causes them to accept a minor surgical intervention into their body, some side effects of varying intensity, and the loss of procreative ability for a period of time.

One cannot predict with certainty how courts would rule on a claim that such a punishment violates the Eighth Amendment. Bodily and reproductive intrusions are clearly disfavored, yet Norplant is not so highly intrusive or shocking, given the restrictions that usually occur with imprisonment, that offering the persons a choice that will temporarily limit their reproductive ability for a period of time as punishment for crime would necessarily be found to be unconstitutional. However, the question is a close one, and cannot be decided without more particular facts. Because the restriction is rationally related to rehabilitation and to preventing the very crimes being punished, the ultimate decision will hinge on perceptions of the need for the state to mandate reproductive restrictions.[38]

In sum, the validity of compulsory contraception for convicted child abusers depends on whether the limitation of procreation must be independently justified or is a rational, nonbarbarous punishment for serious crime. If the former, the state justifications are insufficient. Neither the interest in protecting unborn offspring from harm nor in saving social welfare resources justifies limiting procreation. Only if persons subject to imprisonment but placed on probation have fewer procreative rights would such a condition of probation be acceptable. Even then, one can question whether a technological solution to the problem should be sought.

Compulsory Contraception to Prevent Congenital Disease

The case for compulsory contraception to prevent the birth of offspring with congenital disease is also hard to sustain. One target of such efforts would be couples who are at risk for having children with genetic handicaps and insist on reproducing. Ordinarily, they would have a one in two or one in four chance of having a child with the defect in question. Depending on the disease, the child could die early or have a lifetime of chronic illness and medical care. However, this is a relatively small group, whose overall numbers do not justify such an intrusive intervention.

A more likely target would be women who are HIV positive. They have a 25 to 35 percent chance of passing HIV to offspring.[39] If they do, the child may die early or be maintained at high cost for many years. Even if children are not infected, the parents still are at risk of dying and leaving their children parentless. Indeed, the problem of children who are parentless due to AIDS is a growing social problem, with 80,000 such children predicted by the year 2000.[40]

In either case, however, the compulsory use of Norplant cannot be justified. To begin with, members of both groups have substantial interests in reproduction. The couple that has had a handicapped child may hope for a healthy child, but be willing to raise and care for another child with the handicap in question. Moreover, the risk of a child with handicap will ordinarily be 1 in 4. Preventing the birth of the handicapped child would also prevent the greater likelihood that offspring will not have the disease in question. Avoiding the birth of an affected child may also require prenatal testing and abortion, to which the parents are opposed.

Similarly, women with HIV may still find procreation immensely meaningful, both because it is a prime source of meaning and validation in their social-cultural context, and because it meets their need for continuity after the death looming over them. As Nancy Dubler and Carol Levine note, in the view of these women, "having babies . . . may be the most reasonable and available choice, a natural outcome of all the forces in their lives, in which avenues for self-definition and expression other than mothering are largely absent."[41] Even if particular individuals will not rear affected offspring or will not rear for long, core interests of reproduction are at stake for both groups.

The case for claiming that their reproduction is irresponsible must therefore rest on the burdens which it imposes on offspring and society. The burden commonly cited is that they are knowingly having or risking having children who are born with serious genetic or infectious disease. The children who are born with HIV may face an early death, or a period of health and normal growth until symptoms arise. They will then face repeated hospitalizations and an early death. If they do not themselves have HIV, they are likely to be born into circumstances in which their parents will soon die, and may end up orphaned in foster care or other disadvantageous circumstances.

Similarly, children born with serious genetic handicaps may face repeated surgeries and hospitalizations, significant mortality and morbidity, social stigma, and the suffering that arises from their mental and physical limitations. While their parents may rear them, some of them will be placed in poorly funded state institutions or group homes.

Yet in both cases one cannot say that these children have been harmed by being born, because they have no way to be born free of the congenital diseases or social circumstances that are so disadvantageous.[42] Unlike Parfit's case of the risk of a withered arm, the persons procreating here cannot produce a healthy child by postponing conception. All their offspring are at risk for the conditions of concern. Few of those conditions would make the child's life so horrible that its interests would have been best served by never being born.[43] Thus it is unlikely that the goal of preventing harm to offspring by preventing them from being born would justify a coercive contraceptive policy toward their parents.

Nor will the significant costs that they may impose on the public treasury and charity. In some instances the parents will not impose rearing costs on others, because they will bear the cost themselves, either directly or through insurance. However, in most cases the persons reproducing with this risk will end up requiring large subsidies from the state for medical care and other services for their children. If the children's diseases are serious enough, as AIDS and some genetic conditions will be, they will be demanding subsidies greater than those ordinarily provided to persons who reproduce. In addition, there may be other social costs, from the degradation of many orphans in impoverished settings to the offense felt at the actions of persons who do not attempt to avoid reproduction when the risks of an abnormal birth are great.

None of these costs, however, is sufficient to justify directly imposing Norplant or other contraception on women at risk for offspring with these conditions. Because these women's reproductive interest is generally a strong one, only very compelling needs would justify overriding their fundamental right to procreate. Saving money and preventing offense ordinarily would not rise to the required level. However, a closer analysis of their reproductive interest could on occasion yield a different conclusion. For example, if they lack the capacity or interest in rearing, will institutionalize the child at birth, or face a short life span due to their own illness, required contraception would not violate as significant a reproductive interest than if they intended to rear for long periods.[44] If the bodily intrusion associated with compulsory contraception is relatively minor, it may be that compelled contraception in rare cases could be justified, though such policies would be highly controversial.

At present, however, this discussion is largely hypothetical, because no one has proposed that HIV women or those at genetic risk should be penalized for reproduction or failure to accept Norplant. These remedies seem so extreme because of the seriousness of the intrusion and the lack of sufficient justification for it. They would also be open to charges of racism and discrimination against those who are less than able-bodied.

The more immediate policy question concerns the lengths to which the state may go to persuade these groups voluntarily to avoid reproduction. In both cases the state could support or conduct programs to make sure that persons at risk are aware of the potential consequences of their reproductive behavior, and that contraception and abortion to avert reproduction is available. Included in such information would be facts concerning prenatal or other tests to inform them of their risk status or the status of a fetus.[45]

Much more controversial is whether the state or private parties should engage in directive counseling, urging that they not reproduce because of the risks of affected offspring and the other problems thereby caused. Health-care providers, counselors, and ethicists are currently split over whether directed counseling can be justified in these cases.[46] This debate is largely prudential rather than ethical. As long as directed counseling leaves the woman free to make her own choice, it would not violate her autonomy. Indeed, it may be useful to make her aware of the serious consequences of her actions. However, any mandatory or directive program will be controversial, whatever its ethical or policy justification, because of the perception that it is singling out women who are already stigmatized, and because of the risk that it denigrates the worth of the children whose birth it is trying to prevent.

Welfare Issues

Compulsory contraception through Norplant has also emerged as an issue of welfare policy. Shortly after the FDA approved Norplant, legislators in Kansas, Oklahoma, and Louisiana introduced bills offering financial rewards to welfare mothers who agreed to Norplant implants. The rewards ranged from $100 in Louisiana to $500 in Kansas, with Kansas also offering a yearly maintenance fee of $50. Welfare would also pay the costs of the Norplant. Similar proposals are likely in other states.

Although none of these proposals has passed, the appeal of Norplant as a way to control costly reproduction by poor women is obvious. A common perception is that high welfare costs are the result of poor women having children to cash in on welfare benefits. The editorial board of the *Philadelphia Inquirer* fell prey to this myth when in an editorial entitled "Norplant and the Underclass" it praised Norplant as an answer to problems of welfare associated with a high minority birth rate (when the black community protested, the newspaper quickly apologized).[47] A common sentiment is that poor women are acting irresponsibly when they have children that the taxpayers will have to support. If so, the idea of encouraging them to contracept makes sense.

But is reproduction when one will require public assistance to support offspring irresponsible? A person who intends to rear such offspring, as most welfare mothers do, will have a significant reproductive interest at stake. However, to realize their reproductive goal they will be demanding that the community pay rearing costs that those who reproduce are usually responsible for. Is it unreasonable to ask the community to do so? A good argument can be made that it is, particularly if one has already reproduced and could do so at some point in the future. Only if there are no reproductive alternatives for that person, or avoidance is not reasonably possible, might that action be reasonable.

Yet even if a mild judgment of irresponsibility can be lodged, it would not follow that compulsory contraceptive measures are justified. Indeed, as a legal matter, the state probably could not penalize persons for giving birth to children who need welfare, even if moral culpability could be shown. The injury to the community's resources and norms of proper reproduction is simply insufficient to justify coercive intrusion on a fundamental right. Nor have such proposals been seriously made.

Instead, the focus of policy has been on proposals to encourage women on welfare to use Norplant voluntarily. While no one objects to informing welfare mothers of the Norplant option and providing it free of charge, proposals to pay women to have the implant, or to require it as a condition of receiving welfare, are more controversial. Neither idea unconstitutionally infringes procreative liberty. However, one may question whether the costs of excessive births by welfare mothers are such a serious problem that direct state intervention into reproductive decisions is advisable.

PAYING REWARDS

The idea of paying a reward, whether $100, $500, or some higher sum, to accept and maintain Norplant does not violate the offeree's procreative liberty. In trying to influence or manage reproductive choice, the reward assumes that such choice exists. Although $100 or even $500 may be attractive enough to get a woman's attention and even influence her decision, it does not deny her something that she would otherwise receive, and thus should not be considered coercive. A woman remains free to reject the implant, even though she will not receive the reward or the other benefits of long-lasting, convenient contraception. The idea of manipulating incentives to reduce reproduction is no more offensive than the manipulation of incentives to get welfare mothers to work or marry. No one has proposed so high a sum (say, over $1,000) that would make a charge of exploitation or coercion more credible.

Still, rewards for using Norplant will remain controversial, with groups supportive of welfare rights and procreative choice split on its acceptability. For example, some affiliate chapters of Planned Parenthood of America, a main defender of reproductive choice, have conducted experiments paying teenage mothers a per diem stipend to avoid further pregnancy.[48] Such a policy would implicitly support rewards for accepting Norplant.

Many other liberal groups oppose payments to avoid reproduction, arguing that any reward to impoverished persons is coercive.[49] Even if a $100 or $500 reward is not coercive, it implicitly denigrates welfare mothers by assuming that they cannot rationally weigh the pros and cons of reproduction without the enticement of a reward. Also, such a program has the appearance of buying reproductive potential for money, a practice not acceptable with organ donations. It puts the state in the position of buying their right to have children, and thus paying to avoid poor and minority births.

The question of paying welfare mothers to accept Norplant is less a legal or ethical one than a question of symbols and appearances. Given the symbolic connotations associated with bribing welfare mothers not to reproduce, the preferred strategy is education and counseling about the merits of Norplant and assuring access to all welfare mothers who want it. A concentrated educational campaign might reach most of the target group without incurring the symbolic costs of buying up their right to reproduce. Only if few women respond to that option should a reward system for Norplant be implemented. However, since such rewards can be respectful of reproductive choice, they should not automatically be foreclosed.

AS A CONDITION OF WELFARE

Even more questionable would be a policy that made acceptance of Norplant a condition of receiving welfare payments at all. Proposals linking welfare to sterilization surfaced repeatedly in the 1960s and 1970s but never gained much support. Norplant, however, is less intrusive than sterilization and completely reversible. With renewed interest in tying welfare to education, job training, job seeking, number of children, and even to marriage, it would not be surprising if some states require acceptance of Norplant as a condition of receiving welfare payments.[50]

Legally, such a condition probably would be constitutional. Since a state has no constitutional obligation to provide welfare at all, it would be free to provide it only if certain conditions rationally related to the program are met.[51] A condition relating to contraception, to enable recipients to take care of current children and lower costs, might be found rational in a welfare system that is attempting to reduce costs and help women into the job market. It is clearly distinguishable from unconstitutional welfare conditions that condition benefits on the exercise or waiver of constitutional rights that are unrelated to the purposes of a welfare system, such as one's political party, one's religious affiliation, or the books one chooses to read.[52]

Legality aside, however, one can question whether any state should go so far. Simply making Norplant available will lead many women on welfare to choose it, and a limited reward system would increase those numbers. But making Norplant a condition of receiving welfare seems too strenuous an intervention in reproductive choice. It will also penalize dependent children whose living standard decreases because of their mother's unwillingness or inability to avoid reproduction. Given available alternatives, the case for conditioning any welfare payment on Norplant is not a strong one.

Compulsory Contraception for the Retarded

Controlling the reproduction of mentally retarded persons has a checkered history in the United States. In the early twentieth century the American Eugenics Society actively lobbied to sterilize "mental defectives" and "feeble-minded persons" because of a perceived threat to the gene pool and social welfare. The result was compulsory sterilization laws passed in over thirty states, which the United States Supreme Court upheld in 1927 in *Buck v. Bell*.[53] With this imprimatur, more than 60,000 persons were sterilized over the next thirty years.

In the 1960s a strong reaction to compulsory eugenic sterilization occurred, impelled by awareness of the excesses of Nazi eugenic practices and the scientific unsoundness of the hereditary assumptions underlying these laws. It also became clear that many persons had been sterilized who were neither mentally ill nor retarded, including Carrie Buck, the original plaintiff in *Buck v. Bell.*[54] Although that case has never been reversed, compulsory sterilization is now generally viewed as a gross violation of human rights and no longer performed for eugenic reasons.

In the mid-1970s, however, it became clear that there were some circumstances in which sterilization was justified to protect the retarded from pregnancy rather than to serve eugenics or save money. For example, retarded women in state institutions or group homes are vulnerable to sexual exploitation or rape. Pregnancy, especially in women who lack comprehension, poses serious health risks. Delivery by cesarean section may be necessary. Often parents restrict participation in group homes and other opportunities to avoid having their retarded daughters risk pregnancy.

Faced with parents seeking to have retarded daughters sterilized, state courts began authorizing such procedures. Since few states still had statutes authorizing such sterilizations, the main issue before the courts was whether a probate court's inherent *parens patriae* power over incompetent patients authorized them to order sterilization in the absence of statutory authority when it seemed in the incompetent ward's interest.[55] While some courts preferred to wait for legislative authorization, influential state supreme courts, including those of New Jersey, Massachusetts, and Washington, devised tests that allowed sterilization when it could be shown to benefit the incompetent ward.[56]

Norplant presents an attractive alternative in situations in which sterilization would otherwise be appropriate. Because there is usually no serious reproductive interest at stake, the main question is whether implantation of Norplant will cause harm. If sterilization is justified, *a fortiori* Norplant should be, because it is less intrusive and reversible. Indeed, it would seem preferable to sterilization. Thus parents or guardians who petition for sterilization should show that less restrictive contraceptive measures such as Norplant are contraindicated or not available.

In fact, it may be acceptable for parents or caretakers to have Norplant routinely implanted in mentally retarded and institutionalized women concerned about their risk of pregnancy. Because surgical insertion is required, the consent of parents or guardian is necessary, though the judicial review required for sterilization should not be. Norplant may thus provide a technological solution to the risk of pregnancy faced by mentally retarded women.

Controlling reproduction in severely retarded women with Norplant limits procreation without limiting procreative choice. For the notion of reproductive choice is no more meaningful for severely retarded women than is electoral choice. If they are so mentally impaired that the concept of reproduction and parenthood has no meaning, then limiting their reproduction does not infringe their procreative liberty. The concept of procreative choice simply does not apply to them.[57] If mistakes are made about reproductive interest, the Norplant can simply be removed.

Of course, the retarded do have rights of bodily integrity and rights to be treated with respect. They should not be burdened merely to serve the needs of others. Limiting their reproduction, however, does not harm them, and actually serves their interests by protecting them from the physical risks of pregnancy. If done with a minimal intrusion on their body, as occurs with Norplant, it should be socially acceptable as well. However, careful monitoring of how Norplant is used with this population, including indications, side effects, and length of use, is needed before implantation routinely occurs. With these protections, the use of Norplant with the retarded at the request of parents and guardians may be acceptable.

Norplant and Adolescents

Norplant has also been suggested as an answer to teenage pregnancy. If informed consent is obtained, the use of Norplant poses no issues beyond those raised by teenage contraceptive use generally. The chief issue here is whether teenagers can obtain contraceptives without parental consent or notification. If state law permits adolescent females to obtain medically prescribed contraceptives, then they should be able to obtain Norplant as well.

Also, there should be no barrier to parents or guardians providing Norplant to adolescent girls who desire it. The discretionary power of parents to rear their children entitles them to obtain medical care that is in their child's interests. Postponing pregnancy until a more mature time serves the interests of child and parent. While parents should not be able to have doctors insert Norplant against a teenager's wishes, there should be no objection if the child agrees with the parent's desire for Norplant.

Programs that offer Norplant in school clinics are more controversial, however, because the state appears to be taking a more active role in controlling adolescent reproduction. The Baltimore school system, which now provides Norplant along with other contraceptives, has been careful to preserve choice in offering Norplant to a teenage population with an exceedingly high pregnancy rate.[58] The young women are informed of the risks and benefits of the implant, and are not pressured in any way to accept it. Parents are notified if the teenager consents to such notification. However, some people are troubled by the idea of city authorities trying to influence female reproduction, and doubt whether such programs are truly noncoercive.

A more hypothetical question is whether the state could require that teenage girls have an antifertility vaccine or Norplant implanted shortly after puberty, after one illegitimate birth, or some other risk marker in order to make pregnancy a matter of deliberate choice.[59] This policy would prevent teenage pregnancy, but would not prevent girls who wish to have children from regaining fertility by having the implants removed or the vaccine rendered inactive.

Given the very high rates of unintended teenage pregnancy, such a policy would no doubt have many supporters. Nor would it necessarily violate the procreative liberty of its targets, for it only temporarily postpones pregnancy and is aimed at unmarried adolescents who do not have the same legal right to conceive and reproduce that adults do. If the intrusion is viewed as minor,[60] they will have ample time to have and rear children when they decide to do so. Such a policy would prevent many illegitimate births and the cycle of dropping out of high school, poor employment opportunities, and welfare that adolescent pregnancy often brings. Also, it would prevent the birth of children who themselves are often doomed to repeat that cycle, or who grow up without male authority figures in their life. Although such children are not wronged by being born, society may still prefer that children be born with more advantages.

Although the purpose is commendable and teenagers may lack a right to reproduce, a policy of compulsory contraception will face high constitutional barriers. Teenagers do have a strong interest in bodily integrity. The insertion of the device may be viewed as minor, but the potential side effects are serious enough—many women cannot tolerate Norplant—to make the bodily intrusion substantial. Overriding this interest may be difficult to justify, despite the worthiness of the goal.

A further problem would arise in identifying the target of such an intrusive policy. If directed at all female adolescents, it would be grossly overbroad, intruding upon the many to prevent pregnancy by a few.[61] If targeted to subgroups that have high rates of pregnancy, it risks actual or perceived discrimination on racial or ethnic grounds. In its most defensible form, it would apply only to teenagers who already had a teenage pregnancy and refused to use contraception. Yet even there the intrusiveness of forcing a contraceptive implant on an unwilling subject would be a difficult barrier to overcome, particularly if parents objected.

In short, such an intrusive policy of social engineering sounds too Orwellian to be acceptable, even if the state possessed the raw constitutional power to implement it. As with most instances of allegedly irresponsible reproduction, it is far preferable to rely on education and choice rather than on mandatory measures. Indeed, a fair attempt to encourage contraceptive use by adolescents would probably obviate the need for involuntary implantation.

CONCLUSION

Procreation is a basic right, but it is not an absolute right. Its protected status does not relieve individuals of the moral obligation to reproduce responsibly. When they do not, public pressure arises to use reversible technologies such as Norplant to limit their reproduction.

Unless voluntarily chosen, however, the use of Norplant or other contraceptives can rarely be justified as a solution to problems of allegedly irresponsible reproduction. Its most defensible application is with severely retarded females who are at risk of sexual exploitation or rape. In the other situations discussed, however, its intrusiveness and effect on procreation make it highly suspect. Child abusers, HIV women, welfare mothers, and teenagers have interests in procreation or bodily integrity which mandatory use of Norplant violates. Neither protection of future offspring nor conservation of public funds are compelling enough reasons to justify intrusions on such basic rights. In addition, there is the danger of discrimination or antipathy toward targeted groups.

This conclusion should not prevent the state from informing women of the Norplant option, subsidizing its provision, or even offering financial incentives to use it. If these alternatives are pursued, the need for compulsory contraception through Norplant further weakens. Forcible limitations on reproduction need a much stronger justification than these cases present.

ASSISTED REPRODUCTION

CHAPTER 5

IVF, Infertility, and the Status of Embryos

IN VITRO fertilization (IVF) emerged as a major treatment for infertility in the 1980s. Its reliance on extracorporeal fertilization of human eggs raises questions about the status, control, and disposition of embryos. As a high-tech reproductive procedure, it also presents issues of access, efficacy, and truthful disclosure that test the limits of procreative freedom. To explore these issues, this chapter addresses the conflicts and controversies that arise when husband and wife provide egg and sperm for IVF.[1]

INFERTILITY

IVF and other noncoital techniques are means of treating infertility—a problem for millions of married couples. The most recent national fertility survey shows that 2.4 million (8.5 percent) of married couples between the ages of 15 and 44 are infertile—defined as the inability to reproduce after a year of regular intercourse without contraceptives.[2] These figures underestimate the amount of infertility because they do not cover unmarried persons, or those infertile couples who are using contraceptives. If surgically sterilized married couples are excluded (almost 40 percent of couples in the 15–44-year age group), 13.5 percent of married couples are infertile.

The rate of infertility varies with age and socioeconomic class. Older women have higher rates of infertility than younger women. Excluding the surgically sterile, 14 percent of married couples with wives aged 30–34 are infertile, while 25 percent of couples with wives aged 35–39 are infertile. This is due to the biologic effects of age, as well as to the greater opportunity for environmental and other factors to reduce fertility. Black and poorer women have higher rates of infertility than white, middle-class women, due in part to poorer nutrition and health care, and a higher rate of sexually transmitted diseases.

Infertility is growing in some age groups. The number of infertile women in the 20–24-year age group has grown from 4 percent in 1965 to 11 percent in 1982, due to increased rates of gonorrhea, greater use of intrauterine devices, and increased environmental factors. Since one in three births in the United States occurs in this group, this is an important change. As other members of this age cohort seek to become pregnant, the rate of infertility at later ages will also rise.

For couples who want children, infertility is often a devastating experience. With their normal species urge to procreate frustrated, they are likely to feel inadequate at the core of their being. They often experience guilt, low self-esteem, disappointment or depression, and have higher rates of marital conflict and sexual dysfunction. Couples who seek treatment often find it difficult to stop until they have tried every alternative available.

While demographers debate whether overall—as opposed to age-specific—rates of infertility are increasing, there is little doubt that more and more infertile couples are seeking medical treatment for infertility. With medical insurance covering many infertility services, and fewer children for adoption being available, there is a greater willingness to seek medical help, including high-tech procedures such as IVF. The estimated number of office visits to general practitioners, obstetrician-gynecologists, and urologists for consultation for infertility rose from about 600,000 in 1968 to about two million in 1983, and has continued to increase. Overall, this works out to about one million couples using some form of infertility services annually, with the growth of new cases estimated to be between 110,000 and 160,000 cases a year. With diagnosis and treatment a billion-dollar industry, more doctors are specializing in infertility, thus making fertility services even more widely available.[3] The provision of IVF is a major component of this industry.

IN VITRO FERTILIZATION

IVF treats infertility problems by bypassing the natural place of fertilization in the fallopian tube. It operates by collecting eggs surgically after ovarian stimulation, fertilizing them in vitro in the laboratory, and, after 48–72 hours, placing the cleaving embryos into the uterus.

Originally developed to overcome tube blockage by bypassing the fallopian tubes altogether, IVF is increasingly used to treat infertility due to other conditions, such as endometriosis, cervical mucous problems, and the great number of cases of unexplained infertility. In addition, IVF can be used to treat oligospermia or low sperm count by putting sperm directly in contact with the egg in a dish, where there is a shorter distance to travel to conception. In severe cases, it would enable conception to occur by drilling of the egg's zona pellucida or by microinjection of single sperm into the egg (intra cytoplasmic sperm injection).

The first birth of a child from IVF occurred in 1978 in Great Britain, capping off a long period of research by Steptoe, Edwards, and others.

Since then more than 40,000 children conceived in this way have been born worldwide. The United States has more than 250 programs offering IVF. Over 15,000 children have been born as a result of the procedure in the last four years alone.[4] However, IVF will not provide all patients with a baby. While the best programs have a success rate of over 30 percent per egg retrieval, many programs cannot approach this record.[5] At present women have to undergo on the average two IVF cycles to start a pregnancy, at a cost of $7,000 to $9,000 per cycle. Improvements in success rates will occur as research and experience with the technique grow.

To increase the chances of pregnancy, most IVF programs stimulate the ovaries to obtain multiple eggs, and place several fertilized eggs or embryos in the uterus in each IVF cycle (American programs place on average 3.5 embryos in the uterus per cycle). If too many fertilized eggs are placed in the uterus, there is a great risk of multiple pregnancy, and may create the need for selective reduction (abortion) of the pregnancy. Embryo freezing, now practiced in most clinics, permits extra embryos to be preserved and then thawed for use in later cycles. This will increase the overall efficacy of an egg retrieval cycle and reduce the costs or burdens of later cycles.

Increasingly, eggs are collected by means of ultrasound-guided transvaginal aspiration, which eliminates the need for laparoscopy and general anesthesia.[6] When tubes are patent, the embryos may also be placed directly into the fallopian tube, in a procedure known as ZIFT (zygote intrafallopian transfer). Egg and sperm may also be inserted directly into a patent tube before fertilization occurs (known as GIFT, or gamete intrafallopian transfer). Since the fallopian tube is the natural site of fertilization and early embryo development, these procedures may offer a better chance of success in certain cases.

SHOULD IVF BE DONE AT ALL?

Basic IVF raises many issues that force us to consider the scope and meaning of procreative liberty. At the most fundamental level, the question is whether IVF should occur at all. Engineering conception in the bright glare of the laboratory rather than the dark recesses of the fallopian tube strikes some people as wrong or undesirable. They would deny or severely limit access to this procedure.

Their objection has several strands. One is an antitechnology bias against medical interventions, especially reproductive interventions. A second strand is theological, exemplified by the Catholic position that any separation of the unitive (sexual) and procreative is improper. A third feminist strand sees any reproductive technology as exploiting the socially engrained view that infertile women are inadequate—that women must produce children for their husbands. IVF, which bombards a woman's body with powerful hormones and then invades the body to harvest eggs, is in their view a prime example of such an exploitive technology. It holds out the false promise of success when the chance of taking home a baby is actually quite low.[7] Finally, right-to-life groups would ban IVF because they think that it may destroy the embryo.

Whatever the merits of these objections, they have not dampened demand or had a significant impact on public policy. Although a 1987 Vatican directive urged that civil law be enacted to ban procedures such as IVF, no state has done so and no groups appear to be lobbying for such a measure.[8] Indeed, the incidence of IVF in the United States (and throughout the world) continues to grow. In 1993, 31,900 stimulation cycles for IVF were reported, 27,443 of which went to egg retrieval, with an additional 4,992 retrieval cycles done for gamete intrafallopian transfer (GIFT), in which the egg and sperm are placed directly into the fallopian tube.[9]

If a law banning IVF or GIFT were passed, it would no doubt be found unconsitutional because it directly impeded the efforts of infertile married couples to have offspring, thus interfering with their fundmental right to procreate.[10] The moral objections to IVF made by the Catholic Church, feminists, and others do not constitute the compelling evidence of tangible harm necesssary to justify interference with procreative liberty. Ancillary rules for the conduct of IVF, which are discussed below, should also have to satisfy the compelling-interest test when they substantially interfere with access to IVF.

EMBRYO STATUS ISSUES

IVF is unique because it externalizes the earliest stages of human life, and subjects it to observation and manipulation. Moral and legal controversies over basic IVF concern the control and disposition of embryos created in the process. What is the status of preimplantation embryos?[11] Who has dispositional control over them? What actions may be done with them?

These questions pit deeply felt views about respect for the earliest stages of human life against the needs of infertile couples to create embryos to serve their reproductive goals. Their resolution will have a great impact on the scope of procreative freedom and the use of IVF to treat infertility. The biological, moral, and legal status of the embryo is first discussed before issues of ownership and limitations on what may be done with embryos is addressed.

The Biological Status of Embryos

Conception occurs when a single spermatozoa enters the egg and the chromosomes of each fuse into a single cell of forty-six chromosomes. Fertilization is not instantaneous, but occurs gradually over several hours after penetration of the egg by a single sperm.[12] At this stage a new and unique genome beginning a new generation exists within a single cell.[13]

During the next three days the one-celled zygote divides several times to become an undifferentiated aggregate of two, four, six, or eight cells. In IVF programs the embryo will be transferred to a uterus when it reaches the four-, six-, or eight-cell stage, some 48 to 72 hours after conception. In ZIFT, transfer directly into the fallopian tube occurs via laparoscopy at the one-cell or zygote stage. It is also at this stage that the embryo would be cryopreserved for later use.

Further growth produces the cell clusters of the morula and then blastocyst stage of development. At the blastocyst stage the simple cellular aggregate of the fertilized egg starts to show a central cavity surrounded by a peripheral cellular layer with some distinguishable inner cells.[14] The outer cells develop into a trophoblastic or feeding layer that becomes the placenta rather than the embryo proper. At this time only cells of the inner mass can give rise to an embryo.

The blastocyst stage marks the developing capability to interact with maternal cells of the uterine lining, which is essential for implantation and later development to occur. At six to nine days the developing cellular mass acquires the ability to implant or embed in the uterine wall as the placenta, jointly derived from embryonic and maternal cells, begins to form.[15] Implantation marks the beginning of pregnancy as a maternal state. At this stage the embryonic mass has a clearly distinguishable outer cellular layer which plays the major role in the implantation process. It is the as yet undeveloped inner cell mass, however, that is the source of the embryo proper. It is for this reason that preimplantation stages are more accurately called the "preembryo."

When the blastocyst is well established in the uterine wall (early in the second postfertilization week), the inner cell mass reorganizes into two layers that make up the embryonic disk. This first true rudiment of the embryo is the site of the formation of the embryonic axis, along which the major organs and structures of the body will be differentiated.[16] By the end of the fourth postconception week, the major organs are more fully formed and cardiovascular circulation has begun.[17] By the eighth week an anatomically recognizable human miniature exists, displaying very primitive neuromuscular function but still extremely immature by all structural and functional criteria.[18] The higher parts of the brain do not show any electrical activity or nerve cell connections until twelve weeks after conception.[19] If abortion does not occur, the birth of a newborn infant will complete the gestational process.

The Moral Status of Embryos

While scientists largely agree about these facts of zygote, preembryo, and embryo development, there is also a growing consensus about their moral significance. Three major ethical positions have been articulated in the debate over embryo status. At one extreme is the view of the embryo as a human subject after fertilization, which requires that it be accorded the rights of a person. This position entails an obligation to provide an opportunity for implantation to occur and tends to ban any action before transfer that might harm the embryo or that is not immediately therapeutic, such as freezing and embryo research. Its weakness is that it ignores the reality of biological development just described.

At the opposite extreme is the view that the embryo has a status no different from that of any other human tissue, and can be treated accordingly. Other than requiring the consent of those who have ownership or decision-making authority over embryos, no limits should be imposed on actions taken with them. The problem with this view is that it ignores the fact that a new genome has been formed and that actions with this tissue could affect whether a new child will be born.

The most widely held view of embryo status takes an intermediate position between the other two. It holds that the embryo deserves respect greater than that accorded to other human tissue, because of its potential to become a person and the symbolic meaning it carries for many people. Yet it should not be treated as a person, because it has not yet developed the features of personhood, is not yet established as developmentally individual, and may never realize its biologic potential.[20]

It is noteworthy that law, ethical commentary, and the reports of most official or professional advisory bodies share the view that the embryo has a special moral status less than that of a person. For example, the United States' Ethics Advisory Board unanimously agreed in 1979 that "the human preembryo is entitled to profound respect, but this respect does not necessarily encompass the full legal and moral rights attributed to persons."[21]

In 1984, the Warnock Committee in Great Britain took a similar position when it stated: "The human preembryo . . . is not under the present law of the United Kingdom accorded the same status as a living child or an adult, nor do we necessarily wish it to be accorded the same status.

Nevertheless, we were agreed that the preembryo of the human species ought to have a special status."[22]

The Ontario Law Reform Commission (Canada), which completed an extensive review of the issue in 1985, also took this view, as have nearly all other professional and official advisory bodies that have reviewed the question of embryo status.[23] The most recent pronouncement to this effect came from the Tennessee Supreme Court in 1992 when it overturned a trial court finding that embryos were "children" but held that because of their special status they deserved "special respect."[24]

For the most part, only groups holding the view that "personhood" begins at conception have rejected this middle position. However, Father Richard McCormick, a noted Catholic bioethicist who believes that abortion is immoral, has looked carefully at the biologic facts about the embryo and concluded that because the embryo is not developmentally individual until implantation, it has not clearly been determined to be a person in Catholic theology.[25]

The Legal Status of Embryos

Legal status—position or standing in law—will define what rights, if any, embryos have and what duties are owed to them, thus determining what might be done with these entities, and by whom.

DO EMBRYOS HAVE LEGAL RIGHTS?

The advisory body conclusions parallel the traditional Anglo-American legal view of prenatal life. In that tradition, legal personhood does not exist until live birth and separation from the mother. Common law prohibitions on abortion protected fetuses only after quickening (roughly sixteen weeks of gestation). While many American states did pass restrictive abortion laws in the nineteenth and twentieth centuries, those laws applied only to termination of pregnancy, and thus did not address the status of preimplantation embryos outside the body. Wrongful death statutes did not compensate for the wrongful death of a fetus until the late 1940s, and then only if the fetus was viable at the time of the injury.

At the present time, then, the law does not regard embryos as rights-bearing entities, although it has recognized that prenatal actions could affect the postnatal well-being of persons. In most states the embryo is not a legal subject in its own right and is not protected by laws against homicide or wrongful death, nor is embryo discard prohibited. However, three states (Minnesota, Louisiana, and Illinois) have altered their homicide laws in such a way that they arguably ban the intentional destruction of extracorporeal embryos.[26] Aside from those states, the embryo generally has legal cognizance only if the interests of an actual person are at stake, such as when transfer occurs and offspring may be affected or when someone wrongfully interferes with another person's right to determine disposition of the embryo.

The biology of early human embryo development supports this legal status. Since the embryo does not have differentiated organs, much less the developed brain, nervous system, and capacity for sentience that legal subjects ordinarily have, it cannot easily be regarded as a legal subject. Indeed, the embryo is not yet individual, because twinning or mosaicism can still occur. It is not surprising that the law does not recognize the embryo itself as a legal subject.

This legal status of embryos is not dependent on the continued survival of *Roe v. Wade* and the right to abortion. Because abortion laws penalized termination of pregnancy, they never applied to the destruction of embryos before pregnancy occurred. Thus *Roe* has not been a direct barrier to states wishing to protect embryos in situations other than abortion. A reversal of *Roe v. Wade* is not necessary to have states protect extracorporeal embryos more extensively than they previously have. IVF programs are also free to set their own standards concerning the extent to which embryos will be protected.

DISPOSITIONAL CONTROL OVER EMBRYOS

An important question of legal status concerns the locus and scope of decisional authority over embryos. "Who" has the right or authority to choose among available options for disposition of embryos is a question separate from "what" those dispositional options are.

The question of decisional authority is really the question of who "owns"—has a "property" interest in—the embryo. However, using terms such as "ownership" or "property" risks misunderstanding. Ownership does not signify that embryos may be treated in all respects like other property. Rather, the term merely designates who decides which legally available options will occur, such as creation, freezing, discard, donation, use in research, and placement in a uterus. Although the bundle of property rights attached to one's ownership of an embryo may be more circumscribed than for other things, it is an ownership or property interest nonetheless.

While the individuals who provided the gametes, the couple jointly, their transferees, the physicians or embryologists who directly create the embryos, or the IVF program or embryo storage bank that has actual possession are all possible candidates for decisional authority over embryos, the persons who provide the egg and sperm have the strongest claim to ownership of the embryo. The more interesting questions concern whether and how they have exercised that authority, and whether advance instructions for disposition will be binding if their preferences or circumstances change.

While legislation has not yet explicitly recognized the gamete providers' joint ownership of extracorporeal embryos, it is reasonable to assume that the courts would so hold when confronted with disputes raising this issue.[27] It is also likely that a right of survivorship in embryos would be recognized as well. The Uniform Anatomical Gift Act and other precedents concerning disposition of body parts support that view, even though they do not address it specifically.

Since most IVF programs and storage banks are likely to honor the couple's ownership, the issue would be directly joined only if a program or bank refused to follow the couple's dispositional instructions. The question would also arise if the program intentionally or negligently destroyed embryos.

The two cases that have arisen on these issues support this position. For example, the couple's ownership of embryos was implicitly recognized in *Del Zio v. Columbia Presbyterian Hospital*, a 1978 case that arose before the safety and efficacy of IVF had been established.[28] A New York jury awarded a couple $50,000 for intentional infliction of emotional distress when a doctor who objected to their efforts at IVF without prior institutional review board approval destroyed their incubating preembryo. Negligent or inadvertent destruction of preembryos, due to equipment malfunction or human error, would also be actionable, because of the significant financial, physical, and emotional loss that each imposes. Only difficulties in calculating damages, and not doubts about the ownership rights of the couple, would stand in the way of tort remedies for negligent destruction of preembryos.[29]

York v. Jones, a 1989 case involving one of the largest IVF programs in the United States, illustrates the question of ownership in disputes between a couple and the IVF program.[30] An infertile couple sought IVF treatment at the Jones Institute in Norfolk, Virginia, the first and most successful IVF program in the United States. Three IVF cycles were unsuccessful in achieving pregnancy, but the third produced an extra embryo that was frozen for later use.

The couple, who had moved to California, informed the Norfolk program that they wished to transport their frozen embryo to California to be thawed and placed in the wife by their Los Angeles physician. The Norfolk program refused to release the frozen embryo for shipment to California on a variety of legal and practical grounds, including loss of refrigerant, theft or blackmail of the embryo during shipment, the demeaning effect of shipping human embryos by air "ala [*sic*] cattle preembryos," lack of institutional review board approval, and liability risk of shipping to an unqualified program.[31]

The couple then sued in federal district court in Norfolk for custody of their embryo and won. The district judge found that the Norfolk program was a bailee or temporary custodian of the embryo and had no independent rights to keep it against the couple's wishes. Only if the couple had explicitly agreed at the time of freezing to use their embryos only in Norfolk would the Norfolk program have been entitled to insist on thawing there.

York v. Jones is significant because it is the first case directly dealing with a dispute between an IVF program and a couple over custody of a frozen embryo. The court assumes without question that embryos are the property of the gamete providers, and finds that any transfer of their dispositional authority must be explicitly stated in the documents of participation provided by the program. While a program could still insist that the embryos that it creates not be transferred to other locations, such a restriction would have to be clearly stated at the inception.

An important remaining legal question for couples and IVF programs is whether the couple's joint advance instructions for disposition of embryos will be legally binding, as the *York v. Jones* judge suggested. Binding advance instructions are important both to avoid and to resolve later disputes, and to give both couples and physicians advance certainty about what disposition will occur in case of future contingencies such as death, divorce, passage of time, unavailability, or disagreement among the parties.

Such instructions would ordinarily be given at the time that embryos are created or frozen. As part of the informed consent procedure, the couple will be informed of the dispositional alternatives that are available at that program, for example, whether embryo discard or donation is permitted and the length of permissible storage. In addition, IVF programs may also ask the couple to designate certain dispositional alternatives if contingencies such as their divorce, death, disagreement, or unavailability occur. The couple could reserve the right to change their designated disposition at later times, but until they do, the options selected would be binding when the specified events occurred.

The legal question is whether those designated choices will be legally binding on the couple when the stated contingency occurs and one party now disagrees or wishes to make a different disposition, or when both partners wish to deviate from the conditions and restrictions imposed by the IVF program to which they initially agreed.

The argument for recognizing the binding effect of joint advance instructions and acceptance of IVF program conditions is strong. The right to use embryos to reproduce or to avoid reproduction should include the right to give binding advance instructions because certainty about consequences is necessary to exercise reproductive options. In addition, all parties gain from the ability to rely on prior instructions when future contingencies occur. Finally, it minimizes the frequency and cost of resolving disputes that arise over disposition of embryos.

Although counterarguments against binding oneself in advance exist, the law should recognize the parties' advance agreement with the program and each other for disposition of embryos.[32] The advantages of such a position clearly outweigh the disadvantages, and should be recognized by courts dealing with disputes on these issues.[33] If not, courts will have the much more difficult and expensive task, illustrated by the *Davis* case discussed below, of determining a fair solution in the absence of an agreement.

LIMITS ON THE SCOPE OF AUTHORITY OVER EMBRYOS

Having seen that the gamete providers and their transferees have decisional authority over embryos, we now consider the limits that the state and IVF programs may impose on exercise of that authority. Is the couple's "ownership" of embryos absolute, or may the state qualify or limit it in certain ways? As noted previously, the answer to this question will depend on the reproductive interests implicated and the state's reasons for limiting the couple's ownership. While resolution of some issues will turn on views of embryo moral status, most will turn on the reproductive interests at stake and the degree to which procreative liberty is recognized. The main questions that arise here are limits on discard and freezing of embryos.

Discard or Nontransfer of Embryos

Because most IVF programs hyperstimulate the ovaries and retrieve multiple eggs, couples and programs must decide whether all fertilized eggs will be placed in the uterus, or whether surplus or unwanted embryos may be discarded or donated to others. If all fertilized eggs are to be placed in the uterus, the number fertilized may have to be limited, because of the very serious risks of multiple gestation.[34] Yet limiting the number fertilized might yield too few embryos to initiate a viable pregnancy. Freezing extra embryos may solve the problem in some cases, but not all frozen embryos will be placed in the woman producing them.

The procedure most likely to produce pregnancy is to fertilize all viable eggs, transfer only the three or four embryos that can safely be placed in the uterus at one time, and either freeze the remaining embryos, discard them, or donate them to others. A problem arises when people object to discard of embryos because they believe that embryos are persons with rights, or because they find the symbolic effects of such a practice distasteful and take action to implement their view.

Legally, IVF programs are free to determine their own policy about embryo discard, but must inform couples of their policies before embryos are created. Except in Minnesota, Louisiana, and possibly Illinois, destruction or discard of an embryo is not covered by homicide or other criminal laws.[35] While many programs will allow couples the option of discard, some will apply restrictive policies, either because of their own moral qualms or because of institutional constraints.[36]

An important public policy question is whether couples and programs should be free to decide these matters as they wish, or whether government should intervene to limit their choice. A limitation on embryo discard (by limiting the number of eggs that may be inseminated, banning discard, or requiring donation of unwanted embryos) would interfere with the procreative liberty of a couple that wished to employ this alternative.[37] Would such laws be constitutional? Are they desirable?

The constitutionality of laws that prevent the discard or destruction of IVF embryos is independent of the right to abortion established in *Roe v. Wade* and upheld in *Planned Parenthood v. Casey*.[38] *Roe* and *Casey* protect a woman's interest in not having embryos placed in her body and in terminating implantation (pregnancy) that has occurred. Under *Roe-Casey* the state would be free to treat external embryos as persons or give as much protection to their potential life as it chooses, as long as it did not trench on a woman's bodily integrity or other procreative rights.

Embryo protection laws, however, even if they do not infringe bodily integrity, do interfere with decisions about having biologic offspring and thus limit procreative choice. For example, laws that require donation of unwanted embryos in lieu of discard force people to have biologic offspring against their will, thus infringing the right not to procreate. Even if no child-rearing obligations follow, as would ordinarily be the case if the embryos are donated anonymously to others, the couple would still face the possibility that they had produced genetic offspring. One could argue that genetic reproduction *tout court* is such a significant personal event that it should be included in the fundamental right not to procreate. If this argument were accepted, a state's desire to signify the importance of human life by requiring donation of unwanted embryos would not constitute the compelling interest necessary to justify infringement of a fundamental right to avoid reproduction.

A counterargument to this position is that the Supreme Court is unlikely to recognize the right to avoid biologic offspring *tout court* as a fundamental right, and therefore the state's interest in protecting prenatal life provides a rational basis for embryo protection laws. *Griswold, Roe,* and *Casey* establish a right to avoid reproduction when reproduction is necessarily coupled with gestation or rearing burdens. Laws that mandate embryo donation impose only the psychological burden of having un-known biologic offspring. Such a purely psychosocial interest is not likely to be granted fundamental right status as part of the right to avoid repro-duction. In that case a state concerned with protecting prenatal life would easily satisfy the rational basis test by which such a statute would be judged. The reaffirmation of *Roe v. Wade* in *Casey* does not lessen the state's power to protect extracorporeal embryos, because the right of women to end pregnancy is not at issue.

One could also argue that bans on embryo discard interfere with the right to procreate. By limiting the number of eggs that can be fertilized or requiring that extra embryos be donated, such policies will deter couples from using IVF to treat infertility, thus infringing their right to use non-coital means of procreation. The validity of this argument rests on the degree of deterrence that such policies entail. It is possible that this policy would not "unduly burden" efforts to treat infertility. After all, the cou-ple may still undergo IVF. They just are limited in the number of eggs they can inseminate, or must accept anonymous donation of extras to others. If deemed unlikely to deter resort to IVF, embryo protection policies would not violate the freedom to procreate.

Resolving the question of embryo discard requires coming to terms with two very different value questions. One is the importance of the genetic tie *tout court*—an issue never previously faced in this way. The other is the detriment to values of respect for human life that flow from embryo discard. While the view of many people would be that embryos are too rudimentary to make embryo discard very costly in symbolic terms, some persons—and IVF programs—will hold different views. The values that people hold about these two aspects of reproduction will de-termine what policies ultimately control embryo discard.

Embryo Freezing

Cryopreservation or embryo freezing is a rapidly growing aspect of IVF practice. In 1990 there were 23,865 embryos frozen as a result of the IVF process, an increase of 14,657 over the number reported in 1988.[39] In 1993, more than 6,600 thawed embryo transfer procedures occurred, a 150 percent increase over 1988, resulting in 982 pregnancies and 791 live births. The frozen embryo cycles involved more than 230 clinics, with an overall success rate of 13 percent deliveries per thawed embryo transfer procedure.

Embryo freezing is growing in popularity for several reasons. It could increase the efficacy of IVF by making use of all retrieved eggs. By elimi-nating the need for additional stimulation and egg retrieval cycles, it re-duces the physical and financial costs of later IVF cycles. It also reduces the chance that surplus embryos (those that cannot be safely implanted in the uterus) will be destroyed. Yet many aspects of embryo freezing are controversial and are likely to generate proposals to limit the practice.

Harm to Embryos. Persons opposed to embryo discard also object to embryo freezing on the ground that the freeze-thaw process harms or destroys embryos by damaging particular blastomeres or cells that render the embryo unable to divide further. It is true that frozen-thawed embryos divide and start pregnancies at a lesser rate than do fresh embryos, and that freezing does damage some blastomeres. It is not clear, however, whether the damaged embryos are viable, and thus would have successfully implanted if freezing had not occurred.

A ban on embryo freezing would actually reduce the number of embryos in existence. Rather than risk the possibility of multiple gestation (and the chance of selective reduction of the pregnancy), fewer embryos would be created, since all embryos would have to be placed in the uterus. This reduction might also lead to fewer IVF pregnancies, because one cannot always guarantee that fertilizing three or four eggs will yield three or four viable embryos (the optimal number of embryos to transfer).

Reasonable people, however, could find that embryo freezing is sufficiently respectful of prenatal human life that it should be permitted as an option for infertile couples trying to become pregnant through IVF. Fewer embryos are destroyed than by outright discard. Moreover, it leads to the creation of embryos that would never have existed if freezing were not available. Even if some embryos are harmed by the freezing process, the total number of embryos available for implantation has increased. Even if discard were prohibited, freezing seems more protective than destructive of embryos and should be permitted as part of procreative choice in the IVF process.

Length of Storage. For most infertile couples embryo storage will be temporary, with most frozen embryos thawed within six to eighteen months in efforts to start pregnancy. Technically, however, there may be no outer limit on the length of time that embryos could be frozen before they are thawed and implanted in a uterus. Inevitably, some embryos will end up being frozen for years, as plans change or other factors intervene. An important question for IVF programs and public policy is whether the length of storage should be limited.

Proposals for such limits vary, from set terms such as five to ten years to the reproductive life of the woman providing the egg. Time limits are thought to be easier to administer and more desirable, because it will prevent children from being born to women who are much older.[40] It will also prevent simultaneously conceived siblings from being born years apart.

As a matter of public policy, such considerations are not sufficient to justify time limits on embryo freezing. None of them pose such dangers to offspring—who might not otherwise be born—that the wishes of couples to freeze for longer periods should be infringed. IVF programs should assess more carefully the purposes of time limits on storage, and not impose them unless clearly necessary. If programs adopt such policies, they should clearly inform couples in advance and permit them to remove frozen embryos to other facilities when the period elapses.

Posthumous Implantation.   Embryo freezing also makes possible the posthumous implantation and birth of children conceived before death occurs. While such cases will not be frequent, situations will arise in which the husband or wife dies before previously frozen embryos are thawed and implanted. A surviving wife may request that "her" embryos be implanted in her, so that she may reproduce the "child" that she and her now dead husband created. A surviving husband might wish the thawed embryos be placed in a new partner or in a host uterus engaged for that purpose.

Respect for the procreative liberty of the surviving spouse should permit posthumous thawing and implantation to occur. The survivor has a real interest in procreating, which the frozen embryo serves well. The fear that the child will have only one parent is not sufficient to override the spouse's procreative liberty. Many children thrive with single parents, especially if they have the resources and support to parent, and births to women pregnant at the time of their husband's death occasionally occur. A law that prohibited posthumous implantation would infringe the survivor's procreative liberty, and is unnecessary. IVF programs should not set such a restriction.

The question is somewhat different if both husband and wife die while the embryos are frozen. If the couple has directed that any frozen embryos be donated for implantation, their wishes should be respected. On the other hand, if they directed or accepted the program's condition that remaining embryos would be discarded, that too may be honored. However, a state law that required all frozen embryos remaining at time of death of both to be implanted would probably not violate the procreative rights of the couple, since the prospect of posthumous donation is unlikely to influence their reproductive decision making.[41]

Inheritance Issues.   Posthumous implantation of frozen embryos will also raise some unique problems of inheritance, as the Rios case in 1984 showed. An American couple that had unsuccessfully undergone IVF treatment in Australia had frozen two embryos for later use. A few months later the couple died in an airplane crash, leaving a large estate. The question that captured public attention was whether the frozen embryos, if thawed and eventually born, would inherit the estate. Embryo discard would obviate the question, but Australian authorities passed a law prohibiting discard of that embryo.

An American court quite properly ruled that the embryo could not inherit in those circumstances. The long-standing rule has been that children may inherit if they are born or *en ventre sa mere* at the time of death. Conception alone, without pregnancy, would not count. There is no good reason why this rule should be changed to include embryos *en ventre sa frigidaire* when the decedent leaves no will or makes grants to "heirs" generally and embryos are still frozen at time of death.[42]

A closer question arises, however, if the decedent has specifically named unborn frozen embryos as beneficiaries of her estate. In that case, the decedent's interest in controlling disposition of property may clash with the need for promptness and certainty in the administration of estates. Rather than tie up estates until the last frozen embryo is either thawed or discarded, a rule prohibiting devises to offspring born from frozen embryos that have not implanted at the time of death would seem to be a reasonable solution to the problem, and one that would have little impact on procreative freedom.

Transfer between IVF Programs.   Another policy issue with frozen embryos, already considered in the discussion of *York v. Jones*, concerns transfer to other programs. There is no reason why couples should not have this option, especially in light of modern mobility and the technical feasibility of transfer. They may prefer another storage facility or IVF program; want their embryos to be closer to them when they move; or have other legitimate grounds for transfer.

The case for laws or public policies prohibiting such transfers is very weak. There is no particular danger to the embryos. The couple requesting transfer should bear the risks of mishap, or lack of qualifications in the new facility. The main objection appears to be symbolic. As the Norfolk program put it in *York v. Jones*, it would be "demeaning ala [*sic*] cattle preembryos" to have human embryos shipped transcontinentally or even internationally.

But shipment of embryos from one location to another, at the request of the couple that "owns" the embryo, hardly seems demeaning. Embryos and fetuses are transported in the bodies of women. Human organs are shipped for transplant. Here the couple creating the embryo request shipment so that they will be closer to them, or have thawing occur in a "better" facility. Their judgment of the costs and benefits—minimal harm to embryo vs. greater convenience and ease for the woman—seems reasonable. The woman would be more burdened by a trip to Norfolk and back than the embryo would be by a one-way trip to California. If IVF programs restrict interprogram transfers, legislation protecting this aspect of procreative choice might be needed.

Resolving Disputes over Frozen Embryos. The practice of freezing embryos will also raise questions about embryo disposition when the couple divorces, dies, is unavailable, is unable to agree, or is in arrears in paying storage charges. As noted earlier, the best way to handle these questions is by dispositional agreements made at the time of creation or cryopreservation of embryos. Such agreements should be binding on the parties, and enforced even if their circumstances or desires change. IVF programs that have reasonable grounds for thinking that the agreements were freely and knowingly made should be free to rely on them, without more. This is the best policy to give all parties some control of the process, as well as reliable advance certainty about future outcomes. It also will reduce the administrative costs and difficulty of resolving any disputes that arise.

The advantages of relying on prior dispositional agreements to resolve disputes over frozen embryos is illustrated by the widely publicized 1989 Tennessee divorce case of *Davis v. Davis* concerning disposition of seven frozen embryos. The couple had made no prior agreement for embryo disposition in case of divorce or disagreement. At the time of divorce, the wife insisted that the embryos be available to her for thawing and placement in her uterus or donation to another couple. The husband objected to the idea of children from a marriage that had failed. The trial judge awarded "custody" of the embryos to the wife, on the ground that the embryos were "children" whose best interests required the chance to implant and come to term.

A Tennessee intermediate appellate court reversed the trial court decision, requiring that any disposition of the embryos be jointly agreed to by the husband and wife. The Tennessee Supreme Court affirmed this decision on somewhat different grounds.[43] It upheld advance agreements for disposition in the case of divorce or disagreement, but rejected the notion that the freezing of embryos alone constituted an agreement to later implantation. It also recognized that a right to "procreational autonomy" existed under both the United States and Tennessee constitutions that outweighed the state's "at best slight" interest in "the potential life embodied by these four- to eight-cell preembryos."[44]

In this case, however, the choice of the husband not to procreate conflicted with the wife's desire to use the embryos to procreate. To resolve that conflict, the Court compared the relative burdens and concluded that the burdens of unwanted reproduction to the husband, even if genetic only, outweighed the burden to the wife of not having the embryos donated to another couple, as she now desired. Even if she had wanted them for herself, her claim to have them would be strong only if she had no way to achieve parenthood by other reasonable means. If she could go through another IVF cycle without excessive burdens to her, her interest in procreating with the disputed embryos should not take precedence over the husband's wishes to avoid unwanted reproduction.

The Tennessee Supreme Court's decision is eminently sound and will be a major precedent for the conduct of IVF and the resolution of disputes about frozen embryos for years to come. It nicely illustrates the advantages of relying on a prior agreement in these cases, rather than having to balance the procreative interests anew in lengthy and expensive litigation.[45]

Embryo Research

The couple's dispositional authority over embryos should also give them the right to decide whether research with their embryos will occur. Their power to so decide depends, of course, on whether the jurisdiction permits embryo research. Laws restricting embryo research reflect a more restrictive view of embryo status that is not easily squared with the facts of preimplantation embryo development. However, since embryo research issues are not directly relevant to IVF as a treatment for infertility, further discussion of this topic is postponed to chapter 9, where the production of embryos and fetuses for transplant and research purposes is discussed.

CONSUMER PROTECTION ISSUES

Questions about the control and disposition of embryos have attracted much attention, but questions of safety, efficacy, and access raise equally important policy issues. For most couples, the most important question concerning IVF is whether it will work. The ethical niceties of control over embryos may be much less important.

Unfortunately, IVF does not work nearly as often as people would like. In the very best programs, pregnancy and take-home baby rates are around 20 percent of IVF egg retrieval cycles, which means that fewer than one in ten IVF-created embryos implant and come to term. Only twenty to thirty programs achieve this level of success. Many other programs have much weaker records, and many have very few pregnancies at all. One survey in 1987 found that over half of the then existing American IVF programs had never produced a live birth. Other programs have misstated their success rates to consumers and been the subject of Federal Trade Commission charges of misleading advertising.[46]

The reasons for this relatively poor track record are several. The whole process of IVF is extremely complicated with many unknowns. What eggs best fertilize, what culture medium to use for embryos, when to transfer, what instruments to use, and many other questions will determine the outcome of IVF. Also crucial is the skill and experience of the physicians involved, the reliability of their laboratories, and the age and condition of patients. It is no accident that the biggest and most experienced programs consistently have the highest success rates.

The efficacy situation raises three important policy issues for protecting consumers. One concerns the need to support and fund research to improve success rates. Because of pro-life opposition, the federal government funded no IVF research during the twelve years of the Reagan-Bush administrations. Under the Clinton administration, federal funding of IVF research may now occur, though the amount of funding will have to compete with the many other demands for the federal health research dollar.

A second policy issue is the need to make infertile couples more aware of the varying success rates of IVF programs, so that they can make informed choices about whether and where to seek IVF. Complaints from unhappy consumers about misleading claims by IVF clinics led Congressman Ron Wyden (D-Oregon) to conduct hearings and seek legislation that requires that IVF success rates be uniformly kept and accurately disclosed. Uniform reporting and disclosure will prevent infertile couples from being misled by claims of success rates overall vs. success of the particular clinic, or claims that successful fertilization and even clinical pregnancy is the equivalent of a live-born child, the bottom line issue of interest to patients. Prodded by Congressman Wyden's interest, the American Fertility Society and the Society for Assisted Reproductive Technology began to collect and publish overall and clinic specific data about IVF, GIFT, and ZIFT success rates. The Fertility Clinic Success Rate and Certification Act of 1992 now requires that each IVF program report annually to the Centers for Disease Control their pregnancy success rates as defined in the act.[47]

A third policy issue is the need for oversight of the laboratory settings in which IVF programs handle human oocytes, sperm, and embryos. Laboratories vary widely in the quality and replicability of their procedures, and are thought to be an important factor in the wide variance in IVF success rates. The Fertility Clinic Success Rate and Certification Act of 1992 directs the Secretary of Health and Human Services to develop a model program for the certification of embryo laboratories. This program will be made available to states that wish to adopt it. The act also provides for states to have private accrediting bodies such as the College of American Pathology and the American Fertility Society, which have adopted a joint inspection program, conduct the certification. Greater attention to laboratory conditions and practices should improve the efficacy of IVF.

Questions of IVF efficacy and consumer awareness show that IVF, while a novel reproductive procedure, also presents policy problems typical of most new medical technologies. Medical zeal and interest in self-promotion may mislead patients about its efficacy, and induce women to undergo expensive, invasive procedures that may have less chance of helping them then they thought. A 1992 proposed public offering of stock in IVF America, a chain of IVF clinics that planned to expand across the country, revealed the importance of the profit motive in providing IVF services and the need for ongoing monitoring of the industry.[48] Laboratory certification and accurate disclosure of success rates relative to other clinics is an appropriate policy response to protect the procreative freedom of infertile couples. However, it is they who will have to decide whether the risks and benefits of the procedure are worth it.

FUNDING AND ACCESS ISSUES

Another important policy issue with IVF and other reproductive technologies is cost and access. IVF costs $7,000 to $9,000 per cycle and is often ineffective, with two or three cycles necessary to achieve pregnancy when it is successful. Insurance may pay none or only some of the costs, making IVF a procedure that only wealthier couples can afford. Indeed, the cost may be prohibitive for many middle-class couples.

The high cost of IVF raises questions of access and justice in allocation of health care resources. Given the high rate of infertility, its impact on couples, and insurance coverage of many kinds of infertility treatment, there is a reasonable case for including IVF in private or public health insurance plans. Ten states have laws that require insurance coverage of infertility services. Five of these states (Arkansas, Hawaii, Massachusetts, Maryland, and Texas) currently require health insurers to include IVF as an option.[49] Courts have also ruled that insurance plans that cover surgical repair of blocked fallopian tubes as treatment for an "existing physical or mental illness" must also cover IVF, though other courts have found that IVF is not a medically necessary treatment for illness.[50]

While insurance coverage will increase access to IVF, it also increases the cost of insurance for all policyholders. Depending on the size of the pool, however, this subsidy may not be unfair. Infertility may reasonably be viewed, because of its frequency, expense, and personal importance, as one of the health risks for which people should be insured. Spread over a large group, the cost of IVF coverage is relatively small. It should not be singled out for exclusion if other infertility services are covered.

On the other hand, a policy that covered no infertility services or which excluded IVF and other high-tech procedures might not be unreasonable. At a time of great strain in the health care system, limiting coverage for procedures based on judgments about their cost, efficacy, and benefits to patients is also reasonable. If choices have to be made, people might well prefer coverage for catastrophic or life-threatening illness and preventive services rather than for infertility.

Such a judgment would support exclusion of IVF (and other fertility treatments) from public insurance programs such as Medicaid as well. Despite stereotypes of unrestrained reproduction, the poor actually have higher rates of infertility due to poverty, nutrition, and more infectious disease than does the middle class. If infertility is considered an "illness" for which "medical treatment" is available, existing law would require that Medicaid cover IVF and other infertility treatments.

Yet many people would object to spending increasingly scarce Medicaid funds on IVF when life-threatening illnesses are not adequately covered. It is not surprising that the Oregon health care plan for rationing medical resources for Medicaid patients ranked infertility treatment near the bottom.[51] Such a ranking does deny the poor infertility services available to those who have the means to pay directly. Yet if differences between public and private funding of health care are to exist, one may reasonably conclude that infertility is one place to draw the line. Such a judgment illustrates the limitations of procreative liberty as a negative right that does not entitle people to government resources to fulfill their reproductive goals.

A final issue of access is the control that IVF programs exercise over who receives their services. Many IVF programs will not treat unmarried persons. Nearly all will test couples for HIV, and may refuse the procedure if one or both of the partners test positive.[52] Some may exclude couples whom they think are unstable or unfit parents. The exclusion is usually justified on the "ethical" ground of protecting offspring who would be born in disadvantageous circumstances. However, providing IVF services to these groups would not harm children who have no other way to be born, and thus may ethically be provided if a program is so inclined.[53] Because private IVF clinics have wide discretion in selecting patients for treatment, they may in most circumstances be legally free to set the criteria for selecting patients.

CONCLUSION

This account of IVF shows how different strands of procreative liberty and different views about the status of preimplantation embryos are entwined in the use of this technology. Restriction of IVF to protect embryos will, in most cases, interfere with an infertile couple's interest in procreating and may affect other reproductive interests.

Resolution of the ethical, legal, and policy conflicts that arise in IVF depends, for the most part, on determining the relative importance of these reproductive interests vs. the perceived threat to embryos and respect for prenatal life. The widely held view that the preimplantation embryo is not a person but deserves special respect would resolve most of these conflicts in favor of the infertile couple. However, a more protective view of embryo status would not necessarily exclude central aspects of IVF practice, including embryo freezing, even though it prevents embryo discard from occurring.[54]

A final point to note is how issues of efficacy and access turn out to be as important to IVF as issues of embryo status. The legal right to use IVF is embedded in a set of socioeconomic and structural circumstances that affect exercise of the right. Socially constructed attitudes about the need to overcome infertility will be a main determinant of use. Money also counts when one is seeking access to IVF. IVF shows that procreative liberty is not a fully meaningful concept unless one has the knowledge and means to obtain IVF from the best programs, or the will to resist its allure when its use seems excessive.

CHAPTER 6

Collaborative Reproduction

DONORS AND SURROGATES

ALL REPRODUCTION is collaborative, for no mortal person reproduces alone.[1] The term "collaborative reproduction" is nonetheless useful for describing those situations in which someone other than one's partner provides the gametes or gestation necessary for reproduction, such as occurs with sperm, egg, or embryo donation, or surrogate motherhood. These technologies play an increasingly central role in infertility treatment and raise basic questions about the scope of procreative liberty.[2]

THE DILEMMAS OF COLLABORATIVE REPRODUCTION

Resort to donor gametes or surrogates is not an easy choice for infertile couples. The decision arises after previous efforts at pregnancy have failed, thus confronting the couple with the fact of one or both partners' infertility. A collaborative technique is chosen because it offers an opportunity to have a child who is the biologic offspring of one or, in the case of egg donation and gestational surrogacy, both partners.[3] Yet collaborative reproduction occurs in an uncertain ethical, legal, and social milieu, where social practices and legal rules are still largely unclear.

A basic commitment to procreative liberty—to the freedom to have and rear offspring—should presumptively protect most forms of collaborative reproduction. After all, collaborative reproduction occurs for the same reason as IVF—the couple is infertile and cannot produce offspring. They need donor or surrogate assistance if they are to have children. Even if both rearing partners are not reproducing in the strict genetic sense, at least one partner will have a genetic or gestational relationship with their child. The same techniques may also be sought by a single woman or a same-sex couple that wishes to have offspring. In a few cases, donor gametes are used to avoid genetic handicap in offspring.

Despite its clear link to procreative choice, collaborative reproduction often generates controversy and even calls for prohibition. Collaborative reproduction is problematic because it intrudes a third party—a donor or surrogate—into the usual situation of two-party parenthood, and separates or deconstructs the traditional genetic, gestational, and social unity of reproduction.[4] A child could in theory end up with three different biologic parents (a genetic mother, a gestational mother, a genetic father) and two separate rearing parents, with various combinations among them.[5] Such collaboration risks confusing offspring about who their "true" parent is and creating conflict about parental rights and duties. At the same time, the isolation of the particular components of parenthood tends to depersonalize the contributions of gamete donors and surrogates.

Collaborative reproduction thus poses several challenges for a regime of procreative liberty. On the one hand, it greatly expands procreative options, both for infertile couples seeking to form a family with biologically related offspring, as well as for persons who find satisfaction or meaning in serving as donors or surrogates.

On the other hand, it involves a novel set of practices and relationships in which social and psychological meanings and legal rights and duties have not yet been clearly defined. Given the ample room presented for misunderstanding and conflict, the use of technology to alter fundamental or traditional family relationships seems risky, and should occur only under conditions that protect the welfare of offspring, couples, and collaborators.

Indeed, the decomposition of the usually unified aspects of reproduction into separate genetic, gestational, and social strands calls into question the very meaning of procreative liberty. Are couples who use these techniques "procreating" in a significant way, even though one of them may lack a genetic or biological connection to offspring? Is a collaborator meaningfully procreating if he or she is merely providing gametes or gestation without any rearing role? Do such limited procreative roles deserve the same respect and protection that traditional coital reproduction warrants? This chapter answers those questions and discusses the extent to which such arrangements are permitted, regulated, or prohibited.

Although it appears too late in the game to eliminate most forms of collaborative practice, many ethical, legal, and social questions remain. This chapter addresses the extent to which procreative liberty protects a couple's access to collaborative reproduction.

HARM TO OFFSPRING

Although no organized movement to ban collaborative reproduction exists, many persons—usually those who have not themselves faced infertility—find these practices to be ethically troubling and socially deviant. In

their eyes the central problem is that intrusion of a gamete donor or surrogate into the marital relationship confuses family and lineage in a way
that is ultimately harmful to offspring. To protect offspring from the
problems of multiple parents, they would strictly limit, if not prohibit
altogether, the use of donors and surrogates to treat infertility.

Are Offspring Harmed by Collaborative Reproduction?

The concern about the impact on offspring is an important one. Genetic
and biological ties are so central to our notions of individual identity and
family that the possibility of adverse effects from deliberate separation of
these elements must be taken seriously. Indeed, participants in these en-
deavors are often nervously aware that they are engaged in an enterprise
for which the psychological, social, and legal rules have not yet been
written.

Yet the claim that these practices should be prohibited because they are
so inimical to offspring welfare is not convincing. The chief danger is that
children will be reared by a person who is not their genetic mother or
father, and that they may not know who their "true" father or mother is.
In addition to causing conflict between the rearing partners and collaborator, the nonbiologic rearing partner may subtly or explicitly reject the
child, and the child may experience a sense of loss or abandonment by the
absent biologic parent.

Such experiences, of course, are not unique to donor- and surrogate-
assisted reproduction. More than 25 percent of children are now raised in
a nonnuclear family, and 30 percent of children are now born out of
wedlock.[6] Many children are being raised by adoptive, step, or foster
parents, by relatives or by other persons in situations in which they will
have no or limited contact with their genetic or gestational parents and
have close ties with nonbiologic rearers.

If the phenomenon of split biologic and social rearing is so widespread,
one may question why collaborative reproduction should be of special
concern. Of course, most instances of adoption, stepparentage, and other
forms of blended or mixed families are a postnatal response to death,
divorce, economic travail, abuse, or abandonment. In contrast, collaborative families are intentionally created. The intention is to create a loving
home for a child who has a biological connection to one or both rearing
parents.

The intentional creation of families with an absent genetic or gestational parent is a problem only if being reared in a situation in which one
biologic parent is missing is itself generally harmful. Even if not ideal, we

must ask what the risks of serious psychosocial problems in such families are, and what steps are possible to minimize them. Even then, one must also ask whether the likely problems are so great that offspring of collaborative reproduction, who have no other way to be born, would be better off never existing.

Empirical data is only partially helpful here, because other than some limited studies of sperm donation, no data on other forms of collaborative reproduction are available. The data available on offspring of sperm donation, however, do not show that those families or children are at especially high risk for psychological or social problems.[7] They have fewer problems than adopted children and their families. Healthy adjustment usually occurs, though problems can arise if the parents have not accepted their infertility or worked through the emotional conflicts that donor sperm raises for them. Children who learn of their missing donor father are sometimes angry at their parents for having kept it secret, and may be frustrated at not being able to obtain more information about him. But they typically do not feel rejected or abandoned as adopted children often do, and many express gratitude for the "gift" that made their existence possible. There is no reason to suppose that egg and embryo donation or gestational surrogacy will pose any greater problems. Because of the closer genetic or gestational links that exist in those cases, they may indeed pose fewer problems.

The data on sperm donation suggest that the impact of collaborative reproduction on offspring will depend largely on how well the infertile couple and their family accept and adjust to the situation. If the couple has worked through their depression, anger, and guilt at their own or their partner's infertility, they will have less difficulty in dealing with donor-assisted reproduction. If they are warned about conflicted feelings, given time to adjust to the novelty of the situation, and if their own parents are accepting of their choice for collaborative assistance, they are more likely to have a successful experience.[8] This in turn will make it easier to deal with issues of secrecy, disclosure, and uncertain legal status.

Yet even if couples or offspring have difficulties adjusting to the fact of donor or surrogate assistance, it does not follow that collaborative assistance should be discouraged in order to prevent harm to offspring. But for the technique in question, the child never would have been born. Whatever psychological or social problems arise, they hardly rise to the level of severe handicap or disability that would make the child's very existence a net burden, and hence a wrongful life.[9] Measures to minimize such effects are needed, but their absence alone would not justify banning collaborative techniques.

Protecting Offspring by Disclosure

Given that collaborative reproduction serves individual procreative interests, makes possible children who would not otherwise be born, and does not appear to generate undue psychological or social conflict, such practices should generally be permitted. Rather than try to stop such practices, public policy should focus on preventing the problems that can arise. Legal rules for allocating rearing rights and duties among the participants are discussed in the next section. Later sections also discuss the need to protect collaborators by assuring that they act freely and knowingly. Questions of secrecy and disclosure, which directly affect offspring, are discussed here. This concern raises two questions: (1) should children be told of their donor- or surrogate-assisted birth? (2) What information about donors and surrogates should be provided to offspring?

SECRECY VS. DISCLOSURE OF COLLABORATIVE BIRTH

The usual practice with donor sperm has been secrecy, anonymity, and nondisclosure. Couples usually have had little information about anonymous donors, who have been recruited by physicians or commercial sperm banks.[10] The couple is usually advised to keep the fact of sperm donation a secret from their families and the child. Although psychologists now recommend against secrecy, there is still a strong reluctance to reveal the fact of sperm donation to family and the child.

Secrecy may also inform egg and embryo donation, and even surrogacy, though often surrogates and egg donors will meet the couples whom they help.[11] Even if information is known about the donor or surrogate, the rearing parents may be reluctant to discuss it with the child, though perhaps less so if a relative or friend has helped them. As with sperm donation, the couple may feel shame, embarrassment, or guilt, or simply find it more convenient to say nothing.

As a matter of public policy, the question of secrecy or disclosure to the child is best left to the couple to resolve. Although most psychologists see no good reason for secrecy and emphasize the energy that keeping the secret entails, they recognize that disclosure entails its own complications.[12] At what age to tell the child? What information about the donor is needed? What if the child wants to meet the missing biologic parent? Such questions will recur many times, restimulating the parents' own unresolved conflicts about their infertility, and may take on special urgency during adolescence or times of conflict. The problems presented will vary with the individuals and the particular collaborative assistance involved, and cannot be adequately handled by a law requiring disclosure. Couples, however, do need to be informed of these problems in advance and given the chance to resolve them before proceeding.

ANONYMITY AND INFORMATION ABOUT DONORS
AND SURROGATES

In practice, some families will disclose the existence of a collaborating donor or surrogate to the child. When disclosure occurs, children will be intensely interested in their missing biologic parent. They will need support and understanding in dealing with the emotions that an absent biologic parent may stimulate. Some children might, as adopted children often do, desire to meet that parent and other members of their biologic family. Given these desires, an important policy issue concerns what information should be collected about donors and surrogates, who should maintain it, and when should the child be given access to it.

Since most children who are told of their collaborative birth will desire knowledge of the missing parent, at the very least nonidentifying information about the donor or surrogate should be collected so that parents can provide as much information as possible. In many instances, however, rearing parents willing to discuss the matter may have no information to share, because the transaction was handled anonymously through an intermediary. If the intermediary has kept records, he is likely to keep them confidential out of fear of legal liability. Because *nonidentifying* information about donors will be immensely important to offspring, physicians who perform sperm, egg, or embryo donation should collect this information and provide it to the couple so that they may later inform the child. If private actors do not adequately meet this need, legislation requiring the collection and disclosure of nonidentifying information may be justified.

The more difficult issue is whether *identifying* information about donors and surrogates should also be disclosed. If donors and surrogates prefer to remain anonymous yet the child wishes to learn their identity, a conflict between their privacy and the child's need to know her parentage may arise. Resolution of this conflict requires balancing the importance of knowing one's genetic or gestational parents against the importance to donors and surrogates of avoiding disclosure of their identity to the children whom they make possible.

Individuals and legislatures may well differ on this intensely personal issue. If government chooses to privilege the donor or surrogate's interest in privacy over the offspring's interest in knowing the biologic parent's identity, it appears to have the constitutional authority to do so.[13] On the other hand, if the state chooses to privilege the child's need to know her parent's identity over the collaborator's wish for privacy, that policy too may be constitutional.[14] Some legislatures might reasonably conclude, as Sweden has, that the need of children to know their biologic parents is more compelling than the interest of donors and surrogates in privacy. Options here include a ban on anonymous donation, a registry that offspring might access at age 18, or disclosure only if good medical or other cause is shown. One California sperm bank now permits donors and recipients to agree to have the name and address of the donor disclosed to offspring at age 18, if they request it.

The question of record-keeping and disclosure of both identifying and nonidentifying collaborative information is an important policy issue that has been too long ignored. At the very least, nonidentifying information should be collected and provided to rearing parents, so they may pass it on to inquiring children. Identifying information should also be collected, so that it may be disclosed if a particular jurisdiction determines at a later time that offspring should have the right to know their biologic parents' identity.

REARING RIGHTS AND DUTIES IN COLLABORATIVE REPRODUCTION

A major policy issue in collaborative reproduction is the allocation of rearing rights and duties in offspring. Given that there may be more than two biologic parents and multiple possible social parents, who will have the legal right or duty to rear the child? This issue is of central importance to infertile couples, to donors and surrogates, and to the children born of these arrangements.

While these issues have been largely resolved for sperm donation to a married couple, legal questions remain about the status of sperm donation to an umarried woman and situations where donor and recipient intend to share rearing. The legal status of rearing is even less clear with donor eggs, embryo donation, and surrogacy. A major issue concerns whether the preconception intentions of the parties for rearing shall be determinative, or whether lawmakers should adopt some other system for allocating rearing roles.

In my view there are compelling reasons for recognizing the preconception intentions of the parties as the presumptive arbiter of rearing rights and duties, as long as the welfare of the offspring will not be severely damaged by honoring those intentions.[15] This standard, of course, assumes that the child's best interest does not automatically depend on being reared by a particular genetic or gestational parent.

A main reason for presumptively enforcing the preconception agreement for rearing is procreative liberty. As discussed in chapter 2, the procreative liberty of infertile married couples (and arguably unmarried persons as well) should include the right to use noncoital means of conception to form families. If the couple lacks the gametes or gestational capacity to produce offspring, a commitment to procreative liberty should also permit them the freedom to enlist the assistance of willing donors and surrogates.

Reliance on preconception agreements are thus necessary to give the couple—as well as the donors and surrogates—the assurance they need to go forward with the collaborative enterprise. Without some contractual assurance, the parties may be unwilling to embark on the complicated enterprise of collaborative reproduction. The infertile couple needs assurance that their efforts to become parents, if medically successful, will be legally recognized. Donors and surrogates also need assurance that they will not acquire unwanted rearing duties, or, if they have bargained for a more active rearing role, that their intentions will be honored. Without some advance certainty about legal consequences, they or the couple might be unwilling to collaborate, thus depriving the couple of the ingredients needed to have and rear offspring.[16]

In addition to giving parties advance certainty, honoring preconception intentions will minimize the frequency of disputes and the costs of resolving them if they occur. If preconception agreements concerning rearing are generally binding, there will be less chance that participants will violate them. If disputes do arise, presumptively recognizing those intentions will be the most efficient way to resolve the dispute. Holding the parties to the promises on which the other parties relied also seems to be a fair solution. If enforcement of those agreements does not hurt the child, the only question will be whether the agreement was knowingly and freely made.[17]

The idea of allowing preconception intentions or contracts to control postbirth rearing, however, is objectionable to many people. They point to the rejection of a contractual approach to adoption, the disparities in bargaining position that may exist, and the disregard of the child's best interests. However, the position asserted here is not necessarily antithetical to those points. The parties' preconception agreement about postbirth rearing is not enforced if it was not freely made or if enforcing the rearing provisions will clearly harm the child. However, if the parties who have contracted to rear are adequate child rearers, their preconception agreement should trump the claims of donors or surrogates who later insist on a different rearing role than they had agreed upon. If all parties are equally good child rearers and the collaborative agreement was freely and knowingly entered, the preconception agreement for rearing should be enforced.

In fact, the idea of enforcing preconception agreements for collaborative reproduction is already well accepted with donor sperm. Although not stated in contract terms, a similar result occurs judicially or by statute in over thirty states when the husband consents in writing to artificial insemination of his wife with donor sperm. A similar result presumably would be reached with egg and embryo donation. The main problems with enforcing preconception rearing agreements have arisen with donations to unmarried persons, agreements for greater involvement by the donor, and with surrogacy.

To explore the question of rearing rights and duties in collaborative offspring, it is helpful to distinguish between (1) agreements that exclude donors and surrogates from any rearing role, and (2) agreements that include the donor and surrogate. Within each category, further distinctions based on the collaborative technique involved, the marital status of the parties, and the timing of deviations from preconception agreements may also be relevant.

Agreements to Exclude Donors and Surrogates

The most common arrangement in collaborative situations will be to exclude the donor or surrogate from any rearing role. The infertile couple receiving the third party's gametic or gestational contribution assumes all rearing rights and duties, while the donor or surrogate takes on no visitation, custody, or other rearing rights and assumes no duties of financial support.

The validity of such agreements could be challenged in several ways. The donor or surrogate could, despite his or her agreement, attempt to visit or see the child, or in the case of surrogacy, not relinquish the child to the contracting couple. Such attempts to rear could occur at birth or at some later point. Alternatively, the state or recipient of the collaborative service could seek to impose rearing duties of support on the third party, despite their understanding that they would have no rearing obligations. To evaluate the merits of either attempt to override the agreement, it is necessary to distinguish the collaborative techniques in which these issues might arise.

DONOR SPERM: MARRIED

The validity of preconception rearing contracts excluding the donor is firmly established only in one area—donor sperm to a consenting married couple. Statutes and court decisions in more than thirty states provide that the consenting husband is the rearing father for all purposes, with the donor having no rearing rights and duties.[18] Presumably jurisdictions without statutes or court decisions would also follow this model. Although not worded in contract terms, these laws implicitly recognize the intentions of the parties to exclude the donor from all rearing rights and duties.

DONOR SPERM: UNMARRIED

The situation is more complicated with sperm donation to an unmarried woman (who may be single or cohabiting with a male or female partner). While a few states apply the married person model in this situation and exclude the donor, they may condition legal exclusion on a physician doing the insemination or on compliance with some other condition.[19] Where no statute applies, the question of whether the donor's intention to avoid support obligations will be upheld remains undetermined.

Courts generally do not relieve men of child support obligations even if they were misled by their sexual partner about her inability to conceive.[20] A few cases involving sperm donation to unmarried women have followed this principle when other statutory provisions for excluding the donor, such as physician insemination, have not been met.[21] In most cases, however, no legal attempt to seek support from the donor has occurred, either because the recipient has been able to provide for the child or the donor is unknown.

Resolution of this issue requires balancing financial responsibility for offspring against encouraging or facilitating the use of donor sperm by unmarried women. Holding sperm donors responsible for the costs of rearing offspring would reduce the opportunities of unmarried women to obtain sperm from physicians or sperm banks, thus relegating them to turkey baster inseminations with sperm that has not been screened for infectious diseases.[22] While one can question whether the right to procreate includes the right to impose rearing costs on others, the risk that sperm donation to unmarried women will increase welfare costs is very slight. One could reasonably conclude that this risk does not justify the reduction in reproductive options for single women that imposing rearing costs on sperm donors would create. Until legislation clarifying these issues is passed, complicated questions of inheritance could also arise.

EGG DONATION

Since 1988, collaborative reproduction involving the donation of eggs to women who are unable to produce healthy eggs has been available.[23] The donor goes through ovarian stimulation and has eggs retrieved, as occurs in IVF.[24] In egg donation, however, the eggs are donated to the infertile couple, inseminated with the husband's sperm, and then placed in the uterus of the wife who is unable to produce eggs. The wife carries the embryo to term, and becomes the rearing mother. In this case both rearing parents have a biologic relation with the child, though only the husband has a genetic relation.

As with sperm donation, the egg donor ordinarily will provide eggs with the intention that she will have no rearing rights or duties in the offspring, and the couple will receive them with the intention that they will assume all rearing rights and duties. At present, only Oklahoma, Texas, and Florida have statutes that gives legal effect to such intentions, following the model that they have adopted for donor sperm to a married couple.[25] A similar approach is expected in other states.

There is no good reason why preconception agreements to exclude the egg donor from any rearing role should not be followed. The egg donor who changes her mind has no persuasive claim in her own right to be involved in rearing. She knowingly provided the egg with the intention that she would be excluded from any rearing role. Nor can she argue convincingly that the best interests of the child require that she have contact with her genetic offspring. Whether or not offspring will want to know their genetic mother at a later time, it is unlikely that the child's best interests require contact with the genetic mother at such an early age, especially when the father and gestational, rearing mother object.

By the same token, the genetic mother should not have rearing duties imposed on her that she did not agree to. Because a female parent is usually in the picture to provide financial support, the situation is not like sperm donation to a single woman.[26] Imposing such obligations would greatly deter or discourage egg donation, thus impairing the ability of infertile couples to use this technique to form families.

Nor should the marital status of the recipient matter in this case, as it might with sperm donation to an unmarried woman. Egg donation always involves a woman who is present to birth and care for the child. Enforcing the agreement to exclude the egg donor from rearing rights and duties should not be dependent on marital status, as it sometimes is with sperm donation.

EMBRYO DONATION

A collaborative technique not yet in wide use but that will be sought by a subset of infertile couples is embryo donation. Couples who are unable to produce egg and sperm themselves may form a family by having a donated embryo placed in the wife's uterus and brought to term. Or couples or women who could benefit from egg donation but who wish to avoid the expense of paying a woman to produce eggs might choose embryo donation. Here the wife has a gestational but no genetic connection with the child, and the husband has no genetic connection. In effect it combines egg and sperm donation in the precombined form of an embryo. While neither rearing partner will be reproducing in the strict genetic sense, gestation undertaken with the intent of the woman and her husband to rear deserves respect as an aspect of their procreative liberty.

No statutes or cases yet exist to regulate rearing rights and duties in embryo donation. However, if agreements to exclude sperm and egg donors from all rearing rights and duties are recognized, the same result should apply with persons who receive an embryo donation. Offspring are assured a male and female rearing parent, one of whom—the mother—has a biologic connection with the child. The couple donating the embryo did so willingly, with the clear understanding that they would have no rearing rights and duties. If separate sperm and egg donations would bar donors from a rearing role, there is no apparent reason why combining the donation in the form of an embryo should lead to a different result.[27]

The only situation in which the agreement to exclude from any rearing role might be overidden would be where the donation went to a single woman. In that case, the child would have a female rearing parent but no male rearing parent. If the jurisdiction recognized the sperm donor's obligations to offspring in those situations, then presumably it might do so in similar situations involving embryo donation. However, one can question whether such a policy is desirable for either sperm or embryo donations to single women.

SURROGACY

Collaborative reproduction is also practiced with the assistance of a woman who gestates the embryo of the infertile couple. The wife may have functioning ovaries but no uterus or is otherwise medically unable to carry a fetus to term. Through IVF, she and her husband produce an embryo which is then placed in the uterus of the gestational surrogate. The resulting child is the genetic offspring of the rearing parents, but has been gestated or carried to term by another.[28]

Surrogacy may also occur with the surrogate providing the egg as well as gestation.[29] The collaborator in this case is artificially inseminated with the husband's sperm, and relinquishes the child to the father and his wife at birth. At some point after birth she terminates her parental rights, and the father's wife—the child's stepmother—adopts the child. In this case, the rearing husband will have a biologic connection with the child. The rearing mother will have none.[30]

The question of enforcing preconception surrogacy agreements for rearing is the most controversial issue in collaborative reproduction. Although most surrogates relinquish the child as agreed, widely publicized cases of surrogates seeking custody or visitation in violation of their agreement have arisen. The few courts that have dealt with the matter have usually applied the long standing adoption law principle that preconceptual or prenatal agreements to relinquish for adoption will not be enforced. They reject the notion that the child's best interests can be determined prior to birth or conception by contract, or that women can know their true wishes about rearing offspring before birth occurs. Some persons oppose enforcing surrogate contracts because women may enter into these arrangements under financial pressure, because it is their labor that has produced the child, or because contract law reflects patriarchal notions of rights that use women's bodies for the sake of male reproduction.[31]

In my view, the preconception intentions of the parties should be binding both for gestational and full surrogacy.[32] In both cases the couple will have invested considerable time, energy, and emotion in finding the surrogate and initiating pregnancy in reliance on her promise. In the case of gestational surrogacy, they will also have entrusted their embryo to her. Given these competing interests, it is not obvious that the surrogate's disappointment or loss at having to relinquish the child as promised should be privileged over the loss which the couple will feel if she now insists on rearing. Assuming that both the couple and the surrogate are fit rearers, there is no reason to think that the child is always better off with the birth mother.[33] In addition, overriding preconception intentions interferes with the couple's procreative interest in using this method of forming a family.

The procreative liberty of both infertile couples and surrogates would be advanced by upholding preconception agreements for surrogate services. If the parties have a fundamental constitutional right to use noncoital means of forming families, that right should include enforcement of preconception surrogate contracts.[34] A failure to enforce preconception agreements to rear could block the only avenue open to infertile couples to have offspring genetically related to one or both rearing partners. It may also deny women who wish only to gestate opportunities to do so. Couples who would otherwise engage their services might be reluctant to do so if the the couple's legal right to rear cannot be guaranteed in advance.

While a mix of reasons contribute to the view that the gestational mother's wish to rear should be privileged, they are not sufficient to override the procreative interests at stake. Indeed, in the final analysis, rejection of preconception intentions to fix postbirth rearing rights and duties seems to be based on paternalistic attitudes toward women or on a symbolic view of maternal gestation. Privileging the surrogate's wishes over the reliance interests of the couple assumes that women cannot make rational decisions about reproduction and child rearing prior to conception. It also treats gestational motherhood as a near sacred endeavor, which preconception contracts that separate gestational and social parentage violate.[35] However, paternalistic and symbolic attitudes over which reasonable persons differ do not justify trumping the fundamental right to use collaborative means of procreation.

No court, however, has yet held that enforcement of preconception rearing agreements is required by procreative liberty. The New Jersey Supreme Court rejected it in the Baby M case by characterizing procreation as genetic only, ignoring the rearing relationship that William Stern and most genetic reproducers intend as a result.[36] Most states that have legislated on surrogate motherhood since Baby M also protect the surrogate's right to retain rearing rights, despite her preconception promise to the contrary.[37]

Respect for the preconception agreement however, should fare better in the case of gestational surrogacy, because the surrogate is not then claiming to rear her own genetic child. In *Anna J. v. Mark C.*, for example, the California Supreme Court held that a gestational surrogate had no claim to rear because she was not the genetic parent.[38] Still, many commentators and surrogacy statutes refuse to distinguish the two types of surrogacy because of the value they assign to the gestational bond and the autonomy of birthing women.[39] Questions of custody and visitation then have to be assigned on some basis other than preconception intentions. However, as long as legislators do not prohibit surrogacy altogether (either directly or by banning payments), recognition of the surrogate's legal right to rear may not discourage all uses of surrogacy. Some couples will still proceed with the hope that the surrogate will honor her promise not to seek postbirth rearing.

Agreements to Include the Donor/Surrogate in Rearing Collaborative Offspring

Although most collaborative arrangements will exclude the donor or surrogate from rearing rights and duties, there will be some instances in which the collaborators agree—as a condition of participation—to give donors and surrogates a role in rearing offspring, including joint or limited custody, visitation, or child support.[40] Such reproduction is truly collaborative, for it involves egg, embryo, and sperm donors and surrogates in rearing the "family" that the parties jointly produce.

Such novel familial arrangements raise two separate legal issues: (1) should inclusive collaborative agreements be permitted at all, and (2) should such agreements be enforced?

Laws against such novel intentionally blended families are unlikely, and would probably be unconstitutional.[41] It is no more likely that raising a child openly with several biologic and social parents would be any more or less harmful than raising a child who has no contact with a biologic parent. Either situation may be done well or badly, depending on the parties, their economic and social situation, and their adjustment to the emotional and psychological complexities of these roles. The medical gatekeepers of the reproductive technology who are needed to construct such families may refuse access, but the law is unlikely to be a direct bar.

The second question—should inclusive collaborative rearing arrangements be enforced—will arise when the donor or surrogate wishes to avoid rearing duties that they voluntarily undertook, or the married couple or individual recipient wishes to exclude the donor or surrogate from the rearing role that had been intended.

A commitment to procreative liberty argues for presumptively enforcing these agreements, both against the primary rearing parents who wish to exclude the donor, and against the donor who wishes to escape support obligations. The parties agreed to collaborate on condition that they would have the assigned roles. Denying effect to their agreement may deprive them of parenting experiences that were the reason for their collaboration. It will also deter future collaborations because of legal uncertainty that intentions will be honored. If freedom to use noncoital technologies to treat infertility and to play partial reproductive roles is to be respected, then agreements of donors and surrogates to be included in—as well as excluded from—rearing offspring should be presumptively honored.

Whether courts or legislatures will honor these agreements depends on several factors, including the time at which the rearing claim is made, the presence of male and female rearers, whether the third party is trying to be included or trying to avoid support obligations, and, finally, on whether the aggrieved party has a biologic relation with the child in question.

The timing of the dispute will be key because of the importance of maintaining rearing relationships that have been established with biologic parents. Attempts to exclude a donor or surrogate who has been permitted to visit the child over a period of time will be less successful than attempts to exclude before the child has established a beneficial relationship with that party. If the relationship has already been established, only conflicts deemed detrimental to the child would seem to warrant exclusion of the donor or surrogate from the agreed-upon role. If the relationship has not been established, failure to enforce the agreement may not harm the child, unless a child's access to a biologic parent is deemed important. In any event, donors or surrogates who do not act to assert their contractual rearing rights immediately after birth are in danger of losing them, just as unmarried fathers are who do not timely assert their interest in rearing offspring.[42]

The primary rearing parents' success in excluding the donor or surrogate may also depend on whether a two-parent rearing family is available to the child aside from the donor or surrogate. The couple's claim to exclude is more likely to be successful in those cases because the child's interests in two parents appears to be met, and the presence of a third party could be disruptive.[43] Still, the excluded biologic parent should have standing to raise her and the child's interest in the intended contact, with disposition of the dispute determined by the child's best interests and the excluded parent's constitutional right to rear offspring.

On the other hand, if the recipient of the collaborative service is single, it will be much harder to exclude the donor or surrogate from the agreed-upon role. Courts are then more likely to find that enforcing the agreement serves the child's interest by providing a second rearer, a factor important in cases that have upheld the sperm donor's right to visit the child of a donation to a single woman.[44] This factor could be important in sperm or embryo donation to single women, or in surrogacy involving single men. It is less likely to matter with egg donation or surrogacy to a single women, since a female rearer will be present.

A third factor that will determine whether inclusive agreements are enforced is the nature of the agreed-upon rearing role. Agreements for joint custody or visitation will be more easily revoked and rejected than agreements to provide support, which the donor/surrogate now refuses to pay. As the biologic parent who would ordinarily be liable for support, he or she should still be liable even if conception was noncoital and donors/surrogates are relieved of support obligations if they agreed to be excluded from any rearing role. When they agreed to support the child whom they are directly responsible for producing, it is reasonable to hold them to their preconception promise. Of course, they may then be entitled to some rearing role as well.

A final determinative factor in these cases is whether the party claiming rearing rights pursuant to a preconception collaborative agreement has played a biologic role in the arrangement. If the collaborator is not a gamete donor or gestator, they will not have reproduced and may have little chance of having their rearing role recognized, as recent litigation concerning custody disputes in lesbian families shows.

In the Matter of Alison D. v. Virginia M., a typical case of this sort, involved a lesbian couple who had a child by artificial insemination.[45] The nonbiologic partner obtained sperm from her brother, inseminated her partner, was present at birth, gave the child her last name, and was the main financial support for the family and child for several years. When the couple separated, the nonbiologic parent was allowed to visit the child for a period. After a point, however, the biologic mother barred her former partner from further contact and litigation ensued. The New York Court of Appeals rejected that partner's claim to participate in rearing on the ground that she was not a "parent" within existing law, and thus lacked standing to raise issues of visitation on behalf of herself or the child.

This decision firmly rejects an expanded version of procreative liberty that would include nonbiologic parties who play a central role in arranging the birth of a child, as the plaintiff in *Alison D.* had. No matter what the intentions of the parties or the actual rearing relationship with the child has been, the nonbiologic rearer is not a "parent" and thus has no standing to have the child's best interests in continuing her rearing relationship considered. While the legislature can change this result, legislators appear reluctant to grant nonbiologic rearers parental status in these situations. Such cases directly challenge the importance of bloodline in determining parenting relations, and require us to rethink whether a nonbiologic party should always be barred from a prearranged rearing role when the biologic parent insists.[46]

On the other hand, *Alison D.* implicitly supports the claim of excluded biologic collaborators who are seeking to partake in rearing pursuant to a preconception agreement. They will at least have standing to raise the issue, because "parent" is defined biologically. Whether courts will find the child's best interests served by contact with the excluded biologic parent will depend on the child's need for contact with all biologic parents, on whether some parental relationship has already begun, and on other factors.[47]

Decisions such as *Alison D.* might, if adoption by the nonbiologic parent is not possible, push gay, lesbian, or other nontraditional partners to establish a biologic connection with intended offspring whenever possible, in order to protect their rearing rights in case of death, divorce, or later dispute. Lesbian couples could have one partner provide the egg for the embryo, which is then gestated by the other partner. Each would then be a biologic parent and have standing as a "parent" to protect the child's best interests.[48] Gay couples who form families with the assistance of a surrogate do not have this option. Until techniques for fusing embryos created by gametes from different partners are established, only one man can be the genetic father of a child.

PROTECTING REPRODUCTIVE COLLABORATORS

Collaborative reproduction offers infertile couples, donors, and surrogates the technical means to fulfill their differing reproductive needs in a mutually satisfying way. If done with advance counseling and full understanding of the social, psychological, medical, and legal complications, it may be a fulfilling enterprise for all parties.

But collaborative reproduction may also be frustrating, upsetting, and difficult. Even with sperm donation, which has been practiced since the 1940s, the social, psychological, and legal roles have not been fully defined. The parties will be thrust into new roles and relationships for which there is little guidance and little legal or social approval. Persons embarking on this enterprise may receive little counseling or guidance in how to deal with the complicated emotional issues that may arise. What is proper conduct for a donor or a family that has received a donation? How do they relate to each other? To the child? What do they tell their own parents, siblings, and friends? What do donors and surrogates tell their family, friends, and own children? The opportunities for greeting-card companies and family therapists are endless.

In addition, the parties face an uncertain legal environment. Aside from donor sperm to a consenting married couple where the law is clearest, there is ample room for dispute and litigation, as donors and surrogates change their minds and assert interests that they had not previously envisaged. Also, the procedures sought may be much less efficacious than expected, requiring several cycles of artificial insemination or embryo transfer. Surrogates may miscarry, or have medical complications during pregnancy or childbirth. Donor insemination may transmit cytomegalovirus or even HIV.[49] Egg donors are also at medical risk from hyperstimulation of the ovaries and egg retrieval.

Limiting Collaborative Reproduction to Protect
Donors and Surrogates

Given the problems that could arise in collaborative reproduction, some persons have argued that the enterprise should be banned altogether or greatly limited to protect the participants from pain or later disappointment. However, such paternalism is unwarranted, and would, as discussed in chapter 2, appear to violate the procreative liberty of reproductive collaborators. Rather than discourage collaboration, public policy should focus on making it safe, effective, and rewarding for all the parties.[50]

Indeed, while there are risks of disappointment, emotional turmoil, and perhaps even litigation, these risks are neither so likely nor so substantial that a ban on any particular form of collaborative reproduction is justified. Even surrogacy, which poses the greatest risks to collaborators, usually is successful for the parties, even though some surrogate mothers feel such intense disappointment that they will wish that surrogacy had never been invented. Sperm, egg, and embryo donors may also at times feel a poignant sadness at never knowing their progeny. But these reactions will vary in intensity and permanence with the individuals involved. Later regret does not seem so likely or devastating that collaborative contracts should be prohibited to protect reproductive collaborators. The harm prevented is not so likely or substantial to justify paternalistic interference with the parties' procreative choice.[51]

Assuring Informed Consent and Avoiding Disappointment

An essential step to protect the collaborating parties is to make sure that they are fully informed of the particular risks that they run in participating in collaborative reproduction. In most instances, this will require actions by physicians and other intermediaries. In some cases, laws or professional guidelines will be necessary.

INFERTILE COUPLES AND RECIPIENTS

Couples being treated for infertility often feel that they are riding on an unpredictable roller coaster. In confronting their infertility, they must adjust to the loss of expected children and self-esteem, and the guilt, anger, and depression that these losses usually bring. They may grasp eagerly at the hope that donor gametes or surrogacy will, at last, bring them the child that they so fervently wish.

It is thus crucial that they be fully informed about success rates and about the medical, social, and psychological risks of these procedures, so that they are prepared for later disappointment and complications. The extent of counseling will vary with the program, the parties, and the collaborative technique they choose. Overshadowing the entire enterprise will be the unanswerable questions about the longer-range psychological and social impact of collaborative reproduction.

GAMETE DONORS

Donors of sperm, egg, or embryos also need detailed information, and in some cases counseling, about the social, psychological, and legal ramifications of their role. Sperm donors face no medical risk in masturbating to produce sperm, though they may end up learning disturbing information about their genetic or HIV status.[52] They should be accurately informed of the legal implications of their donation, including any chance that they could be liable in the future for child support or have unwanted contact with offspring. They should also be informed of possible psychological repercussions if they wish to have contact with offspring, yet do not have any recourse. Honest discussion of these issues at the start will minimize later problems.

Egg donors face more medical risks, because they will usually undergo ovarian stimulation and surgical retrieval of eggs. They need accurate information about those risks and the legal ramifications of their donation, and counseling about the unknown social and psychological effects of separating female genetic, gestational, and social parentage. They too should be prepared for the possibility of wanting to know about or make contact with their genetic offspring, yet have no way of doing so.[53] They should also be prepared for genetic offspring seeking to make contact with them. Other complications could occur if they are donating eggs to a family member or friend.

Embryo donors face similar uncertainties. The legal effects of embryo donation are still undefined, so that even reasonable predictions about future rearing rights and duties are necessarily uncertain. In addition, donated embryos will usually have been created as part of an infertile couple's own efforts to form a family. The donor couple may feel a special bond to "their" embryos, and want very much, despite initial feelings to the contrary, to meet or protect "their" child. If their own efforts at pregnancy have failed, these feelings might intensify or even parallel the feelings of abandonment and guilt that persons who relinquish children for adoption sometimes feel. Prospective embryo donors should be informed of these possibilities, and counseling should be provided to help them adjust to these contingencies.

SURROGATES

Special attention must be paid to the needs of surrogates. They will be embarking on a major life event—pregnancy and childbirth—with the intention of then relinquishing the child they have gestated. Accurate information about medical difficulties in initiating and completing pregnancy is essential. Counseling is also essential to prepare surrogates for probable feelings of disappointment, depression, and guilt. Counseling should be provided both prior to conception and after birth to help them adjust to their situation.

A class bias in most surrogacy arrangements may also be inevitable.

While most surrogates are high school graduates, and many will have gone to college, they are more likely to be less educated and less well off than the infertile couples who hire them. Prospective surrogates will be driven by complex motives, including altruism, money, the wish to reexperience in order to master a previous experience of loss, enjoyment of pregnancy, or wanting to reproduce without rearing.[54] Some women may have unrealistic ideas about the experience, or not fully understand their own motivation.

Given the complexity of the situation, some persons recommend that prospective surrogates be screened according to strict criteria of psychological health. They suggest that women with previous psychological problems and women who have not had children not be accepted into surrogacy programs. Others would provide couples with the results of screening tests and leave it to the couple to decide whether to accept a particular surrogate. Still others would formalize surrogacy agreements by requiring that a judge, or alternatively, a review board, examine the prospective surrogate prior to insemination to make sure that she fully understands her rights and duties, and is acting freely.[55] Preconception ratification would bar the surrogate's later claim to custody of offspring contrary to her agreement.

Until regulatory legislation is passed, surrogate brokers have special duties to make sure that the women they recruit are well informed and counseled about the risks they face.[56] Although this has not always been the practice, surrogate brokers should inform prospective surrogates at the earliest possible time in the recruitment process, such as in the material that they send out to women responding to newspaper ads, that surrogacy is disappointing and difficult for some women. Brokers should also make clear to prospective surrogates that they represent the infertile couple, not the surrogate, and advise the surrogate to seek her own legal counsel. They should also screen prospective surrogates psychologically, so that women who appear likely to have problems are excluded or so infertile couples have full information on the psychological profile of the prospective surrogate. They may also have legal duties to make sure that medical tests that protect the surrogate are performed.[57]

Whether privately or publicly imposed, measures to assure that surrogates are adequately counseled and screened will increase costs, and interfere to some extent with the wishes of individuals to engage or function as a surrogate. Such restrictions, however, do not violate procreative liberty, for they are not likely to prevent couples from use of this technique.[58] Moreover, the additional burden they create is justified as a reasonable measure to enhance autonomy and protect the parties in surrogate reproduction.

Paying Money and the Reification of Reproduction

A major concern about collaborative reproduction arises from paying donors and surrogates for their services. Commercializing reproduction is said to exploit and depersonalize women, turning them into mere cogs in the machinery of reproduction. It also risks turning children into commodities that are purchased via the payments for donor and surrogate services that make them possible.

Objections to payment, however, vary with the procedure in question. Some countries, such as France, England, and Australia, have banned payments to gamete donors and depend solely on volunteers. The prevailing practice in the United States is for commercial sperm banks or physician intermediaries to pay sperm donors for their time and effort, thus proving the inaccuracy of the term "donor." Egg donors are also paid on a graduated schedule according to the procedures they undergo.[59] A fee of $1,500 to $2,000 is now common. Some embryo donors have requested compensation to cover the costs incurred in producing the donated embryos. Federal and state laws outlaw the sale of solid organs and nonrenewable tissue, but usually do not apply to the sale of gametes.[60]

Payment to surrogate mothers, however, is much more controversial and is illegal in many states and abroad. Several states have recently passed statutes that expressly forbid commercial surrogacy, banning payments both to surrogates and to the brokers who arrange for their services.[61] Other states reach the same result by construing laws against baby selling, which prohibit payments other than medical expenses for adoption, as prohibiting payments to surrogates. Such laws do not usually distinguish between gestational and other forms of surrogacy. In most states the legal status of payment to surrogates remains uncertain.

One could argue that these laws do not apply to surrogacy because the infertile couple is paying the surrogate for her gestational services, not for giving the child up for adoption. This argument is strongest when gestational surrogacy is involved, and weakest as the contract makes payment conditional on either producing a live baby or on fulfilling the promise to relinquish the child for adoption. Opponents of paid surrogacy, on the other hand, argue that the surrogate contract, no matter how written, is a contract for the sale of a child that falls within laws prohibiting baby selling. The New Jersey Supreme Court adopted the latter view in the *Baby M* case, and it may be followed in other jurisdictions.[62]

Paying surrogates (though perhaps not gamete donors) is probably necessary if infertile couples are to obtain surrogacy services. Although surrogates usually act out of mix of motivations, few women not related to the couple are likely to undergo pregnancy and childbirth unless they are paid for their services. Also, it seems unfair not to pay surrogates for their very substantial efforts, while egg and sperm donors and the doctors and lawyers arranging surrogate services are well paid. If a ban on payment significantly reduced access to surrogacy, it would infringe the infertile couple's procreative liberty, for it would prevent them from obtaining the collaborative services they need to rear biologically related offspring. Such an infringement could be justified only if banning payment prevented a substantial harm that clearly outweighed the burden on procreative choice.

Yet the arguments for banning payment do not appear to reach that level of justification. A main argument is that a ban on payment will prevent exploitation of surrogates, who in most cases will be poorer and of a different social class than the infertile couples hiring them.[63] Exploitation should not be confused with coercion. Women volunteering to be paid surrogates are not being coerced, even if they need the money, because they are not deprived of anything that they are otherwise entitled to if they refuse the couple's offer.[64]

Nor is it clear that they are being exploited to any greater degree than labor markets generally exploit financial need. In this regard, markets for the sale of gestational services are no more exploitive than the sale of other kinds of physical labor. If people are free to sell their labor as petrochemical workers, cleaning persons, or construction workers in the hot Texas sun, why should the sale of gestational services be treated any differently? Much paid labor is equally or even more risky to health.

Proponents of the exploitation claim point to the very different nature of maternal gestation, and argue that women should not be asked to trade their gestational capacity for their need for money. Their argument, in effect, rests on an objection to the perceived risks and demeaning effects of commercializing motherhood. Yet reasonable people have differing moral perceptions about paid surrogacy, with many not finding the symbolic demeaning of motherhood that others see as so glaringly wrong. With such splits in perception, such symbolic concerns alone should not override the couple's interest in having and rearing biologic offspring with the help of a freely consenting, paid collaborator.

A second argument against payment—that it commodifies children and surrogates—also reduces to a perception of the symbolic effects of treating gestation as a product to be sold for money. Professor Margaret Radin has developed this argument more fully than anyone else.[65] But she has failed to show that payment will lead to monetizing or commodifying all children or women, or why certain attributes such as gestation and sexuality may not be sold, while other attributes, such as physical size, skill, attractiveness, and intellectual prowess may be.[66] Her claim that her list of nonmonetizable attributes are more essential "to our deepest understanding of what it is to be human" is not convincing, since one could just as reasonably argue that the physical and mental attributes that drive the market for models, professional athletes, and computer scientists are also essential to "our deepest understanding of what it is to be human."[67]

In short, while some feminist critics stress the harmful effects of paid surrogacy on women, objections to paying surrogates are often more deontological than consequentialist.[68] The exploitation and commodification objections usually boil down to the judgment that it is simply wrong to pay women to gestate, because of the very essence or nature of gestation, regardless of actual effects. The problem with this objection is that perceptions of the wrongfulness of payment vary widely, with surrogates, infertile couples, and many others strongly in favor of payment. Given differing views over the symbolic significance of payment, the need to protect female gestation from the taint of filthy lucre does not seem compelling enough to justify stopping infertile couples from obtaining the services they need to rear biologic offspring. However, until courts and legislatures adopt this analysis, bans on paying surrogate mothers, though arguably a clear interference with procreative liberty, may prevent many infertile couples from using this technique to have children.

THE LOOP BACK TO ADOPTION

Recognition of the right to engage in collaborative reproduction has been grounded in the importance of rearing children who are biologically related to one or both rearing partners. One might question, however, why the biologic tie to one or both of the partners is essential. For medical or other reasons some couples will be unable to establish that tie, yet still have a strong desire to rear children. If couples may resort to donors and surrogates to form a family, why should access to collaborative assistance depend on the couple's biologic participation in the enterprise?

The importance of a minimal biologic connection as a prerequisite to collaborative reproduction may not withstand scrutiny. Adopted children are wanted and loved despite the lack of biologic tie with parents, as are collaboratively produced children who have no biologic tie with a rearing mother or father. Indeed, feminists critical of surrogate motherhood have pointed out that the bias in favor of biology may reflect patriarchal notions of kinship and inheritance that need revision in light of the social realities of rearing families. In forcing us to recognize the rearing interests of both partners, including the partner who may lack a biologic connection with offspring, collaborative reproduction may lead to a reevaluation of the importance of biologic ties in other family arrangements.[69]

Such a reevaluation might show that preconception rearing intentions should count as much as or more than biologic connection. If so, then arrangements in which several persons collaborate to produce a child for person(s) to rear who have no biologic connection with the child should also be presumptively protected.[70] Although it is not reproduction in the strict sense, the rearing couple would be exercising a choice which presumptively deserves respect because of the importance of parenting to persons who cannot themselves reproduce.

If the importance of rearing leads us to privilege rearing intentions and practices over biology, then the existing legal framework for adoption will necessarily be called into question. Under this framework, preconception or prenatal contracts to relinquish children for adoption are invalid, and payments to induce adoption are illegal. Such laws directly conflict with an expanded view of collaborative reproduction that includes a couple's right to form a family with nonbiologically related children, for preconception agreements and money payments will usually be essential to form such families.

If the right to form families is broadened beyond the confines of current adoption law, couples would be entitled to pay women to be artificially or naturally impregnated to produce children for them. The couple would have a presumptive right to rear offspring exclusive of the biologic parents, in accordance with preconception agreements to that effect.[71] After all, they were the prime movers in bringing all the parties together to produce the child, and have relied on the promise of the gamete providers and gestator not to rear in mobilizing the parties to that goal. No doubt brokers adept in finding gamete donors and surrogates and coordinating conception, pregnancy, and childbirth for the sake of intended parents would enter the market. Thus broadened, procreative liberty would lead to a widespread market in paid conception, pregnancies, and adoptions, the very antithesis of the current system.

If collaborative reproduction loops back in this way to undermine the foundations of adoption law, some persons may oppose any use of donors and surrogates. The logic of collaborative reproduction, even when confined to some biologic relation, does challenge the importance of biology. The intended arrangement presumptively trumps the later claims of donors and surrogates, even though they have as strong, or in the case of full surrogacy, arguably stronger, biologic ties to offspring. The theory underlying these practices would logically extend primary rearing rights to the infertile couple who independently recruit sperm, egg, or embryo donor and surrogate to produce a child for them.[72] The need for adoption brokers and payment to collaborators to implement such arrangements would naturally follow. Laws that prevented these arrangements would then need revision.

Yet logic and practice must be distinguished. In the foreseeable future most reproductive collaboration will be for gamete donation or gestational surrogacy, both of which preserve a prime biologic connection. There will be few instances of a couple organizing gamete donors and surrogacy to provide them a child in the extreme way being discussed.[73] The adoption system can be distinguished from these practices and permitted to function independently with its own rules.

In time, however, pressure to change that system might occur. If preconception contracts with donors and surrogates are validated, some persons—infertile couples or entrepreneurs—will no doubt try to extend that principle to commissioned pregnancies and paid adoption. At that point the importance of the biologic gestational connection will have to be directly confronted, and the framework of adoption law reevaluated.[74] In the end, we may come to accept paid, commissioned pregnancies in carefully defined circumstances as another avenue for infertile couples seeking to form a family. Whether or not labeled "reproductive," the interests at stake may deserve equivalent protection. However, fear of that possibility should not prevent the present use of donors and surrogates to form families who are biologically related to one or both rearing partners.

COLLABORATIVE REPRODUCTION AND THE
FUTURE OF FAMILIES

Discussion of these issues inevitably brings us to a recurring concern about collaborative reproduction—that it will accelerate the decline of the nuclear family at a time when that institution is under severe pressure from divorce, teenage pregnancy, single mothers, blended families, gay and lesbian life-styles, and other forces.

Yet such fears exaggerate the effect of collaborative reproduction and do not justify limiting the joint efforts of infertile couples, donors, and surrogates. In most cases, collaborative reproduction enables a married couple to have biologically related offspring, with the gamete donor or surrogate excluded from any significant rearing role. While contracts to include the donor or surrogate in rearing offspring are theoretically possible, they are likely to be rare except where a friend or family member provides the service. Even then, one would expect there to be at most two primary rearers, even if some contact with other biologic parents and their relatives occurs.

Given the great number of families in which nonbiologic parents are primary rearers due to death, divorce, abandonment, and the like, it is difficult to see how collaborative reproduction, with its small number of intentionally blended families, poses a threat to the nuclear family. Indeed, with its emphasis on enabling a married couple to have and rear biologic offspring, it supports that institution more than it diminishes it, despite the social, psychological, and legal complications that might ensue.

Nor would the hypothetical possibility of expanding procreative liberty to include commissioned pregnancies and paid adoptions where there is no biologic connection alter this conclusion. While this practice would increase the number of persons playing partial reproductive roles, its primary aim is to provide a couple with a child to love and rear in a two-parent family. In any event, the numbers involved are likely to be minuscule, relative to the number of births occurring annually.

CONCLUSION

This chapter has shown that collaborative reproduction is an important part of the procreative liberty of infertile couples and the donors and surrogates assisting them to reproduce. Given its increasingly important role in the treatment of infertility, the main policy issues concern how to assure that collaborative reproduction occurs in a safe, effective, and mutually satisfying way. Rather than try to discourage such practices, public policy should insure that the necessary counseling, informed-consent, record-keeping, and legal rules for allocating rearing rights and duties exist.

As collaborative reproductive technologies grow in efficacy, they will be more frequently used, particularly egg and embryo donation and gestational surrogacy. However, the incidence of donor sperm—the most frequent collaborative technique—may diminish, as micromanipulation and intrauterine insemination techniques improve treatment of male factor infertility. Overall, however, collaborative reproduction will remain a subset of noncoital reproduction and a very small subset of reproduction generally. While crucially important for the parties involved, it is likely to have only a minimal effect on female social roles, the vitality of the family, or the shape of society.

In time, acceptance of collaborative reproduction will lead to better definition of the roles and responsibilities of the various participants. This will reduce the social, legal, and psychological uncertainties that now pervade the area, and improve the chances of a satisfying experience for collaborators and offspring. The sooner that collaborative reproduction is woven into the social fabric, the better it will be for all affected parties.

QUALITY CONTROL

CHAPTER 7

Selection and Shaping of Offspring Characteristics

GENETIC SCREENING AND MANIPULATION

EVERY PERSON or couple contemplating children wants healthy offspring, yet knows that offspring characteristics cannot be guaranteed in advance. New screening and selection technologies are now changing this situation. Prenatal diagnosis is occurring earlier and for a wider range of conditions. In the future techniques to alter genes for both therapeutic and nontherapeutic purposes will become available. Whether couples may or must use these techniques raises important questions about the scope of procreative liberty.

EMERGING PRACTICES AND DILEMMAS

Selection techniques now rely on carrier or prenatal screening to identify persons at risk for having handicapped offspring. Carrier screening occurs in high-risk subgroups (blacks, Ashkenazi Jews), but will eventually touch most couples, as carrier tests for cystic fibrosis and other common conditions become routinely available. Couples aware of their carrier status may then decide not to reproduce, use donor gametes, or adopt. They may also seek prenatal diagnosis and terminate pregnancy if they do conceive.

As the ability to diagnose more genetic conditions earlier and less invasively grows, prenatal screening will eventually affect most pregnancies. Chorion villus sampling, which occurs at 10–12 weeks of pregnancy, is replacing amniocentesis at 14–18 weeks as the prenatal diagnostic method of choice for women at risk for chromosomal and genetic conditions. Sixty-five percent of pregnancies in the United States are now screened for alpha fetal protein, an indicator for neural tube defects such as spina bifida and anencephaly.[1] As tests to identify fetal cells in maternal blood are perfected, the genetic condition of every fetus will be diagnosable at 7–8 weeks by a simple blood test. It is likely that such tests will become a routine part of prenatal care, followed often by pregnancy termination when the test is positive. Genetic diagnosis of preimplantation embryos, now occurring in clinical experiments, will also be available.

As advances in genetics grow, persons contemplating procreation will also have more genetic information about potential offspring, including their susceptibility to chronic illness and late-onset diseases as well as the more common autosomal recessive diseases now tested. They may then choose to procreate, avoid conception, or terminate a pregnancy that has already begun. Eventually, they will be able to opt for therapy on the embryo or fetus to correct defects and produce a healthy child. In the more distant future, in utero or in vitro interventions to enhance or improve the characteristics of offspring will also be possible.

Expanded carrier screening, improvements in the timing and scope of prenatal diagnosis, and a greater capacity to intervene at both the fetal and embryo levels are a significant development for reproductive choice. Since carrier and prenatal screening potentially affect every pregnancy, these technologies will have a far greater impact than IVF and assisted reproduction. Given the widespread desire for healthy children, these techniques will be increasingly in demand as part of routine prenatal care. The Human Genome Initiative will accelerate the trend by identifying new genes for carrier and prenatal testing, including, potentially, genes for alcoholism, homosexuality, and depression.

The idea of selecting offspring traits—of quality control of offspring—is both appealing and disturbing. It is appealing because of the understandable desire for a normal, healthy child. Avoiding conception or terminating an affected pregnancy rather than living with the burdens of handicapped birth would appear to be a central part of procreative liberty. So would interventions to treat the affected embryos or fetuses, which will appeal to persons who reject abortion or embryo discard.

Yet there is something deeply disturbing about deliberate efforts to assure a healthy birth, at least when certain means are used. The very concept of selection of offspring characteristics or "quality control" reveals a major discomfort—the idea that children are objects or products chosen on the basis of their qualities, like products in a shop window, valued not for themselves but for the pleasure or satisfaction they will give parents. The danger is that selection methods will commodify children in a way ultimately harmful to their welfare. Carried to an extreme, parents will discard less than "perfect" children and engineer embryos and fetuses for enhanced qualities. A worst-case scenario envisages repressive political regimes using these techniques to create a government-controlled Brave New World of genetically engineered social classes.

Even if such futuristic scenarios never occur, the focus on offspring quality alters the experience of human reproduction. At the very least, pregnancy becomes in Barabara Katz Rothman's evocative term "tentative"—not disclosed or accepted until prenatal tests certify the acceptability of the fetus.[2] Although selection techniques will permit some defective "products" to be repaired before birth, most affected fetuses will be discarded based on a judgment of fitness, worth, or parental convenience. In addition to destroying prenatal life, these actions may convey the view that persons with handicaps should never have been born. It may also create pressure for all couples to use these techniques to avoid saddling the public with the high cost of medical care for children with genetic disease. When positive actions to shape offspring become feasible, couples may feel compelled to engineer offspring according to predetermined criteria of acceptability. If such practices become widespread, they could fundamentally alter our views of ourselves, our children, and human reproduction.

The development of quality control or offspring selection techniques thus raise ethical, legal, and policy issues that deserve careful attention. One set of issues concerns assuring access for those who wish to use them.[3] Here we must distinguish positive from negative selection techniques, and ask whether the technique is used for therapeutic or nontherapeutic purposes. In each case we must first establish whether the central concerns of procreative liberty are involved, and then whether the use in question harms the interests of others sufficiently to justify restriction. A second set of issues concerns protecting the choice of those persons who do not wish to engage in prenatal selection. This issue is most salient with carrier and prenatal genetic screening and is discussed in that context only.

As with other reproductive technologies, procreative liberty would entitle most couples to use—or not use—negative and even positive selection techniques as they choose. The perceived dangers of "quality control" appear to be insufficient to remove these choices from the discretion of persons planning to reproduce. This is clearest with negative forms of selection because of their close connection with the right to avoid reproduction. Prenatal interventions to cure disease or defect at the fetal or embryo level should also be permitted. However, positive interventions purely for enhancement purposes present a more complex problem, as do cloning and other techniques that go beyond assuring the birth of a normal, healthy child for rearing.

SELECTION OF OFFSPRING CHARACTERISTICS AND PROCREATIVE LIBERTY

Whatever reservations one has about technologies that shape or select offspring characteristics, their use or nonuse would appear to be centrally involved with procreative liberty. While the main focus of this chapter is on the right to engage in selection, procreative liberty should also protect the right to refuse to use these techniques. As the discussion in chapter 4 made clear, bringing unavoidably handicapped offspring into the world does not harm them because there is no way for them to be born healthy, and in most cases no wrongful life is involved.[4] As long as persons who choose to ignore genetic information in reproducing are able and willing to rear affected offspring, the costs of their reproduction are unlikely to be sufficient to support a charge of reproductive irresponsibility.[5] Public action to prevent the birth of genetically handicapped offspring by mandatory means is thus not justified.

However, mandatory use of carrier screening or prenatal diagnosis poses a different issue. Requiring that such techniques be used does not interfere with a person's right to procreate as long as they are free to ignore test results. Mandatory carrier or prenatal tests would, however, interfere with privacy or liberty rights not to know certain information. Any mandatory test more invasive than a simple blood test is also likely to violate rights of bodily integrity. Even if the state has the power to mandate such tests, there is widespread agreement that requiring such tests would be unwise policy. It is unlikely to decrease appreciably the incidence of handicapped births beyond voluntary measures and will incur a heavy cost in personal liberty. Given these legal and policy reservations, mandatory carrier and prenatal screening policies are unlikely to be adopted.[6]

On the other hand, the interest in using technologies to select or exclude offspring characteristics is directly involved with procreative liberty. Selection decisions are essential to procreative liberty because of the importance of expected outcome to whether a couple will start or continue a pregnancy. Because expected outcome is so material to reproductive decison making, it implicates the liberty interest both in avoiding and in achieving reproduction.

As discussed in chapters 2 and 3, persons have a right not to procreate because of the physical, psychological, and social burdens that reproduction entails, with the person directly affected the best judge of when reproduction is too burdensome. If a person has the right generally to avoid procreation, then she should be free to reject reproduction because of the burdens that particular reproductive outcomes impose.[7] The right to use carrier or prenatal screening techniques to determine whether those burdens exist thus follows.

Selection of offspring traits might also be viewed as an aspect of the right to procreate. As noted in chapter 2, there is a presumptive right to procreate because of the great importance to individuals of having biologic offspring—personal meaning in one's life, connection with future generations, and the pleasures of child rearing. If a person thought that she would realize those benefits only from a child with particular characteristics, then she should be free to select offspring to have those preferred traits. The right to procreate would thus imply the right to take actions to assure that offspring have the characteristics that make procreation desirable or meaningful for that individual. On this theory, both negative and positive means of selection would be presumptively protected.

Arguments against recognizing selection of offspring characteristics as part of procreative liberty exist, of course. One argument asserts that particular selection techniques should not be permitted because of the harm that they will cause embryos and fetuses. In that case, the problem is not selection per se, but particular means or circumstances of selection, such as abortion or embryo discard. This argument would deny that because there is a right to abort generally, there is a right to abort for reasons such as gender, sexual orientation, hair or eye color, or a disease susceptibility trait. The validity of this argument will turn on the grounds that justify abortion.[8] It is dealt with in greater detail in the discussion of prenatal diagnosis below.

Another argument would deny that the right to reproduce implies the right positively to engineer offspring traits. On this view, the right to reproduce is the right to give oneself over to the natural process of reproduction, not to guarantee its outcome. Yet we may ask why giving oneself over to the natural process is ethically necessary. If any interference in nature is inappropriate, then this argument proves too much. Any attempt to avoid reproduction or treat infertility would also be illegitimate, because one would be interfering with nature for selfish purposes. Such a view is Luddite in the extreme, and would ban almost all forms of medical care as well as myriad other activities of daily life, all of which interfere with nature.[9]

On the other hand, if the claim is that positive selection actions are not part of protected procreative liberty because they will ultimately harm offspring, the argument confuses the existence of a presumptive right to control offspring traits with whether the effects of control are so harmful that such a right can be justly limited. As noted in chapter 2, procreative liberty requires a high standard for determining when harmful consequences justify overriding reproductive choice. The question in each case is whether the harm is severe enough to override the presumptive right to procreate. The risk of harmful effects does not undercut the presumptive importance of selection as part of reproductive choice, even if analysis of particular cases shows sufficient harm to justify limiting the right to select.

Finally, some but not all selection activities may be central to procreative liberty. Some selection activities may not be determinative of decisions to procreate. In addition, extreme measures such as cloning or nontherapeutic enhancement may violate widely shared notions of what makes procreation important. Still, a wide range of negative and positive selection activities are likely to fall within the bounds of procreative freedom.

SELECTION BY NEGATIVE MEANS

Most selection activities in the foreseeable future will occur negatively by decisions aimed at preventing the conception or birth of offspring with undesired characteristics. In most instances the undesired condition will be severe handicap or disability, usually genetic in origin, though gender, late onset disease, or disease susceptibility traits may come to play a role. Given a presumptive liberty right to reproduce or to avoid reproduction, the right to use or to avoid using selection techniques should be presumptively recognized.

Preconception Methods of Selection

The desire not to have a child with severe defects is not itself immoral, and actions to avoid such a reproductive outcome should be respected as an important aspect of procreative liberty.[10] The question then is what means to achieve that goal are acceptable. Preconception means obviously pose fewer problems than postconception efforts. Preconception selection by voluntary selection of mates or gametes raises the fewest problems. Although we do not ordinarily select mates explicitly on the basis of genetic fitness, genes clearly affect many elements of attraction. Concern with the genetic fitness of a prospective mate may not be romantic, but it is rational if one is concerned about the health of spouse and offspring. Mate selection should thus be left to the individual. Similarly, the selection of a gamete donor should be left to the couple that needs this service.

Selection of offspring characteristics through prenatal carrier screening will have a much greater impact on reproductive choice. By determining in advance their heterozygote carrier status for common autosomal recessive diseases such as sickle cell anemia, Tay-Sachs disease, and cystic fibrosis, a couple contemplating procreation will gain information important to their procreative choice. If both carrier tests are negative, they may be encouraged to conceive. Positive tests, on the other hand, may lead them to refrain from conception, to adopt, or to use donor gametes. It may also lead to prenatal diagnosis and abortion of fetuses with the disease in question.

Access to carrier screening is thus an essential aspect of procreative liberty. Indeed, a case for banning voluntary carrier screening cannot be persuasively made. It provides couples with information essential to their reproductive decision making, and does not in itself lead to abortion. The main issue in coming years, now being played out with cystic fibrosis carrier screening, will be determining when a carrier test is sensitive and specific enough that it should be routinely available to those for whom it is of interest. For example, should couples have access to a carrier test that may not yet be ready for population screening, if they are willing to accept the uncertainties the test poses?[11] Legal recognition of remedies for claims of wrongful birth will help determine whether couples are informed of all opportunities for carrier screening prior to conception.[12]

On the other hand, carrier screening should not be imposed on people without their consent. In the late 1960s and early 1970s several states adopted mandatory carrier screening laws for sickle cell anemia. Because of inadequate counseling, the carrier trait was often confused with the disease. Some persons with the trait were fired, denied insurance, and stigmatized.[13] This experience has led to a strong presumption against any mandatory carrier screening program, and resistance to voluntary screening programs that do not have strong counseling components built in to prevent misunderstanding and stigma. As carrier testing for cystic fibrosis has shown, without the resources and infrastructure for such counseling, adoption of such programs is premature.[14]

Despite these reservations, mandatory carrier screening would not infringe procreative liberty as long as freedom to decide whether or not to reproduce remains. Such a law could be justified as a means to assure that people who are likely to reproduce are aware of their risk of producing diseased offspring so that they might make a more informed choice, and in the process, avoid giving birth to offspring who will require extensive medical care. Although one might disagree with such a policy, it would not directly violate procreative choice.

Postconception Methods: Screening Embryos

Although now experimental, it is likely that screening of preimplantation embryos for genetic disease will become an available option. Embryo screening will occur by removing one or two cells of an early preimplantation embryo in order to assess its genetic makeup. If the result is negative for disease, the embryo can be transferred to the uterus in the hope of starting a pregnancy. If the test is positive, the embryo can be discarded or not transferred. In the future, a positive test could lead to gene therapy on the embryo.

Once established as safe and effective, embryo biopsy will be sought by couples undergoing IVF who are at risk for genetic disease or who wish to select the healthiest embryos for transfer. In addition, it will be sought by couples who are known carriers of genetic disease who wish to avoid prental diagnosis and abortion.

No strong ethical argument exists for denying couples access to embryo biopsy as a diagnostic technique.[15] A main objection is that it will lead to the destruction or discard of embryos. Compared to abortion of fetuses, however, selection of embryos should be more acceptable because the excluded entities—preimplantation embryos—lack defined individuality and differentiated organs. Although some persons view embryos as a powerful symbol of human life, only a small minority of persons view them as moral subjects with a right to life. If discard of unwanted embryos is accepted, discard on the basis of genetic traits should also be acceptable.

Unless one views all embryos as having rights to be placed in a uterus, arguments against embryo selection must rely on the burdens on women who would choose to undergo IVF rather than conceive coitally so that embryos can be screened prior to pregnancy, or on the dangers of opening the door to more positive engineering of offspring characteristics.[16] However, it is difficult to see why a couple at risk for a severe genetic disease should not be free to prefer IVF and embryo discard over coital conception and later abortion. Couples choosing this option are likely to have had prior births or family experience with the diseases screened, and know full well what is at stake.

However, we should recognize that embryo selection for less serious conditions, for susceptibility traits, or even for gender may occur once screening of embryos for more serious conditions is established. Yet because the embryo is so rudimentary in development, selection for less serious reasons should be less objectionable than screening of fetuses for those same reasons. If one has to choose three out of seven embryos to place in the uterus, it is not irrational to exclude those which have genetic markers for susceptibility to major disease. Even gender selection might be acceptable at this stage because the expense and burdens of the practice make it unlikely that this technique would ever be so widespread as to alter societal sex ratios—a main concern with gender selection.[17]

A final concern with embryo biopsy is the slippery slope—the fear that it will open the door to more problematic forms of embryo engineering. As we will see below, the fear that something will occur in the future is rarely a sufficient reason to stop an otherwise acceptable action from occurring in the present. In most instances there is no certainty that the future use will ever occur or that it could not be stopped by other means if it were clearly unacceptable.

Postconception Methods: Screening Fetuses

The main method of negative screening for the foreseeable future is pre-natal diagnosis followed by abortion. Two technological developments will greatly increase the demand for prenatal screening of fetuses. One is the rapidly growing number of genetic conditions that can be identified at the carrier and fetal stage. As knowledge of the human genome grows, carrier tests for many more autosomal recessive traits will become available. Couples at risk who decide to conceive may then seek prenatal diagnosis to screen out affected fetuses.

The second development is the likelihood that prenatal diagnosis will be routinely available at very early stages of pregnancy by minimally invasive means. As previously noted, maternal blood is now routinely screened for alpha fetal protein to detect neural tube defects. More informative diagnostic tests on fetal cells recovered from a pregnant woman's blood in the first trimester should be available in the next three to five years, thus making early abortions for a growing range of genetic conditions more widely available.[18] If routinely available, such a test will make all pregnancies "tentative" until prenatal screening certifies the fetus as healthy.

Assuming that these technical developments occur, it will be important to safeguard the freedom of individuals and couples to avoid or to use these screening techniques as they choose. Personal liberty is not well protected if women are routinely subjected to prenatal genetic screening without their consent or made to feel irresponsible if they say no. By the same token, they are deprived of procreative freedom if the state bans use of prenatal screening techniques because of objections to abortion.

THE RIGHT TO REJECT PRENATAL DIAGNOSIS

The availability of early prenatal diagnosis through a simple maternal blood test will create pressure on all pregnant women to have their fetuses screened prenatally. In most instances the pressure will come from physicians who view such tests as a routine way to assure a healthy birth. They may simply perform the test without discussing it, or pressure women into accepting it "for their own good." Without having freely chosen to be in this situation, women may end up with pressure from providers, spouses, or others to terminate a wanted pregnancy.

Alternatively, one can imagine government programs that require all women to undergo routine prenatal testing. The policy goal would be to have all pregnant women be aware of the genetic traits of their fetuses, so that they may make an informed choice about continuing the pregnancy.

As noted earlier, such a requirement would not directly interfere with procreative liberty as long as the decision whether or not to continue the pregnancy is left to the woman. However, such a policy would set up strong pressure to terminate pregnancy, and would in any case violate autonomy, privacy, and possibly even bodily integrity. The wisdom of such a policy is questionable.

The possibility of routine genetic screening of fetuses via maternal blood samples thus presents the question of whether the right to reject such screening should be protected. If personal choice about prenatal diagnosis is to be respected, then action beyond rejecting government-mandated programs is also needed. The greatest pressure for testing is likely to come from a medical profession acting out of malpractice fears, profit motive, or a sense of helping women. To protect a woman's right not to be screened, doctors should inform women of the decisional risks and benefits of such tests before doing them, including the decisions they face if the test is positive. Autonomy is important, even when it is not directly involved with reproduction.

THE RIGHT TO USE PRENATAL DIAGNOSIS

On the other hand, the right to use prenatal diagnosis and terminate pregnancies should also be protected. Restrictions on prenatal diagnosis interfere with procreative choice by depriving a woman of information material to a decision of whether to continue pregnancy.[19] The main argument against use of prenatal diagnosis is that it leads to the destruction of fetuses. However, if abortion is morally acceptable and legally available, then prenatal diagnosis is not objectionable because it might lead to abortion.

Although people disagree about the morality of abortion, the case for previability abortions rests on the view that a previable fetus has not yet reached a stage of development at which it has interests in itself. Prior to viability, it lacks the neurological capability for sentience. Despite its potential, it thus is not owed any moral duties in itself. Continuing a pregnancy is thus a matter of personal choice, and not a moral duty owed the fetus.[20]

Although abortion may still be a symbolic devaluation of human life, these symbolic losses can be justified by the burdens on the woman who chooses to abort. Faced with an unwanted pregnancy, abortion offers her relief from the burdens of unwanted gestation and child rearing. On this argument, her freedom from those burdens trumps the symbolic cost of ending a fetus's life.

If a woman has a moral right to end an unwanted pregnancy when the fetus is healthy, she would also have a right to terminate a pregnancy when the fetus has a genetic defect. Freedom to abort a normal pregnancy implies an equal freedom to abort to avoid the special burdens of having a handicapped child. This practice need no more devalue the life of handicapped persons than carrier screening to avoid their birth does, or than aborting a normal fetus devalues children generally. If abortion is accepted generally, then it should be available for genetic selection reasons as well.

This argument holds even where the genetic indication appears less serious or even trivial. For example, some couples might abort fetuses with cystic fibrosis or phenylketonuria, even though those conditions vary widely in their seriousness or are treatable. Some couples might also abort for reasons of gender or for trivial indications such as disease susceptibility traits. As long as the termination occurs at a stage at which the fetus itself has no interests, such terminations would violate no moral duty to the fetus, and thus be within the moral rights of the woman who does not wish to continue such a pregnancy.[21] In any event, most of the indications for prenatal diagnosis and abortion involve serious conditions that clearly fall within the woman's prerogative.[22]

A person who rejects the idea that abortion is ethically permissible because previable fetuses lack interests or rights should also reject abortion for serious genetic anomalies. If normal fetuses cannot be aborted because of their inherent value, and both normal and handicapped newborns must be treated at birth, then it is inconsistent to permit abortion only of handicapped fetuses. An exception for severe deformity when abortion is otherwise unacceptable devalues fetuses because of their handicap, not their stage of development. Only in cases of anomalies totally incompatible with life, such as anencephaly, would abortion of the severely handicapped fetus be morally defensible. In that case, death of the newborn is inevitable, and nontreatment at birth is also permitted. The claim that abortion of handicapped fetuses is permissible because of the great burden on the parents overlooks the great burdens that parents may experience even when the fetus is normal.

Legally, under *Roe v. Wade* the reason or indication for the abortion is irrelevant—abortions may occur for strong or weak reasons, for major or for trivial genetic defects. Thus laws that banned abortion for sex selection purposes or for genetic reasons perceived as trivial would most likely be struck down if ever challenged.[23] The woman is the final judge of the importance of the pregnancy to her.

If *Roe v. Wade* were reversed, it is likely that wide room for prenatal screening and abortion on genetic grounds would still exist. Many states would continue to make abortion available for any reason. Despite the inconsistency of such exceptions with the state's general protection of prenatal life, even restrictive states would probably recognize exceptions to a general ban on abortion for severe handicap or fetal deformity.[24] Polls consistently show that around 70 percent of respondents say that they are in favor of abortion for severe deformity, with only the strictest right-to-life groups opposing it.[25] If exceptions for genetic handicap are recognized, the availability of abortion for selection purposes will depend on how exactly the exception is phrased and interpreted. Treatable genetic conditions such as phenylketonuria might not qualify as "severe fetal deformity," though Down's syndrome and cystic fibrosis might. However, Huntington's disease and other late-onset disorders or genetic traits that increase the risk of heart disease, cancer, or diabetes probably would not qualify.

Even if abortion is legally available, a residue of ethical concern will remain if the abortion occurs for gender or other seemingly trivial reasons. The willingness of physicians to screen pregnancies and perform abortions will vary with the perceived importance of the goal sought as well as the stage of the pregnancy. As the reason moves away from the impact of a serious handicap, there will be greater hesitancy to screen or end pregnancy on genetic grounds, even though the law permits such selection to occur. This is evident in the reluctance of physicians to perform prenatal screening for sex selection.[26] The scope of legal remedies for wrongful birth will affect physicians' behavior in this regard and women's access to prenatal screening for controversial indications.[27]

POSITIVE INTERVENTIONS

As medical technology progresses, prenatal screening of embryos and fetuses will lead to treatment of genetic defects. Rather than abort or discard affected embryos, couples may request that in utero or in vitro treatments be done when postnatal treatment is not effective. As techniques improve, couples might request genetic interventions for enhancement purposes—to make a normal child even better.

Like the difference between killing and letting die, the difference between positively and negatively selecting offspring traits seems morally weighty. After all, one is not merely deciding whether to accept the results of nature, but is trying positively to alter them. While such intervention seems acceptable when it enables a child who would otherwise be aborted or born damaged to be born healthy, such interventions carry a risk that the child will be viewed as a product or commodity engineered to satisfy parents. Embryo alterations will most likely affect the germ cells as well, thus affecting future generations who have not given their consent to this intervention. Despite these implications, respect for procreative liberty should protect many positive interventions from state prohibition.

To assess the permissible scope of positive interventions, we must examine more closely the competing interests in two situations. One situation involves therapeutic interventions, where the intent is to correct a disease or defect which the child would otherwise have. The second situation is one where the positive intervention is to enhance or make an otherwise normal, healthy child even better. Finally, two situations that do not fit into either category—cloning and intentional diminishment—are discussed.

Therapeutic Interventions

Therapeutic interventions are intended to treat a disease in the embryo or fetus which will affect the welfare of a subsequently born child. Because seeking to have healthy children is a central aspect of procreative liberty, prenatal actions designed to prevent serious disease or defect in expected offspring is part of that liberty. In assessing competing concerns, interventions at the fetal and embryo stages should be distinguished.[28]

IN UTERO INTERVENTIONS

In utero interventions would occur in cases in which prenatal diagnosis reveals a defect and the couple is against abortion. A medication given to the mother might correct a congenital heart condition in the fetus. Or in utero surgical intervention could repair a urethal blockage that will cause severe kidney damage. Fetal surgery might occur in utero through a catheter, or the fetus could be removed from the uterus and replaced when the surgery is over.[29] Although the original high expectations for in utero surgery have not been borne out, more effective operations can be expected in the future.

The availability of prenatal medical or surgical intervention for couples who reject abortion should be decided on the medical merits alone.[30] If deemed safe and efficacious, there is no morally or legally relevant ground for rejecting in utero treatment merely because it is a positive prenatal intervention.[31] Even if the affected fetus could have been legally aborted, parents should certainly have the right to bring their fetus to term in a healthy state. If abortion is rejected, in utero interventions may be the most effective way to protect offspring health.

The major concern with in utero therapies is that they will turn out to be more risky and less beneficial than envisaged. Women might then submit to expensive in utero surgery with high complication rates, thinking that it will solve their expected child's medical problems. The intervention might fail or be only partially successful, enabling children who would otherwise have died to survive with severe handicaps.[32] But this is a problem of experimental vs. established therapy generally, and should not prevent use of positive interventions when the risk/benefit ratio is favorable.

THERAPEUTIC EMBRYO INTERVENTIONS

Interventions at the embryo level for therapeutic purposes, though more problematic because of germ cell effects, should in principle also be acceptable. Germline gene therapy is likely to be available in the next decade. The need for it would arise with couples at risk for genetic disease who request preimplantation embryo biopsy. When one or more embryos are found to have a genetic defect and fetal or postnatal therapy is not effective, the couple might request gene therapy because they have few healthy embryos to transfer or because they have moral objections to embryo discard. Because their interest in reproducing is directly involved, the couple should be free to take steps to have all their embryos come to term in a healthy state.[33]

Assuming safety and efficacy, the main objections to therapeutic interventions on embryos are effects on the gene pool and later generations and slippery slope fears that it will lead to more dangerous interventions. However, neither harm is sufficiently weighty to deny parents this path to healthy offspring.

Germline and Gene Pool Effects

A frequently asserted fear about germline therapy is that it will eliminate from the gene pool a gene that is beneficial to future generations. Of course, such a fear would require that the genetic intervention replace defective genes, not merely add functional ones. It also requires that the deleted harmful genes turn out at some future time to be beneficial, and that the replacement occur on such a frequent or large scale that the gene is effectively lost. But these fears appear too speculative to justify denying use of a therapeutic technique that will protect more immediate generations of offspring.

Another alleged harm is that germline therapy constitutes experimentation on future generations without their consent. But if no harm occurs, because the inserted gene overrides a defective one, this is just a theoretical objection. In any case, but for the genetic alteration in question, later generations allegedly harmed without their consent may not have existed at all. Different individuals would then exist than if the germline gene therapy had not occurred.[34]

Germline gene therapy should not, of course, be undertaken lightly. More work on gene insertion and expression is needed before it is clinically available, and it may never be available to any great extent. Existing regulatory mechanisms, such as the National Institutes of Health Recombinant DNA Advisory Committee, are in place to assure that the techniques work well, for example, will express the gene product in sufficient quantities without causing other disruptions.[35] Other national review bodies may also be called to review the need for germline gene therapy before it becomes clinically available. But if the clinical science has progressed to the point that genetic interventions on embryos are permitted, then speculative concerns about the loss of genes and potential harm to unknown future generations should not prevent couples from using germline gene therapy to prevent severe harm to their offspring.

Slippery Slope Concerns

A main objection to therapeutic alteration of embryos is the fear that it will irreversibly open the way to widespread genetic interventions for nontherapeutic purposes, both voluntary and governmentally imposed. The main slippery slope fear is that parents will want genetic interventions not only to prevent severe defects, but to enhance offspring characteristics as well.[36] Once therapeutic germline therapy occurs, it is said, it will not be possible to deny parents genetic alterations for nontherapeutic enhancement purposes. Such practices could then lead to widepread abuses and even governmental engineering of offspring traits. To prevent these situations from occurring, all gene therapy at the embryonic level should be prohibited.

Like all slippery slope arguments, this argument rests on three questionable assumptions. First, there is no certainty that the predicted undesirable outcome will actually come about. Second, the feared extension may not be as undesirable as presently envisaged. Third, even if it is, there may be ways to prevent that use without foregoing beneficial uses. Finally, if all conditions are met, one would still have to show that future harms discounted by their probability of occurrence outweigh present benefits of gene therapy. With this immense hurdle to overcome, it is unlikely that slippery slope concerns will justify denying germline gene therapy to parents for clearly therapeutic purposes.

First, it is very uncertain whether genetic enhancement will ever occur. At present, somatic gene therapy is still rudimentary, and germline interventions have not yet occurred in humans. If germline therapy is ever perfected for single gene insertions, it is still a long march to the multifactorial gene alteration necessary for nontherapeutic enhancement.

Suppose, however, that either single or multigenetic interventions were available to make otherwise normal, healthy children taller, stronger, brighter, or more beautiful.[37] Some parents might seek to engineer such traits in order to benefit their children by giving them as many advantages in life as possible. Is nontherapeutic enhancement so terrible that all therapeutic alterations of embryos should be banned to prevent any enhancement from ever occurring?

The answer to this question is not obviously yes, for parents now have wide discretion to enhance offspring traits after birth with actions that range from the purely social and educative, such as special tutors and training camps, to the physio-medico as occurs with orthodontia, rhinoplasty, and exogenous growth hormone. Such actions may give the child advantages over other children, exacerbate class and socioeconomic differences, and risk treating the child like a product or object to serve the parent's interest. Yet they fall within a parent's discretion in rearing offspring, and could not constitutionally be banned.[38]

Given wide parental discretion in rearing offspring, it is difficult to see why prenatal enhancement should be excluded from parental choice. Of course, genetic enhancement might have a far greater effect on offspring than postbirth efforts. If widely practiced, prenatal enhancement might also exacerbate class and social disparities in the population. Others will object to genetic enhancement because it violates religious or moral notions of accepting the vagaries of fate when reproducing—a question over which reasonable persons in a pluralistic society may well differ. In short, nontherapeutic enhancement is not so clearly horrific, given postbirth enhancement practices, that preventing it justifies denying parents the right to alter embryos for therapeutic purposes. But even more work is necessary to make the slippery slope argument against therapeutic germline therapy persuasive. Even if enhancement interventions were available and were clearly evil, one would still have to show that there is no effective way to stop the evil uses short of banning all therapeutic uses. But if the evil of enhancement is so clear, the weight of public opinion would be strongly against it, as would the ethical standards of those in control of the technology. Even if some slippage in the control apparatus occasionally occurred, it would most likely not produce such widespread harmful use of nontherapeutic enhancement that beneficial therapeutic uses should also be prohibited.

Finally, one would still have to show that this harm clearly outweighed the good that therapeutic gene alteration would bring. With these hurdles to surmount, it is unlikely that parents could be denied this technology to prevent nontherapeutic enhancement from occurring. By the same token, research into therapeutic germline therapy should not be hostage to the fear that it will lead to nontherapeutic alteration of embryos.

Government Use of Enhancement

A related slippery slope concern is that private enhancement will inevitably lead to mandatory governmental enhancement programs. This fear suffers from the same defects as the private enhancement scenario.

The prospect of mandatory government use for nontherapeutic reasons—the Brave New World scenario—is much more fanciful, and for that reason even less compelling a reason to ban voluntarily sought therapeutic uses. A government bent on engineering docile and submissive social classes through control of reproduction would have to monopolize or control most instances of reproduction, a Herculean task for any government. Also, a radical change in society's sense of civil liberty, democracy, and relation to government would have to occur. Such speculative possibilities are too far-fetched to constitute a compelling case against voluntary parental use of gene therapy to prevent serious genetic harm in offspring. The slippery slope argument collapses here as well.

Nontherapeutic Genetic Interventions

While even therapeutic interventions will be relatively rare in the foreseeable future, three nontherapeutic scenarios—enhancement, cloning, and the Bladerunner problem—deserve attention. Although they are highly speculative, they or variations on them are frequently mentioned as likely horrific endpoints if any positive selection of offspring characteristics is permitted. Discussion of them will illuminate the outer bounds of procreative liberty and parental control of offspring characteristics.

NONTHERAPEUTIC ENHANCEMENT

Although nontherapeutic enhancement has been discussed in terms of a slippery slope argument against therapeutic alteration of embryos, it deserves attention in its own right as an aspect of procreative liberty. Suppose that a gene for height, intelligence, coordination, beauty, or some other desirable characteristic could be inserted in an embryo or fetus to enhance those characteristics in an otherwise normal, healthy child. The parents take this step out of love and concern for their offspring—they want to give their child every advantage. Does the couple's procreative liberty protect their freedom to select or shape offspring characteristics in this way? If not, should it nevertheless be permitted as part of parental discretion in rearing offspring?

Is Enhancement Harmful?

Before addressing whether parents have a right to enhance offspring characteristics, let us first consider whether prenatal enhancement would in fact harm offspring. The genetic manipulation could go awry and lead to embryo or fetal demise or cause physical effects that make the manipulated child worse off. In addition, parents might have unrealistic expectations of children who have been subject to efforts to make them superior.

This could create an unhealthy psychological environment, engender disappointment if the child is merely normal, or affect the child's self-esteem and self-concept in unforeseen, harmful ways.[39]

One can only speculate about whether genetic enhancement, if ever feasible, would help or hurt children. If physical safety and efficacy has been established, the main danger would be the psychosocial impact on offspring and family. Even then one might expect counseling and preparation of the parents to minimize those effects. If the enhancement were sought primarily out of love and concern for the child's welfare, adverse psychological sequelae could be minimized. Enhancement could be seen as an act of love and concern, rather than a narcissistic effort to make the child a product or commodity. Indeed, one would expect that parents would not pursue this option unless they thought that it was a reasonable alternative for protecting their child's welfare.

The main problem with genetic enhancement then might be the disparities in life chances that parents are able to provide offspring. Those with the money and inclination to give their children extra height, intelligence, or pulchritude would be giving their offspring advantages that other children would not have. If this occurred to any significant extent, it would exacerbate class differences, creating more unfairness than the natural lottery already creates. If it occurs sporadically, it would be more tolerable—simply another instance in which wealth gives advantages.

Is Enhancement Part of Procreative Liberty?

But even if genetic enhancement clearly benefited offspring, it would not follow that it falls within the scope of procreative liberty. Enhancement efforts might occur after one has decided to reproduce anyway. But if not determinative of the decision to reproduce, prenatal enhancement would not fall within the core interests protected by procreative liberty. If this is true, the couple could not claim a presumptive right to enhance their children's characteristics based on procreative liberty. Concerns about social unfairness and commodification of offspring would then suffice as a ground for restrictive state action, even though they would not satisfy the strict scrutiny required if core interests of procreative liberty were involved.

What, however, if the couple seeking prenatal enhancement insists that they won't reproduce unless prior to birth they can use genetic techniques to give their child all possible advantages? In that case they could argue that enhancement is central to procreative liberty because it will determine whether they reproduce at all. As long as serious harm to offspring cannot be shown, prenatal enhancement would then be protected as part of their right to reproduce.

Such a claim forces us to confront the outer limits of procreative liberty in a way not previously required in our tour of reproductive technologies.

If everything material to a decision to reproduce is part of procreative liberty, then its scope would extend to enhancement, cloning, and the Bladerunner scenario discussed below. Yet can we not posit a core view of the goals and values of reproduction such that all actions that affect the decision to reproduce are not protected? On such a view, procreative liberty would protect only actions designed to enable a couple to have normal, healthy offspring whom they intend to rear. Actions that aim to produce offspring that are more than normal (enhancement), less than normal (Bladerunner), or replicas of other human genomes (cloning) would not fall within procreative liberty because they deviate too far from the experiences that make reproduction a valued experience.

One problem with such a view of procreative liberty is that it might exclude use of any reproductive technology which deviates from traditional coital conception. But such an implication does not necessarily follow. Noncoital forms of conception, including even the more exotic forms of collaborative reproduction, still aim to produce healthy, normal children for rearing, which is not the situation with enhancement, cloning, or diminishment interventions. It is this interest which gives the freedom to reproduce its value.[40]

Although it may not count as part of core procreative liberty, nontherapeutic enhancement may nevertheless be protected. A case could be made for prenatal enhancement as part of parental discretion in rearing offspring. If special tutors and camps, training programs, even the administration of growth hormone to add a few inches to height are within parental rearing discretion, why should genetic interventions to enhance normal offspring traits be any less legitimate? As long as they are safe, effective, and likely to benefit offspring, they would no more impermissibly objectify or commodify offspring than postnatal enhancement efforts do. Indeed, prenatal enhancement might turn out to be preferable, because an existing child will not be the immediate object of the efforts.[41] If prenatal enhancement becomes technically feasible, its acceptability may depend on the relative risks and benefits of prenatal vs. postnatal enhancement, and not on procreative liberty per se.

CLONING

Cloning a human being would involve creating an exact genetic replica of another human genome. The individual cloned could be living or dead. A sample of his or her DNA, available from any cell of the body, would be placed in the nucleus of an egg or embryo which was then implanted in a uterus and brought to term like any other child.

Cloning is not now practiced nor is it likely to be in the foreseeable future except in the limited form of embryo splitting. Enormous advances in enucleation of eggs or embryos and control of DNA, far beyond present capabilities, would be necessary. Nor are the needs or advantages of cloning, other than in certain IVF micromanipulation procedures to increase the number of embryos, apparent.[42] The prospect of cloning humans seems so far-fetched and bizarre that ethics advisory commissions have an easy time decrying cloning and recommending that it be prohibited.

To test our understanding of procreative liberty, however, let us assume that micromanipulation of cells, embryos, and DNA has progressed to the point that it becomes feasible to clone humans. Suppose then that a couple wishing to have children requests cloning by nuclear transplantation.[43] The genome sought for their offspring might have special meaning (a previous child or respected family member) or be deemed especially advantageous for offspring (Nobel Prize winners, Olympic gold medalists). They assert that they wish to gestate and rear a child who will be benefited by having the desirable genome,[44] and that they would not produce offspring unless they can clone the sought-for genome.

Like most selection/shaping technologies, cloning may be viewed as either a negative or a positive intervention, though here the positive aspects seem to be dominant.[45] The couple is choosing the specific genome of offspring and taking positive steps—having an egg or embryo enucleated and the genome of choice inserted—to bring that result about.

Is Cloning Harmful to Offspring?

While some persons would object to cloning because of the intense engineering involved, a major objection would be the harm predicted to befall offspring who have been intentionally given the genome of another person (or persons, if many clones are made). One could argue that cloning is harmful because it violates a basic notion of human dignity—the right to have one's own unique identity.[46] It could also lead to unrealized parental expectations, invidious comparisons with the cloned individual, or simply identity confusion.

As with genetic enhancement, however, we can only speculate as to whether these expected harms would be realized, and whether they would outweigh any advantages that cloning might confer. In our scenario, couples are seeking a rewarding family experience, not a pack of psychological problems. While the dangers are obvious, it is unclear how severe the problems would be, and whether counseling of all parties could minimize them. Although the child will not have a unique genome, he may still be treated as an individual, indeed a unique one precisely because his entire genome was selected.[47] In addition, the power of genotype alone, relative to nuture, may be overestimated. Environmental and family factors might be more determinative than genes, with significant phenotypic variation even among clones. Finally, there may be benefits from being given a desirable genome by loving parents, and even the special bond, akin to the genetic bond of identical twins, of being the clone of a living individual.[48]

But there is another problem with assessing harm here that goes beyond the psychosocial and familial problems of a child who is a clone of another. The problem—a recurring one with engineering of offspring characteristics—is that the potentially harmful effects of cloning cannot truly harm the clone, because there is no unharmed state, other than nonexistence, that could be achieved as a point of comparison. If cloning did not occur, the cloned individual would not exist. If she had been given a different genome, that is, not been cloned, she would not be the same individual.[49] Thus even if the clone suffers inordinately from her replica status, there is no alternative for her if she is to live at all. Unless the life of a clone were so full of unavoidable suffering that her very existence were a wrong (an unlikely scenario), cloning would then—whatever its psychosocial effects—not harm offspring.

Cloning and Procreative Liberty

As with prenatal enhancement, even if cloning does not harm the resulting person, it may still not fall within the couple's procreative liberty. Unless they were using their own DNA or that of previous offspring, they would not be reproducing at all. Even if the wife's gestation of the cloned embryo were viewed as a form of reproduction, reproducing with a cloned embryo may deviate too far from prevailing conceptions of what is valuable about reproduction to count as a protected reproductive experience.[50] At some point attempts to control the entire genome of a new person pass beyond the central experiences of identity and meaning that make reproduction a valued experience.

Cloning may thus be distinguished from other technological interventions that aim to produce healthy offspring. Coital reproduction is not essential to a valued reproductive experience because noncoital and even collaborative reproduction also produces a new, biologically related individual for rearing. Positive and negative selection techniques also aim to produce a healthy normal child, even if they sometimes trim nature's excesses or improve its bounty. By contrast, cloning exerts such a pervasive influence over the new individual that it violates a basic sense of what makes reproduction valuable.

It is a question of degree. The wrong of cloning is not that it harms offspring, but that it breaks the constitutive rules of protected reproduction by going far beyond what is essential to assure a normal, healthy birth. If a couple's wish to clone is to be respected, it must find its protection elsewhere than under the canopy of procreative freedom. Unlike nontherapeutic enhancement, however, cloning has no analog to common rearing practices, and thus may have no independent protection. If so, cloning could be banned on a lesser showing than restrictions on reproduction usually require.

INTENTIONAL DIMINISHMENT: THE BLADERUNNER SCENARIO

Another selection dilemma arises when shaping techniques are used to make offspring less healthy or whole than they could be. One can imagine a sadistic scientist who delights in genetically engineering misshappen and bent human beings. She could have created healthier persons, but then they would have been different persons, so no individual has been harmed. If she were not permitted her evil experiments, she would not create them at all.

Or consider a more utilitarian scientist in the employ of a large corporation that specializes in producing human laborers for work on distant planets. As presented in the 1982 Ridley Scott film *Bladerunner*, genetically engineered human "replicants" are created to do dirty and dangerous work "off-planet." They resemble persons in all respects, including having memories of family and childhood, but have been genetically programmed to die within four years. The film concerns the efforts of one "replicant" to find the scientist-creator who has the key to reprogram them to live full, human lives.

The ethical issue in this fanciful scenario is whether there is a moral duty when altering or engineering human beings to make them as healthy and normal as possible. The intitial response might be that respect for human dignity requires that we give them at least the minimum needed to lead a species-typical satisfying life. In that case, however, they might not be created at all. If they were created with healthy traits, they would be different individuals than those who are allegedly harmed by being less than they could be. Is it not in their interest to be created in a lesser form than not at all?

The paradox of harm and nonexistence does not entirely settle the matter. The individuals in question have no way to exist but in their limited form, preventing such fabrications does not harm or violate the rights of the "replicants" who would not then exist, because there is no existing individual to be harmed by the policy that prevents their creation with lesser traits. Decisions to prevent the birth of possible people do not harm them if they never exist, even if they would have been grateful for very limited lives once they did exist.

The fabricator's procreative liberty would not include the right to create offspring who have fewer capacities than they could otherwise have had.[51] First, reproduction by an individual would not be occurring unless the genes or gestational capacity of the fabricator were directly involved. Second, even if the lesser fabrication were in some sense deemed "reproductive" or "procreative," it still does not follow that such actions would fall within the core concept of procreative liberty. As noted with enhancement and cloning, procreative liberty is a protected activity because of the importance of reproduction to personal identity and meaning. When one deliberately tries to have a less than healthy child to serve extraneous goals, the reproductive interests that are ordinarily valued are so diminished that a meaningful conception of the values underlying procreative liberty appear to be absent. Indeed, the scenario here treats the engineered individual as an object or thing to serve the fabricator's interests, rather than a new person desired in part for her own sake.[52] Even if no harm accrues to the lesser engineered person (who has no alternative unharmed way to exist) and the fabricator would not otherwise have created a healthier or more whole individual, one can still conclude that the interests and values that underlie respect for procreation do not attach in the Bladerunner scenario.

A real-world setting for this problem would exist if persons with disabilities such as deafness or extreme short stature would wish their offspring to share their disabling condition. Suppose they believe that their child will be happier if she shares her parents' condition, and take action to prevent her from developing normally, for example, not giving the growth hormone that will make her taller, or not providing a cochlear implant that might overcome a mild form of congenital deafness. Such actions would arguably harm the child and constitute child abuse, for the child would be denied a treatment essential for future functioning in society.[53]

If this judgment is correct, then the parents should have no greater right to produce that handicapping condition by prenatal genetic alteration just because they would not otherwise bring the child into the world.[54] In that case they would be using their reproductive capacity to produce a less than healthy child when a healthy normal child was possible. Unless it could be shown that children born to such parents are in fact better off if they share the parents' disability, stopping parents from prenatal lessening of offspring abilities would not, under the view presented here, interfere with their procreative liberty.

CONCLUSION

This chapter has dealt with screening and selection technologies that enable parents to have healthy offspring. In it I have argued that procreative liberty includes the right to select or shape offspring characteristics because of the great importance that outcome has on decisions regarding reproduction.

Selection decisions are thus a core part of procreative liberty and should be respected as such. If it is legitimate for parents to want healthy children, then it should be legitimate for them to use both negative and positive techniques to achieve that end. Thus access to information about the genetic status of partners, embryos, and fetuses should be protected, as should selection activities based on that information. The right to intervene positively to assure healthy offspring should also be respected, because having healthy offspring is so central to reproductive choice.

Yet there are limits here as well—limits that recognize the profound ambivalence that arises when one talks so starkly of shaping or selecting offspring characteristics. One such limit is the right of people not to use these technologies if they find the enterprise offensive or inimical to their own reproductive project. Even if they could be required to confront their and their partner's genetic status when they reproduce, they should not be prevented from reproducing because of that status.

Another limit arises from a physician's discretion not to make technologies available for prenatal screening and abortion which physicians view to be trivial or less important than the prenatal life that will be sacrificed to achieve that goal. Procreative freedom does not entitle one to the services of providers who profoundly disagree with the means that one is willing to use to achieve procreative goals. However, providers have the obligation to make their disagreement known in advance, so that consumers may seek services elsewhere.

A third limit will arise if positive alteration of genes ever becomes a reality. In that case, prenatal interventions for nontherapeutic enhancement, cloning, or diminishment of offspring will not be protected by procreative liberty because these actions conflict with the values that undergird respect for human reproduction. Even if those activities determined whether a new person were born, they could be banned on grounds that would not suffice if core reproductive values were involved.

At present, selection technology can do no more than screen fetuses and embryos and prevent them from being born. Although in utero and in vitro genetic interventions will eventually be feasible, concern about their possible extension should not be a dominant factor in determining the scope of therapeutic research and practice. Fears about Brave New Worlds and abuses of genetic engineering should not prevent steps now within reach to help couples give birth to healthy offspring.

CHAPTER 8

Preventing Prenatal Harm to Offspring

ISSUES of quality control and public policy also arise with prenatal conduct that risks harm to offspring. Persons who reproduce want healthy, normal children and may go to great lengths to achieve that goal. Pregnant women often change their diet, work, and drinking habits, and religiously follow their physicians' advice. They may undergo prenatal screening and abort affected fetuses, or risk experimental surgery to have a healthy child.

Yet some persons who reproduce are unable or unwilling to avoid risky behavior that harms their children. Some pregnant women take drugs, drink heavily, or behave in other ways that risk damage to offspring. Their spouses or partners may encourage or acquiesce in the harmful behavior. In other cases, they omit medical care or refuse medical treatments that will prevent handicaps. Because of the seriousness of the harm threatened, some persons have urged that such women be punished or seized prior to birth to prevent them from causing harm to their children.

In such cases a strong argument can be made that persons who intentionally or negligently engage in prenatal conduct that risks harming offspring are acting irresponsibly. In these instances, the harm to offspring is avoidable. If the woman or man acted differently they could still procreate and rear healthy offspring. Unlike the question of unavoidable harm to offspring discussed in chapter 4, offspring are harmed by the prenatal conduct because they could be born free of the harm. In addition, there are significant costs to the public in caring for children who have been harmed prenatally. Thus these cases present a strong case of reproductive irresponsibility. The question then is what actions, if any, the state should take to discourage such activity.

Yet public policy proposals to limit or discourage such activity have been extremely controversial. Feminist and civil liberties groups have protested any attempt to punish prenatal conduct, and many courts have found ways to avoid holding women legally responsible for their prenatal conduct.[1] Yet the idea that personal autonomy allows pregnant women to disregard the risk of prenatal harm to their offspring seems wrong. Autonomy is limited by the harm principle—the duty to avoid harming others, and clear harm often results from the prenatal conduct in question.

However, because this conduct occurs prenatally when only a fetus exists, the conduct seems less dangerous than harmful actions occurring after birth. Also, because the fetus is inside the woman, prenatal actions to protect offspring necessarily restricts her freedom. Opponents of such policies have argued that coercive remedial actions violate the rights of pregnant women by treating them as vessels or containers to reproduce healthy offspring. They also believe that punitive policies will not help offspring and will have other undesirable side effects.[2]

THE SCOPE OF THE PROBLEM

A variety of medical, legal, and social developments have brought this issue to the fore. Rising rates of birth defects (due to genetic and teratogenic factors) has focused attention on prenatal behavior. Drug and alcohol abuse during pregnancy has risen dramatically. There is greater consciousness of fetal toxins in the workplace. Also, pregnant women occasionally refuse cesarean section and other medical treatments that appear necessary for their children's health.

The issue of prenatal obligations first became visible in the early 1980s when cases of women refusing cesarean section reached the courts and in utero fetal therapies were being developed.[3] Advances in obstetrics and reproductive medicine had enabled the fetus to be visualized and treated in utero, making fetal medicine an obstetrical subspecialty. The fetus that was going to term came increasingly to be viewed as a patient in its own right. When conflicts developed between the wishes of the pregnant woman and the needs of the fetus, physicians often acted to protect the fetus.

In the mid- and late 1980s the issue took on renewed urgency as crack cocaine use by pregnant women began affecting offspring. One study estimated that 158,400 children are born each year exposed to cocaine, at a cost to the medical care system alone of over $500 million.[4] Infants exposed to cocaine in utero are more likely to be born premature, have lower birth weights, be irritable and have learning problems. Similar problems have been found with prenatal exposure to heroin and marijuana.

Newborns with a positive drug test were routinely reported to social service agencies. Some agencies started neglect proceedings to protect the child. Others referred cases to district attorneys, who brought prosecutions for prenatal child abuse, fetal abuse, delivery of drugs to a minor, or homicide. With the drug use epidemic continuing and few drug treatment facilities that take pregnant women, the birth of children suffering the prenatal effects of cocaine and other drugs is likely to continue.

Alcohol and tobacco use during pregnancy also focused attention on the issue. Many studies have found a correlation between smoking during pregnancy with lower birth weight, though permanent damage has not been shown.[5] The devastating effects of large quantities of alcohol at certain stages of pregnancy are better established. Fetal alcohol syndrome is now a well-established condition, noted by its effects on facial features, head size, mental retardation, and severe, irreversible learning disabilities. The devastating effect of alcohol abuse during pregnancy is vividly documented in Michael Dorris's *The Broken Cord*, an account of raising a Native American boy with fetal alcohol syndrome.[6]

Since alcohol is the most widely used drug, it poses the greatest danger to newborns, yet the prosecutorial response seen with cocaine and heroin use by pregnant woman has been missing. This is due in part to alcohol's legal status, and because dose-response curves for deleterious effects, except in large quantities, have not yet been clearly established. Still, pregnant women now shy away from drinking, and may feel guilt if they have a glass of wine or drink at any time during pregnancy. Signs warning of the dangers of alcohol during pregnancy now appear in bars and on liquor bottles, and incidents of waiters refusing to serve alcohol to pregnant women have occurred.[7]

Adding to the controversy over prenatal harm have been the practices of some companies to exclude women from the workplace, ostensibly to protect future offspring, but also to protect the company from tort liability for prenatally caused injuries. In the late 1970s and 1980s, lead and chemical manufacturers that had only recently hired women adopted employment policies that excluded women of childbearing age from certain jobs, because of the threat of preconception or prenatal exposure of prospective children to workplace toxins. To retain these often higher paying jobs, women had to be sterilized. Although evidence of reproductive effects on men also exists, men have not been excluded. A court challenge to these practices under federal occupational health and safety laws was unsuccessful, and lower courts split on whether such practices were gender discrimination.[8] In 1990 in *United Auto Workers vs. Johnson Controls*, the United States Supreme Court held that a battery maker's practice of excluding women of childbearing age from certain jobs violated existing federal sex discrimination laws.[9] However, the decision left open the extent to which Congress could permit employers to reach a different trade-off between offspring welfare and parental and family interests in employment.[10]

Medical treatment during pregnancy, drug and alcohol use, and employment practices have thus combined to make the question of moral and legal duties to avoid prenatal harm to offspring an important public issue. The scope of the problem—thousands of children are at risk—and the intrusiveness of preventive remedies have made the subject of prenatal duties a highly charged and contested area.

After clarifying some important distinctions, I argue in this chapter that procreative liberty is not directly implicated in harmful prenatal conduct, though other liberty interests are. I then discuss public policy options for minimizing such behavior, ranging from education and services to postnatal sanctions and prenatal seizures. I close with a discussion of how the prenatal duty issue is better viewed as an aspect of more general parental duties that should apply to both men and women.

PRENATAL RESPONSIBILITY: CRUCIAL DISTINCTIONS

The ethical, legal, and policy evaluation of this issue turns on whether persons who engage in conduct that risks harming offspring are acting responsibly or irresponsibly. To address this question, however, several distinctions are crucial. The first distinction is between avoidable and unavoidable damage to offspring. The question of prenatal duties concerns those actions/omissions that cause a child who would otherwise be born healthy to be born handicapped or damaged. The damage is avoidable, because the child could have been born without the harm that he now suffers. If the avoidable damage is irreparable and could have been reasonably avoided, a serious wrong to offspring has occurred.

Thus this situation is to be contrasted with the situations discussed in chapter 4, in which offspring born with congenital disease or in disadvantageous circumstances were said not to be harmed by parental action bringing them into being. In those cases, the damage to the child is unavoidable, because there is no way that the child can be conceived or be born and not be damaged.[11] Except in rare cases of wrongful life, bringing a child into the world in those circumstances does not harm the child, for it has no way to be born free of the conditions of concern. By contrast, in situations of prenatally caused harm, the child could be born healthy if the harmful prenatal conduct did not occur. The most controversial issues of prenatal conduct concern actions that cause avoidable harm, not that cause the birth of a child that is already or inevitably harmed.

The second crucial distinction is between fetus and offspring. The controversy in this area is usually termed one of "maternal-fetal" conflict or "fetal protection" policies, because the activities of concern arise during pregnancy and directly affect the fetus. Unless these terms are used very precisely and narrowly, however, this terminology risks confusing the issue, and subtly biasing evaluation in favor of the mother's liberty. For in nearly all cases (the exception is with viable fetuses), the real party in interest is not the fetus itself but the child that the fetus will become.

The damage experienced by the fetus is of concern not for the fetus's own sake, but because the fetus will go to term and the resulting child, who could have been born healthy, will be harmed. The term "fetal protection" thus subtly shifts the focus of concern from the child—harmed by avoidable prenatal conduct—to a fetus that ordinarily, because it is located in the uterus at the time, has no rights to be born, and indeed, may be aborted. This formulation has also injected pro-choice and pro-life sentiments into an issue that exists independent of rights to abortion. The question of avoiding prenatal harm to offspring arises when a woman has decided or might decide to give birth to a child who could be born healthy, and thus will have rejected abortion.

In a few cases, however, fetal rights are directly involved, for example, when the action in question will cause a viable fetus to die in utero or be stillborn, as might happen with refusal of cesarean section. But in most cases the fetus is of moral interest because it is going to term, and a child will be born who could have been healthy but for the prenatal action in question. Since the use of the terms "fetal damage," "fetal protection," and the like is now so firmly entrenched, clarification of ethical, legal, and public discourse on this topic will be difficult. As long as the reason why the fetus is so valued—because it will go to term and become a child—is kept clearly in mind, the use of "fetus" is not inaccurate. However, language that specifies prenatal duties to expected offspring is preferable.

A third set of distinctions concerns the difference between moral and legal duties, and the different public policies that recognize or implement those duties. Moral rights and duties are, of course, distinct from legal rights and duties. Finding that there are moral duties to avoid harmful prenatal conduct does not mean that those duties should always have legal standing. If legal duties are to be recognized, distinctions between civil and criminal remedies and between postbirth sanctions and prebirth seizures are also relevant. Public policies designed to prevent prenatal harm to offspring may take a variety of forms, from providing medical services and education, to coercive measures involving sanctions and seizures.

PRENATAL HARM, PROCREATIVE LIBERTY, AND PROCREATIVE DUTIES

A basic question concerning prenatal conduct that harms offspring is whether such conduct falls within a pregnant woman's procreative or other liberty, or whether persons who engage in reproduction have prenatal duties to avoid harm to offspring.[12]

In the case of unavoidable harm, procreative liberty is directly and explicitly involved. The choice is either to have the affected child or not give birth at all. While the couple may be free to avoid reproduction of such children (by not conceiving or aborting), the basic right to reproduce would appear to give couples the right to conceive and give birth to unavoidably handicapped offspring. Despite the child's handicaps, parents may still have strong reproductive interests in rearing and caring for offspring. State polices that attempted to discourage such reproduction by mandatory contraception, abortion, or sterilization would interfere with the right to procreate.[13] Because antinatal policies in these cases "protect" offspring by preventing them from being born, they cannot be justified on the basis of protecting offspring from harm. As a result, to discourage such births the state is largely limited to education, access to services, and incentives rather than coercive sanctions.

In situations of avoidable damage to offspring, however, the conduct in question is not conceiving and continuing a pregnancy, but rather behaving in the course of continuing a pregnancy in ways that will make the child worse off than she would have been.[14] The question posed for an investigation of procreative liberty is whether the right to procreate includes the right to engage in any conduct during pregnancy regardless of the consequences for offspring. If not part of procreative liberty, does autonomy or bodily integrity protect the woman's choice?

Behavior during pregnancy that causes offspring who could have been born healthy to be born damaged is not part of procreative liberty, and should not be regarded as an aspect of that liberty. Except for postviability actions that cause fetal demise in utero, the conduct in question does not involve a choice of whether or not to procreate.[15] By rejecting abortion and going to term, the woman has decided to procreate. Rather, the asserted liberty interest is the freedom to act as one wishes in the course of reproduction, regardless of the effect on offspring.

Two possible claims of liberty *in*, but not *of*, reproduction may be noted. A claim that a woman is free to make offspring less healthy than they would have been—a right to engineeer or create a less than normal child—was discussed in chapter 7. Even if determinative of a decision to reproduce (which is not the case in these prenatal situations), neither the core values that underlie procreative liberty nor any other protected liberty includes the right to make offspring less than healthy and normal, when a healthy birth is reasonably possible.

The second claim is that a woman's right of liberty and bodily integrity give her a right to behave as she wishes in the course of reproduction, not because it is reproductive, but because it is her body and liberty that are involved. Thus she is free to use her body as she wishes during pregnancy and may resist medical intrusions for the sake of the fetus and potential offspring because they intrude on her body.

But while liberty in the course of procreation and bodily integrity are important rights, they are not unlimited. At a certain point one's right to use one's body as one wishes, including resisting medical intrusion into the body, must take account of the interests of others whose needs those decisions directly impinge.

This point is but another application of the harm principle. One cannot use one's body to injure another. Because the fetus is inside her and she is going or may go to term, a pregnant woman's actions may affect the child that the fetus, through her own choice, will become.[16] She may then reasonably be held to have a duty to avoid harm to her expected offspring. If her actions have very little benefit to her and pose great harm to offspring, they could be proscribed under the harm principle. Similarly, if a medical procedure is moderately or minimally risky and intrusive, but will prevent great harm to offspring, it may reasonably be demanded of her, because of her obligation to act for the good of the person that she is choosing to bring into the world. This obligation exists even with behaviors that have a probability, rather than a certainty, of causing postnatal harm. If the risk of harm to offspring is high enough, a person engaging in potentially harmful conduct has an obligation to alter her behavior accordingly.

Thus pregnant women and others who threaten prenatal harm to offspring may reasonably be said to have moral duties to avoid prenatal actions that have a high risk of harming the child that the fetus will become. Unless the action served a compelling need of hers, for example, chemotherapy for her own life-threatening cancer, she ought to avoid it, because of impact on expected offspring. Activities like drug, alcohol, and even tobacco use should be avoided if they pose signficant risk to offspring. The benefits to her of the activity seem clearly outweighed by the impact on expected offspring. A similar judgment could be made of workplace hazards. The benefits to her and other children of the job vs. the actual prenatal hazards and alternatives must be weighed. At some point, it would be immoral to engage in conduct—whether drugs or jobs—that clearly will harm offspring.[17] Of course, more discussion and analysis may be needed to know whether that point has been reached in any given situation.

In some instances there may also be a duty to accept medical intrusions for the sake of the child to be. The woman has either chosen to become pregnant, failed to take steps to avoid contraception, or at least decided to continue the pregnancy to term. While people may differ over whether she has a moral duty not to abort, if she decides to go to term, one may reasonably argue that she has a duty to accept minimally invasive or minimally risky medical treatments that will prevent severe harm in offspring. She is responsible for the child's medical need by choosing to continue the pregnancy and giving birth to a child whose suffering could be averted by prenatal medical intervention. Thus imposing a duty on her to accept necessary medical treatments that will prevent that harm is morally defensible. Neither her procreative liberty nor right of bodily integrity give her the right to cause or avoid preventing reasonably avoidable harms to offspring that she chooses to bring into the world. Of course, the scope of her duty will depend upon the risks and burden to her of the intrusion and the ease of obtaining it. She would, however, ordinarily have a duty to accept medical treatments that impose little or moderate risk, when doing so will prevent substantial harm to offspring.

Questions will arise concerning the point in pregnancy at which these duties attach. The clearest case is late in the pregnancy after viability, when the woman knows that she is going to term. But duties to avert harm could also arise early in pregnancy. For example, if abortion were not available, actions occurring after conception could affect the welfare of expected offspring, so duties could attach prior to viability. Indeed, in certain rare instances American tort law recognizes preconception duties to foreseeable offspring as well, though there may be few circumstances in which such a duty would apply to persons procreating.[18] If abortion is available, a woman's previability actions could still affect offspring, if she rejects abortion and decides to go to term. Anyone at risk of getting pregnant and continuing the pregnancy would then have a moral obligation to take into account how her actions could affect offspring who might be conceived and come to term.

POLICY ISSUES

Given the foreseeable impact of certain prenatal acts or omissions on the welfare of offspring, one cannot reasonably argue that women and men have no prenatal obligation to avoid harm to children they choose to bring into the world. The more contested question is what public policies and legal options should be pursued to prevent prenatal harm to offspring. The choice ranges from education and access to treatment to postbirth sanctions and prenatal imposition of treatment on pregnant women. Because procreative liberty is not involved, and because the conduct in question poses serious harm to offspring, coercive sanctions are not in principle excluded. However, as we shall see, the better policy in most cases will be to rely on information, education, and access to treatment.

Noncoercive Policies: Education and Services

The most effective measures to prevent prenatal harm to offspring are likely to be noncoercive policies that educate women and men about prenatal risks and provide services and treatment essential to offspring welfare. In many cases, children are injured by prenatal conduct because of the parent's unawareness of the danger, or lack of access to the treatment or other services needed to prevent the harm.

For example, better prenatal care, including access for all pregnant women, would greatly reduce the incidence of premature births which contributes so highly to infant mortality and morbidity.[19] In addition, the dearth of substance abuse programs for pregnant women should be rectified. Ironically, at the same time that cocaine use by pregnant women is widely decried, most pregnant addicts cannot find a drug treatment program that will take them. If only for the sake of offspring, all pregnant women who abuse drugs or alcohol should be given access to drug and alcohol treatment.

Policies to inform women of the dangers of drugs, alcohol, tobacco, and other activities during pregnancy are also desirable. Since they are relatively inexpensive and may prevent the need for medical treatment from developing, one might expect them to be uncontroversial. However, feminists have opposed notices in bars and on liquor bottles warning of the dangers of drinking while pregnant as unduly emphasizing the interests of fetuses and engendering guilt for otherwise legal activities. Indeed, the National Organization for Women joined with the tavern industry in New York to oppose a state law that would have required that bars post warnings about the effects of alcohol on developing fetuses.[20] Given the dangers of alcohol, this position seems short-sighted. Surely informing pregnant women of the dangers of their behavior so that they can choose accordingly should be an acceptable policy.

Workplace Issues

There are many steps short of excluding workers that could render the workplace reproductively safe—for men, women, and offspring. Occupational health and safety standards should require employers to reduce to an acceptable level the risk to reproductive health. Once those levels have been reached, employees—both men and women—should be informed of the remaining risks to them and to offspring, and be given the opportunity to switch to other positions during pregnancy or other risky periods.

Fair notice and free choice should greatly reduce workplace hazards to future offspring and eliminate the need for exclusionary policies.

Whether public policy needs to go further will have to be determined by future experience. For example, if cleanup efforts and fair notice fail to protect offspring from workplace hazards, legislative consideration of limiting workplace exposure should occur. The *Johnson Controls* decision, while finding that current anti-sex discrimination laws banned gender-based exclusionary practices, gives Congress the authority to change the law to permit some exclusions. Until there is more experience with other options, one cannot say whether congressional action to permit exclusions of men or women only would ever be justified. If harm to offspring is inevitable, this harm will have to be balanced against the benefits to the worker and his or her family of the jobs in question, given the alternatives. At a certain point allowing one sex to continue in such a risky job might be more likely to harm expected offspring than would allowing the other sex.[21] If these facts are established, any legislative authority for excluding workers to protect offspring should be narrowly drafted, and be clearly necessary as a last resort to prevent great harm to offspring.[22]

Criminal Sanctions

The most controversial policy issues in this area concern the use of coercive measures, either postnatal sanctions or prenatal seizures (discussed below). Postnatal sanctions usually involve criminal prosecution for conduct occurring during pregnancy which has harmed or which risked great harm to offspring.[23] To date most prosecutions have involved illegal drug use of some sort, with over sixty prosecutions brought in nineteen states and the District of Columbia since 1987.[24] While most have been unsuccessful, convictions have occurred, and more prosecutions can be expected.

Most prosecutions have resulted from perinatal evidence of illegal drugs in the mother's or the newborn's blood or urine that is reported to child welfare or law enforcement authorities. Since few states have had statutes specifically penalizing conduct during pregnancy, charges have been filed under such statutory rubrics as child abuse and neglect, delivery of drugs, and even homicide.

The two most widely publicized prosecutions illustrate many of the problems of prosecution. In the Pamela Rae Stewart case in San Diego in 1986, a woman gave birth to a severely brain-damaged child, who died within a month.[25] When traces of marijuana and amphetamines were discovered in her baby's urine, the case was reported to the district attorney.

His investigation revealed that in the ninth month of pregnancy her doctor, after diagnosing a complete placenta previa, advised her to take medication, refrain from sex and illegal drugs, and go immediately to the hospital if bleeding began. She allegedly ignored all these instructions and delayed going to the hospital for 7–8 hours. She was charged with failure to provide a child with necessary medical care. After wide publicity, a court dismissed the charges prior to trial on the ground that the statute in question did not apply to prenatal conduct.

The case of *State v. Johnson* involved prosecution of a woman who used cocaine on a daily basis during pregnancy, including the day of delivery.[26] She was charged with delivery of drugs to a minor, a serious felony, on the theory that drugs passed through her umbilical cord to the infant in the few minutes after birth before the cord was cut. She was convicted at trial, and sentenced to one year in a rehabilitation program and fourteen years probation. The conviction was affirmed on appeal by an intermediate appellate court, but eventually reversed by the Florida Supreme Court on the ground that the legislature did not intend the prohibition on delivery of drugs to a minor to apply to transfer through the umbilical cord.[27] To criminalize maternal drug use during pregnancy, the state would have to pass new legislation.

Prosecution or punishment of a pregnant woman for drug use during pregnancy may take other forms as well. In a few cases women have been charged with drug possession based on finding drug traces in the blood or urine of newborns.[28] In one case, a woman was charged with manslaughter based on the postnatal death of her child allegedly due to prenatal use of cocaine.[29] In another case, a judge imposed a jail sentence on a pregnant woman convicted of forging a check in order to prevent her from continuing to use cocaine, even though probation was ordinarily given for the crime in question.[30]

The idea of prosecuting women for conduct during pregnancy is highly controversial, and opposed by feminist, civil liberties, and medical groups. Both the American Medical Association and the American College of Obstetrics and Gynecology have issued policy statements opposing criminal prosecution.[31] However, at least twelve states have expanded their definitions of child abuse to include fetal drug exposure, and prosecutions are likely to continue. Although courts may continue to reject prosecutions under broadly drawn statutes that were not written with prenatal conduct in mind, statutes specifically intended to apply to prenatal conduct may well lead to convictions.

One can question the wisdom of prosecution on many grounds. If the statute under which the charge is brought does not apply specifically to prenatal actions, questions of fair notice and legislative intent will arise, as occurred in *State v. Johnson*.[32] Then too there are serious questions of culpability. Not only may drug-using pregnant women be unaware of the dangers to offspring, but they may lack the ability to control their conduct because of their drug or alcohol addiction. Indeed, some women prosecuted have been turned away from drug treatment programs, on the ground that they do not treat pregnant women.

In addition, such prosecutions may end up hurting children more than they help them. Conviction might deprive newborns of access to their mother. Also, the threat of prosecution will deter some drug users from seeking prenatal care, because of the risk that they will be reported to the police. To avoid prosecution, some pregnant women will have abortions, thus preventing the birth of the very children that prosecution is meant to help.

Opponents of prosecution also see a grave threat to personal privacy and civil liberties. If illegal drug use during pregnancy is independently punishable, then anything with the slightest prenatal risk to offspring could be punished as prenatal child abuse. Women could be prosecuted for smoking or drinking even moderate amounts of alcohol at any time during pregnancy, because even a few drinks might lower IQ points, and smoking increases the risk of prematurity and low birth weight.[33] In the worst-case scenario, special pregnancy police will be commissioned to monitor women for pregnancies, and then surveil their behavior. If they err, they are then stigmatized, shamed, fined, or incarcerated. Margaret Atwood's *The Handmaid's Tale*, a chilling novel of women forced to serve the reproductive needs of a repressive dictatorship, starts sounding much less fanciful than it appears to be.[34]

A final ground for opposition is that the impact of criminal prosecution for prenatal harm is likely to be felt most by lower income and minority groups, who are more likely to be prosecuted and may have less chance to avoid the harmful occasions. A Florida study, for example, found that although rates of drugs in newborn urine was as high among whites as among blacks, only blacks were referred to prosecution or child welfare authorities.[35]

All these points deserve considered attention. They explain why prosecutions have been largely unsuccessful, are widely opposed, and are unlikely to be a key factor in preventing prenatal harm. They also show why education, treatment, and services are the more desirable and most effective avenue for public policy.

Despite the drawbacks of a criminal approach, however, these criticisms do not establish that criminal sanctions should never be imposed on persons who culpably harm offspring by prenatal conduct. When culpability is established, criminal law theory easily includes prenatal as well as postnatal conduct that harms offspring. For example, Lord Coke in the seventeenth century recognized criminal liability for prenatal actions that caused postnatal death, a precedent now accepted in every American jurisdiction in cases of homicide.[36] The same principle could apply to any prenatally caused harm. Under these precedents, there would be no violation of notice requirements if general statutes, such as child abuse statutes, were applied to prenatal conduct that culpably caused postnatal harm. In any event, statutes that penalized specified prenatal conduct would not raise problems of notice.

However, culpability would also have to be established, as for any crime. A woman who was unaware of the harmful effects of her conduct, either because she did not know that she was pregnant or that her actions could harm the fetus, would lack the *mens rea* usually necessary for guilt. However, a woman informed and notified of the risky impact of her behavior could not make that claim. Since drug addiction is no defense to selling or possessing drugs or theft or burglary to buy drugs, the addicted status of the pregnant woman should not prevent conviction for prenatal actions that harm offspring. Nor is the fact that minorities are disproportionately prosecuted, as long as no invidious purpose to that effect is shown. Minority children, who may be at increased risk from prenatal conduct, also deserve protection, a point overlooked by those critics who claim that prosecution of minority women for prenatal drug abuse is racist.[37]

But will criminal prosecution do any good? This is a pragmatic policy judgment over which reasonable people may well differ. At the very least, prosecution will fulfill the law's function of enunciating minimum acceptable standards of conduct to which all citizens of the state, regardless of cultural affiliation, must conform. In this case, the standards are enunciated for conduct during pregnancy that risks avoidable harm to offspring. In denouncing unacceptable conduct, legal proscription and prosecution might encourage women to refrain from harmful prenatal conduct, or to seek help, if they know that they are at risk of causing harm to offspring. In any event, it will announce the community's condemnation of such conduct, deter some injuries to offspring, and generally contribute to community norms of acceptable behavior.

In any event, the practical effects of criminal prosecutions may turn on the frequency of prosecution and the merits of the cases chosen for action. The benefits of prosecution may be greatest and the costs least in egregious cases of culpably caused harm. If prosecution is reserved for the most egregious cases, it may serve useful purposes without undesirable side effects.

The costs and benefits of limited prosecution will have to be tested empirically. For example, the fear that prosecution will drive drug-using women away from prenatal care altogether, to the detriment of their children, may be exaggerated. A similar claim used to oppose enactment of postnatal child abuse reporting laws turned out to be unfounded. The threat of being reported has not stopped parents who batter their children from bringing them to hospital emergency rooms for treatment. Similarly, fears of racial discrimination require further proof of discriminatory purpose, not just disparate impact. Also unclear is whether prosecution for crimes of prenatal harm would increase abortions. If so, and if one is against abortion, this is a serious cost. But such abortions would not violate the rights of the children who then are never born, because there is no existing person to be injured.[38] On the other hand, a punitive policy leading to abortion will not protect children from prenatal harm, because it prevents their birth altogether.

In my view, the case for criminal sanctions is closer than the opponents make it out to be. They focus too much on the fact that the conduct affects a "fetus," and on the alleged procreative liberty of the pregnant woman, ignoring the interests of the child who is born damaged as a result of avoidable prenatal conduct. They point to side effects that are more speculative than established, and which do not prevent prosecution in many other contexts. To immunize from prosecution egregious, culpable conduct just because it occurs prenatally does not give adequate respect to the children who are avoidably and irreversibly injured.

Criminal law enforcement, however, should not detract from or replace education and services as the primary focus of public policy. But criminal sanctions are appropriately invoked in egregious cases of culpable conduct, in which injury clearly caused by prenatal conduct has occurred. Men who contribute to or who cause the harmful conduct should also be prosecuted.[39] Limited use of criminal sanctions is necessary to respect the rights of children born injured who, with reasonable care, could have been born healthy.

Prenatal Seizures

Even more controversial than criminal sanctions is the direct imposition of treatment or preventive measures on pregnant women to protect viable fetuses from death or prospective offspring from avoidable harm.[40] Ordinarily in these cases the woman's body is not actually "seized" and treatment imposed while she is physically resisting. Rather, doctors tell her that she has no choice, or a judicial order that the surgery be performed is issued, and under threat of sanctions she submits. Only in cases of incarceration does an actual physical restraint ordinarily occur.

What kinds of seizures are at issue? One is incarceration, which occasionally occurs to prevent women from getting drugs or other substances that will cause the harm. However, the most common seizures involve the direct imposition of medical treatment, as might occur with mandatory in utero treatments or cesarean section. Starting with *Jefferson v. Griffin Spalding Memorial Hospital* in 1980, there have been over fifty cases of court-ordered cesarean sections.[41] Most notorious was the *In re A.C.* case in Washington, D.C., in which a woman twenty-six weeks pregnant and in the late stages of cancer had a cesarean section done ostensibly against her will. Neither she nor the baby survived.[42] The specter of mandatory interventions is a real one.

Cases of this sort have provoked outrage from feminists and civil libertarians who decry direct government impositions on the body of women for the sake of "fetuses." Indeed, discussions of prenatal duties often confuse prenatal seizures and postnatal sanctions, and assume that if the latter occur, the former must as well. Although both sanctions and seizures are coercive, there are important differences between them.

Prenatal seizures have one clear advantage over sanctions and other policies. The advantage is that, unlike postnatal sanctions that are applied after the harm has occurred, they attempt to intervene before the damaging event has occurred, and thus enable the child to be born healthy. The ethical justification for seizures has previously been discussed. Having placed her expected child in peril by her prenatal behavior, the mother has a duty to incur the physical intrusion necessary to protect the child's well-being. On this theory a properly authorized physician who intrudes on her body against her will does not violate her rights, because she has effectively waived them by becoming pregnant, choosing to go to term, and engaging in harmful conduct.

There are, however, several problems with prenatal seizures that should greatly limit though not totally eliminate their use. A major problem is the uncertainty of predicting the occurrence of the harm that ostensibly justifies the intrusion. There is no certainty that the child would not have been born healthy anyway, nor that the intervention will necessarily be successful.

For example, cesarean sections, which are the procedure most frequently imposed on pregnant women, appear to be highly overprescribed by doctors, for reasons ranging from malpractice fears to convenience and higher fees.[43] A doctor's prediction that a mandatory cesarean section is necessary to protect the child may simply be wrong. In the *Jefferson* case, for example, the mother, diagnosed with a complete placenta previa, left the hospital before the court-ordered cesarean section could be done. To the surprise of her doctors, the condition righted itself spontaneously and she had the child safely elsewhere.

A second major problem is the degree of bodily intrusion that seizures might entail. Mandatory cesarean section entails general anesthesia and surgery. It increases the morbidity and mortality of childbirth, and is painful. Other seizures could be shorter in duration and less risky, but an unconsented-to injection, blood transfusion, or in utero catherization is still a significant intrusion. Less intrusive seizures, such as incarceration, may not directly intrude into the body, but they significantly interfere with bodily movement.[44]

Direct seizures also raise serious problems of due process. Cesarean sections have been mandated under general *parens patriae* court powers, not pursuant to legislation specifically authorizing them. They may be imposed in circumstances in which a preseizure hearing with counsel and cross-examination cannot effectively be held. In *A.C.*, for example, a rushed hearing with lawyers was held in the hospital, but there was not enough time to give due regard to the complex issues in the case, nor appeal fully to the higher court that later found the judicial order for the surgery to be erroneous.

There is also a problem of substantive due process. Even with carefully drawn statutes, notice, and hearing, the direct imposition of treatment appears to violate a fundamental right of bodily integrity. Is prevention of harm to the expected offspring a compelling enough reason to justify such an intrusion? Although courts have split on this issue, there is implicit support for certain mandated intrusions in *Roe v. Wade*'s holding that if a woman has continued a pregnancy to viability, a legal duty to continue the pregnancy to term can be imposed. If this bodily imposition is justified by the interests of the fetus, more limited physical intrusions to prevent harm in offspring should be as well.

A special problem with prenatal seizures is the danger that they will be used disproportionately against minorities. A 1986 study of court-ordered cesarean sections found that 81 percent of the women subject to cesarean section were of a minority ethnic group, 24 percent did not speak English as their primary language, and 100 percent were clinic patients.[45] While this disparity might not be intentional and may reflect cultural patterns of refusal, it still must give us pause. Doctors may be more willing to request court authority when lower-status women refuse treatment than when private or higher-status patients do. If such a disparate impact is inevitable, perhaps direct seizures should not figure into public policy. However, one cost of protecting minority women from possible discriminatory seizures will be minority children who are born damaged rather than healthy as a result of the refusal to intervene.

Despite these problems, the case against all direct seizures must rest on grounds of policy rather than principle. Seizures, after all, have the great advantage, if successful, of preventing the very harm at issue, rather than merely punishing after the fact when the damage is done. Moreover, if authorized by a specific statute in carefully defined circumstances for a compelling need, they would probably meet substantive constitutional standards. If the intrusion is minimal, has great benefit, and the need is a direct result of the woman's actions or choices, a statute authorizing it may well be constitutional.[46]

Although not excluded in principle, the policy question is whether direct seizures will provide policy benefits at acceptable costs not attainable in other ways. Good programs of education, counseling, services, and treatment will greatly reduce the need for any coercive intervention. In cases where those measures fail and some coercive sanctions are sought, postnatal sanctions are preferable to prenatal seizures, for the harm would have clearly occurred and the full panoply of due process can be accorded to the actor charged with abuse. Like the strong First Amendment presumption against prior restraints of the press, postnatal sanctions are almost always preferable to prebirth seizures.

However, just as prior restraints of the press can be justified in very extreme circumstances, direct seizures may occasionally be acceptable. The clearest case would be where the intrusion is minimal, the benefit to offspring clear and substantial, and all lesser means of persuasion have failed. The great benefit to the expected child, whose need has been caused by the woman refusing treatment, would justify the intrusion. If relatively infrequent, such cases could occur without incurring the very real costs of error and abuse that direct seizures threaten.[47]

Consider how frequently the most likely candidates for prenatal seizures might occur.[48] With in utero fetal therapy, the case for mandatory treatment will arise only if the treatment is clearly safe and effective, and is minimally intrusive. A one-time blood transfusion or injection that prevents serious and otherwise irreversible damage in the offspring might fit that model. More complex procedures, such as in utero catheterization to drain urethral blockages or hydrocephalus, or ex utero fetal surgery for repair of diaphragmatic hernia and pulmonary hypoplasia, are still too risky and experimental.[49] Even if established as safe and effective, they may be too uncertain in any given case to be the subject of mandatory orders, though they clearly should be within parental discretion.

Mandatory cesarean section is the most likely candidate for occasional direct imposition. If the indications for cesarean section are accurate, the procedure will be necessary to prevent the child's death or serious brain damage. Although the intrusion is significant, the net burdens of surgical delivery, especially where vaginal birth is also risky for the mother, may not be that much greater. However, courts should not order cesarean sections unless statutes authorizing their imposition in narrowly defined circumstances have been enacted. Legislative unwillingness to give this specific authority will indicate the prevailing social assessment of the competing interests. In any event, the unreasonable refusal of a recommended cesarean section that does cause severe damage to offspring might still be punished as a form of prenatal child abuse.

Even prenatal incarceration of pregnant women to prevent access to drugs or to restrict diet might seldom be justified.[50] In this case, the imposition does not intrude into the body, though it limits liberty and bodily movement in significant ways for several weeks or months. A major difficulty with incarceration to prevent prenatal harm to offspring is establishing the efficacy of such a remedy. By the time proceedings to authorize incarceration have begun, prenatal damage to offspring from drugs or alcohol may already have occurred. The incremental protection from incarceration might not justify the significant loss of liberty.

In sum, direct seizures have many problems that make them an acceptable policy alternative only in a small number of cases. Reasonable people may well differ over whether the benefits outweigh the risks and harms of even limited seizures. If used at all, direct seizures of pregnant women to protect their offspring from prenatal harm are likely to be rare.

THE FEMINIST CRITIQUE AND EXPANDED PARENTAL DUTIES

The debate over prenatal obligations of pregnant women has become a feminist cause célèbre that is being fought to prevent further expropriation of women's bodies. Feminists object to any public or political view of pregnant women as having obligations to limit their freedom of choice over work, leisure, or sexuality in order to produce healthy offspring. They argue that such a view reinforces the sexist view that women are primarily childbearers, and treats them as fetal vessels or containers whose own needs can be sacrificed to bring healthy children into the world. As medical technology renders fetuses more visible and subjects the uterus to greater threats of public control, the struggle for control over reproduction will grow more intense.

As this chapter as shown, however, this is a very partial, if not distorted, view of the issue. Women are in a special relationship with the fetus and potential child, because of its location inside their bodies. Moreover, the pregnant woman has, in an important sense, acceded to or chosen this relationship, either in getting pregnant or in continuing the pregnancy.[51] Usually her own freely chosen behavior poses the risk that calls for restriction or intervention. Rhetorical claims that restrictions on pregnant women treat them as "fetal vessels" or "containers" thus obscure women's actions in creating the situation and how, under widely shared moral principles of responsibility, they may be obligated to avoid prenatal harms to offspring.

Moreover, neither moral analysis nor public policy views the woman solely as a "fetal container." Her legitimate needs and interests must also be given their due in protecting offspring from avoidable prenatal harm. She is not required to risk her own health substantially or to forgo her own needed medical treatments to produce a healthy child. In situations of great uncertainty about potential harm, her freedom should ordinarily prevail. But where her actions clearly threaten offspring, the child's interests should take priority.

The feminist critique of prenatal duties is nonetheless powerful in reminding us that public policies to implement these duties apply to a woman with a body, a history, a social context, and separate interests, which should be given due regard in seeking to protect the prenatal interests of children. Rational policies often have unintended consequences, and might produce fewer benefits and greater harms to women and offspring than the theory behind them envisages. The temptation to punish and blame the pregnant woman rather than deal with the complex social, economic, and medical problems that produce the problem in the first place should also be resisted.

An important, though perhaps unintended, implication of the feminist critique is to expand the focus of the debate from pregnant women to the males and other actors who threaten prenatal harm. Because of the fetus's location within a pregnant woman, there is a natural tendency to focus on the duties of women and to direct legal measures at them alone. But male actions also affect the welfare of offspring, and they too should, in appropriate cases, be repositories of prenatal duty.

For example, in the Pamela Rae Stewart case, there was evidence that her husband knew of the risks of ignoring the medical advice, yet chose to have sex, gave her drugs, and made no effort to get her to the hospital once bleeding commenced. Yet she, not he, was charged with crime. Similarly, men who encourage their pregnant partners to smoke crack or drink should also be liable as joint actors or coconspiritors in causing prenatal harm to offspring.[52] Workplace restrictions, if they are ever valid to protect potential offspring, should also apply to men, whose sperm might be equally affected by workplace conditions.

A larger sense of prenatal duty thus emerges here. The issue becomes not just the pregnant woman's duty, but the duty of all persons to avoid unreasonable conduct that will prenatally harm offspring. While this duty is well recognized with certain third parties in tort and criminal law, this chapter has shown how the pregnant woman herself can be found to have a duty. If she does, then there is no reason why the relevant male cannot have a duty as well. Both mothers and fathers have duties to protect their offspring from avoidable prenatally caused harmed.

But the issue is even broader. In focusing on the duties of mothers and by extension fathers, we are really grappling with the larger question of parental duties—both prenatal and postnatal—for the welfare of offspring. Viewed broadly as a question of the parental duties of both men and women, attention to prenatal conduct during pregnancy seems less discriminatory, because this is a period of such crucial importance to offspring. To the extent that men also cause prenatal harm or are in a position to make a physical contribution to avert harm, they too should be held to have prenatal duties to protect offspring.

The larger question is what society may reasonably ask parents, by virtue of their decision or actions causing reproduction to occur, to provide both before and after birth to insure the welfare of their offspring. If we ask the woman to bear physical burdens for the sake of the child, then we should be willing to place similar burdens on fathers when the need is shown. Whether the need arises before or after birth should not matter if the offspring's health and welfare are significantly threatened. A community judgment, constitutive of our understandings of parenthood, could reasonably be made that parents must accept both prenatal and postnatal physical intrusions for the sake of offspring.

Consider two hypothetical situations, one prenatal and one postnatal, that illustrate this point. The prenatal situation involves a woman seven months pregnant with a fetus that has been diagnosed as lacking an essential blood component, which the father alone can provide. Ordinarily, the father is willing to provide the blood product, and the mother to have it injected transabdominally into the fetus, so that the wanted child will be born healthy.

Suppose, however, that the father is willing to provide the blood, but the mother is unwilling to have the procedure done to her, even though the child will be saved from almost certain brain damage. Whether the mother could be ordered to have the injection or penalized if she refused has been discussed earlier. The case would appear to be a strong one for mandatory intervention, if the risks to the mother are small. If the mother could be penalized for refusing the injection, then a father who refused to provide the needed blood product should be penalized as well.[53] In either case, our constitutive sense of voluntarily chosen parenthood could include both men and women having prenatal obligations to incur some physical burdens for the sake of offspring whom they knowingly choose to bring into the world.[54]

Now consider a postnatal case, in which a five-year-old child suffers from acute leukemia or liver disease. The doctors would like to do a bone marrow or liver transplant, but no donor other than the parents is available. Either the mother or father could, at minimum or moderate risk but with substantial physical intrusion, serve as a donor. Ordinarily, parents would gladly undergo the rigors of bone marrow or partial liver donation to save their child.[55]

If they both refused, however, should the state nonetheless require that they donate the needed organ or tissue? Given the physical burdens that we expect women to undergo during pregnancy for the sake of offspring (which could be extended where appropriate to fathers), one could reasonably argue that they both have postnatal moral obligations to donate tissue when the risk/benefit ratio justifies the intrusion.

Of course, the question of making postnatal moral obligations legally required is troublesome. No doubt we would shrink at the thought of the state requiring that parents undergo bone marrow, kidney, or liver donation, merely because they chose to have children. But if we recall the physical burdens legally demanded of pregnant women, including continuing a postviability pregnancy to term and accepting surgical and medical interventions for the sake of the child, the idea is not so outlandish. One could even argue that fairness to pregnant women requires that both men and women have such postnatal physical obligations. Indeed, given the physical contributions the woman makes during pregnancy, some might argue that the father has the primary obligation to donate tissue.

Such a question is instructive for elucidating how questions of prenatal obligation might be seen as part of a larger question of parental responsibility for the welfare of offspring. The mandatory transplant scenario is highly speculative, but advances in medical technology may well pose it in real life. Indeed, parental donation of liver for transplant is now commonly practiced. Interestingly, it is the mother who in the most publicized cases to date has contributed the liver.[56] If neither parent is willing to donate, the question of establishing legal duties will eventually have to be faced. When that issue arises, it should be resolved, not solely by transplant norms that require a consensual donor, but also by comparison to the physical burdens demanded of men and women during pregnancy.

Thus in defining the prenatal duties of women and men toward offspring, we may be implicitly defining their postnatal duties as well. If we hesitate to impose postnatal physical duties, then we must ask why women should have prenatal duties either to carry a viable fetus to term or to permit unwanted medication or surgery. If we shrink from requiring the father in a prenatal scenario from providing the blood factor against his will, then we must ask why women could be forced to undergo cesarean section or other fetal therapy for the sake of offspring, or indeed, carry any pregnancy to term.[57] The issue, in short, forces us to consider the physical scope of parental duties. If we accept them prenatally for women, then they must be accepted prenatally for men, and possibly postnatally for both men and women as well.

CONCLUSION

The question of prenatal obligations to avoid serious harm to expected offspring is a matter of great controversy. The issues here move beyond the basic question of procreative liberty—whether to procreate or not—to second-order questions of liberty in the course of procreation. If a decision to proceed with reproduction has been made or is likely, then moral duties to avoid prenatal harm or to accept surgery or medical treatments for the sake of the child may attach.

Whether the state should adopt coercive sanctions or seizures to enforce those duties is an entirely separate matter. Education, counseling, and treatment are clearly the most fruitful policy alternative. A limited role for sanctions and seizures might exist in egregious cases, or where great harm to offspring can be prevented at relatively little cost to the pregnant woman. However, the focus should be on freely chosen measures, education, and services.

The feminist critique of prenatal obligations is important for focusing attention on the many problems that coercive measures might cause, but does not settle the matter as a question of principle. It does, however, raise the larger question of the scope and content of parental obligations to offspring, including both prenatal and postnatal physical obligations. After considered reflection, we may decide that parental roles require physical contributions as well as financial and social ones. If so, these physical burdens should be imposed on both men and women, both prenatally and postnatally as appropriate. Women should not be the sole subject of physical obligations to offspring.

EXTENSIONS AND LIMITATIONS

CHAPTER 9

Farming the Uterus

NONREPRODUCTIVE USES OF
REPRODUCTIVE CAPACITY

REPRODUCTIVE technologies prevent or enable reproduction to occur, and they select or shape the characteristics of offspring. In the late 1980s and early 1990s, however, major controversies arose about using one's reproductive capacity for other purposes, such as a source of tissue or organs for transplant or for medical research.

The use of reproductive capacity for nonreproductive goals raises important questions about the scope of procreative liberty. Even if not directly tied to the usual goals of reproduction, freedom in use of the body is involved and the purposes sought are themselves important. On the other hand, the nonreproductive use of reproductive functions treats the body and its intermediate reproductive products as instruments or means. This usually entails the creation and destruction of embryos and fetuses to serve other ends. Many persons would argue that proper respect for prenatal human life and the dignity of women and the body require that such uses be strictly limited.

This chapter sorts through these issues first by assessing their connection to procreative liberty. It then examines four situations of current controversy: (1) production of embryos for research purposes; (2) selective termination of multifetal pregnancies; (3) conception and abortion to produce fetal tissue; (4) conception and childbirth to produce bone marrow tissue for transplant.

PROCREATIVE LIBERTY AND PRODUCING
EMBRYOS, FETUSES, AND OFFSPRING FOR
NONREPRODUCTIVE PURPOSES

A major question is whether these activities involve procreative liberty at all. With the exception of having children so they can be tissue donors, basic procreative liberty does not appear to be directly involved. The technologies in question are not used to produce offspring, but to start and then interrupt the reproductive process for motives unrelated to the usual reasons for terminating pregnancy. Does procreative liberty entitle people to use their reproductive capacity to produce products or material to serve nonreproductive ends? Is there a liberty right to begin the reproductive process knowing that it will be intentionally interrupted?

In answering these questions, we cannot rely on the values associated with reproduction, because the intent is not to produce live offspring for rearing.[1] The embryos and fetuses in question are necessary for procreation to occur, but they are created for nonreproductive purposes, thus severing them from the procreative value that usually envelops them. In cases where the technologies at issue depend on abortion or embryo discard, those acts were planned prior to conception as ways to procure tissue or products to be used for other ends, a situation materially different from the usual situation of avoiding unwanted offspring.

One could argue that all use of reproductive capacity should be protected, whatever the intent, because selective protection will ultimately undermine protection of reproductive capacity in instances central to procreative choice. Indeed, drawing lines between reproductive and nonreproductive uses of the same capacity is difficult, particularly when conception and pregnancy are conditional on other events and needs. Also, inroads on one use of reproductive capacity will make further inroads easier to accomplish, just as any restriction of the content of speech makes the legitimacy of other speech restrictions more easily tolerated.[2] However, one might also find that clear distinctions can be drawn and that respect for the basic components of procreative choice need not shelter uses of reproductive capacity that are clearly abusive or offensive.

Even if reproduction per se is not involved, the use of reproductive capacity may serve other important personal and societal interests, including liberty in use of one's body, promoting biomedical research, and protecting the life or health of loved ones. Since these are legitimate goals, the case against the nonreproductive use of reproductive capacity should depend less on whether the "procreative" label properly attaches and more on the substance of the competing concerns that such uses present. In the end the question may turn on whether largely symbolic moral claims on behalf of embryos, fetuses, offspring, and women should limit the free use of one's reproductive capacity.

EMBRYO RESEARCH

IVF technology—hyperstimulation of the ovaries and fertilization of eggs in a laboratory dish—is most noteworthy because of the aid it provides infertile couples. However, access to the early preimplantation embryo also opens doors to research in infertility, contraception, reproductive medicine, genetics, cancer, and embryology. Yet embryo research has been so ethically controversial that until 1994 federal funding was not available, and little embryo research was conducted with private funds.[3]

The main ethical concern has been the alleged immorality of using embryos for research purposes. By treating embryos as means rather than ends, such research is said to denigrate the importance of human life. There has also been concern that embryo research could harm children, if the embryos used in research are then placed in a uterus. As a result, persons have urged limts on the purposes of embryo research, on transfer to the uterus after research, on keeping embryos alive in vitro for more than fourteen days, and on the creation of embryos solely for research purposes.[4]

Despite these concerns, a consensus has emerged that many kinds of embryo research are ethically acceptable when done with the consent of the gamete providers and approved by an institutional review board. The symbolic costs of using embryos as mere means are outweighed by the importance of improving IVF and infertility treatments.[5] If the embryo will be placed in a uterus with the intent of initiating pregnancy, research could be beneficial for the child that might be born. If the embryos are not going to be transferred, research on them before discard cannot harm them, because they are too rudimentary to have interests that can be harmed.[6] Only if one takes a strict right-to-life view that the embryo is itself a person from the time of fertilization, do near total prohibitions on embryo research make sense.[7]

This view is shared by nearly all of the ethical review boards that have addressed the issue, including the Ethics Advisory Board in the United States, the Warnock Committee in Britain, the Ontario Law Reform Commission in Canada, the American College of Obstetrics and Gynecology, and the American Fertility Society.[8] In addition to the limitations already discussed, these bodies also agree that embryos should not be kept alive in the laboratory for more than fourteen days for research purposes. They also generally approve the creation of embryos for research knowing that they will then be discarded.

These parameters have been largely accepted throughout the world, with the exception of Germany and several American states that ban all embryo research. The German policy is a reaction to that nation's sorry history of human experimentation during the Nazi era.[9] The restrictive American legislation, on the other hand, is a largely unintended by-product of a movement in the 1970s to ban fetal research. Although embryo research was not then contemplated, broad language used in those statutes sometimes extended to embryo research as well.[10] For example, Pennsylvania, in its 1989 restrictive abortion legislation that was upheld in *Planned Parenthood v. Casey*, banned all nontherapeutic experiments on an "unborn child," which it defined as "an individual human organism from the time of conception."[11] Such legislation would appear to prohibit research use of nonviable embryos even though embryo discard itself is not banned. Similar statutes have been struck down on grounds of vagueness and interference with procreative liberty, yet several states have restrictive embryo research laws still on the books.[12]

Even though most jurisdictions, commissions, and commentators now accept a wide degree of embryo research, ethical controversy continues to surround the production of embryos solely for research purposes—a non-reproductive use of reproductive capacity.[13] For example, this issue split the influential Warnock Committee in 1984, with only a narrow majority approving of creating embryos solely for research purposes. Legally, only a few European nations and Victoria, Australia, prohibit the creation of embryos solely for research purposes.[14] However, when Australian researchers pointed out that this ban would interfere with research on the viability of egg freezing and thawing and micromanipulation of eggs and sperm, Victoria altered its law to allow deliberate creation of embryos to the point of syngamy (some twenty-four hours after fertilization) to occur.[15]

The question of producing embryos solely for research poses a direct conflict between use of reproductive capacity for nonreproductive purposes and respect for prenatal human life. The need would arise presumably because the wide availability of cryopreservation would leave fewer embryos available for donation to research.[16] The gamete source is willing to provide egg and sperm to create embryos for valid research purposes. Ordinarily the eggs would be obtained from women going through IVF, but it would be possible to recruit women to donate eggs for research alone. Sperm could be obtained from sperm banks, separate donations, or the partner of the woman going through IVF. The resulting embryos would then be subject to manipulation, study, or observation and then discarded. However, no research procedure would occur that could not be done on spare embryos discarded in the IVF process, if they were available.[17]

We may ask two questions: (1) does procreative liberty protect creating embryos for research purposes as opposed to creating excess embryos for reproductive purposes? (2) Even if not part of procreative liberty, should it nevertheless be protected on other grounds?

Creating embryos solely for research does not involve procreative liberty, for there is no intention that the entity resulting from the union of egg and sperm be placed in a uterus, much less that it produce offspring. A step necessary for reproduction does occur—a human egg is fertilized with sperm—but the purpose is to produce embryos for research which will then be discarded, not to produce offspring. This is not an act of procreative liberty, but an act of liberty in the use of one's reproductive capacity.

Because a procreative interest is not directly involved, creating embryos for research and then discard deserves protection only if other important interests are served that justify whatever symbolic costs deliberate creation and discard of embryos entails. The purpose here is to increase knowledge of how to treat infertility, improve contraception, and treat or prevent cancer or birth defects.[18] With cryopreservation of extra embryos limiting the number donated for research, a policy against creating embryos solely for research and discard could greatly limit the amount of embryo research. Research with embryos would then occur only with spare embryos created as a by-product of IVF treatment of infertility, which may be too few to meet all research needs, with the result that important research across a range of fields is lost.

The symbolic benefits of protecting embryos from being created solely for research purposes does not appear to justify this loss. If the embryo is so rudimentary that research on excess, discarded embryos does not harm them and is permissible, there would appear to be no additional harm to embryos from creating them for this purpose only. In both cases research will occur at the same stage of development, and thus no added harm would occur from deliberate creation of embryos for research purposes.

Opponents, however, would argue that additional symbolic harm arises from creating embryos solely to be vehicles of research and then discarded. Additional symbolic harm results because creating embryos with the intent to discard them demonstrates a profound disrespect for the earliest stages of human life. This practice permits human life to be created, manipulated, and discarded for utilitarian purposes, without regard to the embryo's own interests or potential. The deliberateness of the act—creating new human life only to destroy it—is thus viewed as symbolically more offensive than research on excess embryos created as a by-product of the IVF process of treating infertility.

Reasonable persons who value respect for human life could differ over whether there is a significant moral difference between research on embryos created solely for research purposes and research on spare, discarded embryos. If one accepts that research on spare, discarded embryos is ethically permissible, then creating embryos solely for research and discard may reasonably be viewed as not substantively so different as to justify the loss of biomedical knowledge that banning such research would entail. While some persons will disagree, researchers who create embryos solely for valid research purposes would then not be acting unethically, and should be permitted by institutional review boards and other ethical oversight bodies to proceed.[19]

Of course, resolution of the controversy will depend on how essential this source of embryos is for legitimate, meritorious research. If other sources of embryos are available, they probably should be used first. If there are no other viable sources, however, creating embryos solely for research and then discard should be permitted. The incremental symbolic harm that arises from creating embryos solely for research is too slight to justify the loss of this important avenue of research.

An intermediate position that draws the line at syngamy is not a satisfactory solution. The law of the Australian state of Victoria permits eggs to be fertilized outside the body for experimental procedures "from the point of sperm penetration to the point of syngamy"—defined as "the alignment on the miotic spindle of the chromosomes derived from the pronuclei."[20] This line allows experimental procedures that test or develop the fertilizing power of egg freezing and thawing. It also allows research to determine whether micromanipulation of egg and sperm via partial zona dissection and subzonal insertion of sperm will produce fertilization up until syngamy. Its ethical rationale is that until syngamy, an entity with a unique genome is not involved and thus can be manipulated and discarded without harming a uniquely new prenatal entity.

The syngamy line does permit some research that would otherwise be prohibited to occur. It also opens the debate over the status of the earliest stages of human life to more biologic detail and sophistication than has formerly been the practice.[21] However, it still would eliminate large areas of potentially very useful research, on the basis of a symbolic line that reasonable persons could view as only marginally different from what is permitted with excess embryos remaining from IVF treatment. While better than a complete ban, it limits the full scope of embryo research that should be available.

In the United States, the legality of embryo research laws, like many issues in the use of reproductive technology, is independent of *Roe v. Wade* and the legal status of abortion. Because the embryo is outside the body and no right to terminate a pregnancy is involved, *Roe* would not directly limit a state's power to restrict embryo research, just as it does not appear to limit its power to prohibit embryo discard.[22]

Some constitutional constraints, however, may still exist. Distinctions between permissible and impermissible embryo research cannot be arbitrary and must be precisely drawn. In addition, if restrictive research laws prevented research that would develop better ways to achieve or avoid pregnancy, those laws might unconstitutionally interfere with rights of procreative liberty that exist independently of *Roe*.[23] In that case, legislation restricting embryo research will need a stronger justification than preventing the symbolic costs of creating embryos solely for research. These considerations, however, do not limit the state's power to refuse to fund research with embryos created solely for that purpose.

SELECTIVE REDUCTION OF MULTIFETAL PREGNANCY

The growing practice of selective reduction or termination of multifetal pregnancy is another reproductive technology that forces us to confront the limits of procreative liberty. It is now common for women who are carrying quintuptlets, quadruplets, or even triplets to have the number of fetuses reduced to two or three by selective abortion of the excess fetuses.

Ironically, the need for selective reduction usually arises iatrogenically from medical efforts to overcome infertility. Suddenly a couple that was having great difficulty having any children is faced with the prospect of so many that selective abortion must be considered. For example, couples going through IVF may, in order to increase the chance of starting a pregnancy or to avoid discard of extra embryos, have four or more embryos placed in the wife's uterus, which greatly increases the chance of a multifetal pregnancy and the need for selective termination. An even more likely cause of selective reduction is the use of "fertility" drugs like pergonal to stimulate the ovaries prior to intercourse or therapeutic insemination. This practice may lead to mulitple eggs being fertilized and result in multifetal pregnancies, which then need to be selectively reduced. A need for selective termination may also arise if one of two fetuses has a genetic abnormality that in the case of one fetus would lead to termination.[24]

A woman faced with a pregnancy of three or more fetuses has three options. She could carry all to delivery, but there is a high risk of fetal mortality and severe morbidity. If there are more than four or five fetuses, the likelihood of any surviving is very small. Even quadruplets will have severe problems, while the evidence is more mixed about the outcome with triplets. Delivery is very likely to be preterm and probably by cesarean section. The fetuses will require long stays in neonatal intensive care units, and even then may face permanent disabilities. Also, continuing the pregnancy poses serious health risks for the mother.[25]

The alternative option of terminating the entire pregnancy to avoid these burdens is also unattractive. The pregnancy was very much wanted, and likely the result of expensive and demanding infertility treatments. Selective termination, on the other hand, is an attractive alternative, because it reduces risks to surviving fetuses and the woman and still allows her to have children.

By mid-1990 over four hundred selective terminations had occurred in the world. The safest and most effective technique involves transabdominal injection of potassium chloride directly into the heart or thorax of unwanted fetuses at 10–12 weeks of pregnancy.[26] The choice of which fetus(es) to terminate is strictly a technical issue of which fetuses are easiest to reach. The procedure can be accomplished in 100 percent of the cases. As a leading practitioner of the procedure put it, "With patient cooperation and good visualization, we have reduced septuplets to twins in less than 30 minutes."[27] The remaining pregnancy then proceeds to term as normal.

A major issue for couples and practitioners is how many fetuses to leave. The answer is determined by the safety and efficacy of neonatal intensive care and obstetrical practice. Because a twin pregnancy is more easily handled, the current practice is to reduce multifetal pregnancies to twins. However, some physicians believe that a reduction to triplets is sufficient to minimize dangers, and therefore ethically preferable. While the couple will ultimately decide, most obstetricians agree that the risks of triplets is so significantly greater than twins that a reduction to twins, at the couple's request, is justified. However, these judgments may change as obstetrical and neonatal technology improve outcomes for triplets or more.

The ethical and legal status of multifetal pregnancy reduction depends largely on views of the morality and legal status of abortion, and the importance of using pergonal and IVF to treat infertility. A person totally against abortion would probably be totally against selective reduction, especially if the need were iatrogenically caused. However, persons who would permit abortion only when necessary to protect the life or health of the mother might accept selective reduction, at least to triplets, because of the serious threat to maternal health of carrying quadruplets or more to term. Less clear is whether persons holding such views would permit selective reduction in order to maximize the survival of the remaining fetuses.[28] They might also oppose the practice because the woman knowingly used an infertility treatment that risked creating the need.

A person opposed to abortion unless there is a very good reason for it, such as rape, incest, genetic abnormality, or serious health impact, will have fewer problems with selective reduction to triplets or even to twins, especially if the reduction occurs during the first trimester. The need both to protect the mother and to enhance the chance and quality of life of surviving twins is a substantial reason for abortion, given the alternatives of delivery or abortion of all. A person who believes that a woman may abort whenever a pregnancy is unwanted would not have serious moral objection to selective reduction, and might even have few qualms about treating infertility in ways that created the need in the first place.

If abortion is legal for any reason, there should be no legal barrier to selective reduction. If a singleton pregnancy could be aborted simply because it is unwanted, then triplets could be reduced to twins and twins to

singletons. If one believes that previable fetuses have no rights or interests, then no moral wrong is done by reduction of any number of fetuses,
or even of knowingly using techniques that create the need for selective
termination. Such action might symbolize disrespect for prenatal human
life, but that symbolic cost would have to be weighed against the need for
the reduction and the infertility treatments that created the multifetal
pregnancy.

If previability abortion were illegal except to save the life or health of
the mother, then some selective reductions might nevertheless be permitted. The clearest cases would be from five or four fetuses to three or even
two, if a serious risk to the mother's health could be shown.[29] The fact
that reducing quadruplets to twins will greatly improve the chances—for
example, reduced morbidity—of the surviving fetuses would not under
most restrictive abortion statutes, justify abortion of the other two. Only
if a choice among lives had to be made would this possible justification
arise. However, as a practical matter, if one jurisdiction prohibited reduction, the couple could go elsewhere for the procedure.

In addition to views about abortion, selective termination is ethically
controversial because of the perceived callousness of the procedure and
because the need for reduction was a calculated risk which the couple
took in choosing to treat their infertility. The directness of the procedure—the deliberate selection of some fetuses for intentional death—does
sound stark and callous, yet by the time the pregnancy is established,
there is no preferable alternative (at least with more than three fetuses).

The avoidability of the need, however, poses more difficult issues. As
noted, the need for selective reduction is largely iatrogenic, a result of
suboptimal use of drugs to stimulate the ovaries or the transfer of a large
number of IVF-created embryos to the uterus. If one undertakes X knowing that there is a high or an unreasonable risk that an undesirable event
Y will occur, then could not one be prevented from doing X in order to
prevent the need to do Y? Is not this claim all the stronger if the need to
do Y itself, once it arises, is compelling? If so, could not infertility practices that risk creating the need for selective reduction be limited, given
that once there are multiple fetuses, the right to terminate selectively
seems so compelling?

Efforts to prevent the need for selective termination could take several
approaches. One approach, recommended by the Vatican and ethicists
who think that no intervention for infertility is justified, would be to prohibit any technological intervention for infertility. This approach would
obviously interfere with the right of infertile couples to procreate. Because it would ban all use of IVF and pergonal, it cannot be persuasively
defended.

A second approach would be to limit strictly the use of the infertility techniques that are most likely to create the need for selective reduction. For example, laws that restricted the number of embryos that could be placed in the uterus at one time, or that required only minimal doses of pergonal, would greatly reduce the risk of multifetal pregnancy. Yet either limitation, by reducing the efficacy of treatment for infertile couples, would appear to limit their procreative liberty.

Consider, for example, a law that limits the number of IVF embryos that can be placed in the uterus to three in order to reduce multifetal pregnancies.[30] Such a ban would require either that extra embryos be discarded or cryopreserved for later use or that the number of eggs fertilized be limited to the number that could be transferred. Since some couples will prefer to avoid discard or the cost and psychosocial implications of cryopreservation, the effect would be to limit the number of embryos that are inseminated to those that can be transferred at any one time. Such a policy could result in too few embryos to start a pregnancy, since not all inseminated eggs may fertilize or cleave. The price of minimizing the chance of a multifetal pregnancy and selective reduction would thus be a higher cost and lower efficacy of basic IVF, and interference with the couple's right to procreate. Preventing the symbolic effects of selective reduction of a multifetal pregnancy is an insufficient ground for restricting such a basic right. A preferable policy is to have the couple understand the risks and permit them to choose the alternative that seems best for their situation.

Consider also restrictions on prescribing pergonal to treat infertility. Women with ovulation problems who are treated with pergonal often end up producing multiple eggs and thus multifetal pregancies. A restriction on the use of pergonal to prevent the need for selective reduction would deprive 20,000 women a year of the drug of choice for their infertility.[31] Yet a restrictive law is unnecessary because the threat of malpractice suits from improper monitoring of women treated with pergonal and the burden on women and fetuses of multifetal pregnancies alone seems sufficient to encourage proper use by physicians. Although multifetal pregnancies would still occur, a total ban on pergonal is overkill that would interfere too much with procreative liberty.

In sum, the conflict between efficient assisted reproduction and the symbolic losses involved in multifetal pregnancy reduction is multilayered. Once a multifetal pregnancy arises, reduction to two or three fetuses is clearly the most desirable outcome, and should be respected as an exercise of the right to avoid procreation. But that need arises only because of a prior decision to use infertility treatments that cause multifetal pregnancies. The underlying moral and policy issue is whether some reduction in the efficacy of assisted reproduction is justified to prevent multifetal pregnancies. Since the participants have ample incentives to transfer fewer embryos or to monitor the use of pergonal, prohibitory laws to achieve that goal are unnecessary. If enacted, they would probably be an unjustified intrusion on the right to procreate.

ABORTION AND FETAL TISSUE FOR TRANSPLANT

The use of reproductive capacity for nonreproductive purposes arises most clearly with abortions that produce fetal tissue for transplant. This issue became controversial in the late 1980s when the possibility of transplanting fetal tissue into persons with Parkinson's disease, diabetes, and other serious conditions appeared to be a promising treatment.

Since these diseases are caused by a deficiency in certain cell products, injection or transplantation of cells that produce the missing substance might relieve symptoms of the disease. Fetal cells are especially promising for this job, because they are fully functional and pose few of the histocompatability problems that complicate transplantation in other settings. When animal studies showed that human fetal tissue was effective in relieving experimentally produced Parkinson's disease in monkeys, clinical trials in humans with fetal cells obtained from induced abortions were proposed.[32]

The National Institutes of Health were prepared to carry out such research on Parkinson's disease when a bitter controversy broke out over the ethics of such research. Opponents argued that the use of aborted fetal tissue was inherently immoral and would encourage abortions, and therefore should not be supported by federal funds. An interdisciplinary ethics panel appointed to review the matter found by an 18–3 vote that experimental use of fetal tissue was ethically acceptable in carefully limited circumstances (the tissue was otherwise available, no sale or conception for research puposes, and consent for abortion separated from consent to donate).[33] However, Secretary of Health and Human Services Louis Sullivan rejected this advice and refused to allow "federal funding of research in which human fetal tissue from induced abortions is transplanted into human recipients."[34]

This decision was widely criticized (except by right-to-life groups), and efforts to lift the moratorium on federal funding moved to Congress. After hearings and debate in 1991, both the House of Representatives and the Senate passed legislation that authorized federal support of such research with safeguards to prevent abortions solely to produce tissue for transplant.[35] However, President Bush in 1992 vetoed the bill and a veto override failed in the House by twenty votes.

Congress made another attempt in 1992 to overturn the ban. President Bush attempted to scuttle the effort by proposing a federally sponsored bank of fetal tissue collected from spontaneous miscarriages and ectopic pregnancies but not from induced abortions.[36] Even though researchers criticized this proposal because of the poor quality of tissue from those sources and Congress again voted to overturn the ban on federal funding, Bush's veto of the bill was narrowly upheld. On January 22, 1993, President Clinton used his executive authority and finally ended the moratorium on federal funding of transplantation research using fetal tissue from induced abortions.[37] Congress has since codified authority for federal funding of fetal tissue transplant research with limits akin to those initially recommended by the NIH adivsory panel.[38]

As the battle for federal funding went on at the national level, researchers at Yale, Colorado, and other centers carried out fetal tissue research with nonfederal funds. Initial reports from these studies and studies abroad have been encouraging. Although no Parkinson's patient has been completely cured, nearly all have some improvement and many have gotten dramatically better.[39] These results suggest that research should continue with fetal tissue transplants for Parkinson's disease, as well as for Huntington's disease, diabetes, and Alzheimer's.

Ethically, the fetal tissue transplant controversy has centered over whether use of tissue from aborted fetuses can be sufficiently separated from the underlying abortion producing the tissue to be ethically acceptable to those who would oppose abortion in order to obtain tissue for transplant. Although some opponents of abortion believe that the two issues can be separated, many think that the two are inextricably intertwined. They see any support or acceptance of fetal tissue donations as giving direct or implicit encouragement to abortion, as well as making the user complicit in the underlying abortion.[40]

On the other hand, the proponents of fetal tissue transplantation deny moral complicity with the underlying abortion and claim that the use of tissue and its underlying production can be clearly separated. They argue that tissue from induced abortions that are otherwise occurring should not be wasted when they might save the life or preserve the health of seriously ill patients. With rules concerning when consent is obtained, against payment for donation, and against donor designation of recipients, the underlying decision to abort can be insulated from the decision to donate tissue, and fetal tissue can be used without encouraging abortion.

At this level of debate both opponents and proponents share the assumption that abortions performed for the purpose of obtaining fetal tissue for transplant is ethically unacceptable and should be discouraged, if not prohibited altogether.[41] This view is also frequently expressed by ethical commentators and by other bodies that have reviewed the issue.[42] The main point of political controversy has been whether any use of fetal tissue from induced abortions that are otherwise occurring will encourage more abortions, and therefore should not be supported by federal funds.

While only the first issue—abortion to procure tissue for transplant—directly involves use of reproductive capacity for nonreproductive purposes, the two issues are sufficiently intertwined to warrant discussion of each. If any use of fetal tissue did encourage or lead to abortion to get tissue, then it would violate the widely voiced assumption that abortions to produce tissue for transplant are unacceptable.[43] Whether that assumption is valid also needs discussion. Each issue is addressed in turn.

Does Use of Fetal Tissue Encourage Abortion?

Would use of tissue from abortions that are already occurring encourage women to abort? The opponents of federal funding claimed that therapeutic uses of aborted fetuses will make it easier for women who are ambivalent about ending a pregnancy to do so, if they know that the tissue will be donated to save lives. They also think that rules designed to insulate the abortion decision from use of the resulting tissue are unworkable.

This position is evident in Secretary Sullivan's reasons for continuing the moratorium against federal funding of fetal tissue research:

> I am persuaded that one must accept the likelihood that permitting the human fetal research at issue will increase the incidence of abortion across the country. I am particularly convinced by those who point out that most women arrive at the abortion decision after much soul searching and uncertainty. Providing the additional rationalization of directly advancing the cause of human therapeutics cannot help but tilt some already vulnerable women toward a decision to have an abortion."[44]

Evidence for this position, however, is difficult to find. At issue is what motivates women to terminate pregnancy. The NIH Advisory Panel heard evidence that the primary factor in a woman's decision to have an abortion was the fact that the pregnancy was unwanted. While a significant number of women undergoing abortion experience ambivalence, and a minority of them might even change their mind several times before the abortion, the key factor remained whether the pregnancy, in light of the totality of their circumstances, was wanted. Accordingly, the panel concluded that a request shortly before the abortion occurred for consent to use the resulting tissue for anonymous use in transplantation research or therapy would not lead women not otherwise willing to abort to do so. Donation might, of course, make them feel somewhat better about their abortion experience, but given the separation of the abortion decision and the request to donate, and the fact that donation is anonymous and uncompensated, it is reasonable to think that fetal tissue transplants will not affect the abortion decision itself.

Secretary Sullivan and his allies, in taking a different view, did not always distinguish what is importantly at stake here. His argument basically was that tissue donation will provide an "additional rationalization" for abortion which "cannot help but tilt some already vulnerable women toward a decision to have an abortion."[45] But this assumes that they will know and expect to be asked to donate fetal tissue before they have finally decided to have an abortion. Both the NIH Advisory Panel and Congress had made clear that the decision to abort must come first. Only after the woman has signed the consent for the abortion and is present in the clinic where the procedure will be done may she then be asked to donate tissue.[46] While a few women might still have not gone through with the abortion at this point but for the request to donate, there is no reason to think that this number will be significant. Moreover, there is no particular reason to think that general public awareness that fetal tissue is obtained from abortions will, by assuaging ambivalence before a pregnant woman reaches the clinic, greatly increase the number of abortions.[47]

In the absence of data, however, there is no clear empirical way to resolve the question. One can only make a judgment about which scenario about a pregnant woman's decision-making process appears to be more accurate. The proponents of fetal tissue use cannot prove that there will never be a woman for whom the possibility of donating, even anonymously, will not be the determinative factor in her decision to abort. A few women who are highly ambivalent about aborting may decide to abort because the prospect of donation makes the abortion just palatable enough to be undergone.

Opponents, on the other hand, fail to recognize that the number of women so affected will be vanishingly small. The chance to help science or unidentified, anonymous patients may make women who abort and donate tissue feel better, but this factor is unlikely to be determinative in the vast majority of cases. Surely it is more reasonable to believe that the wanted or unwanted status of the pregnancy and the woman's marital, social, economic, and physical situation will dwarf whatever effect the possibility of anonymous tissue donation for research or therapeutic purposes would have. Whether a pregnancy is wanted or not will continue overwhelmingly to determine whether an abortion occurs.

Because it is reasonable to assume that a very small number of additional abortions might occur if fetal tissue from induced abortions is used, the controversy is really over what public policy stance to take if even a small number of abortions occur because tissue will be donated. Proponents of use argue that the increase is nonexistent or so small as to be *de minimis*. Opponents, on the other hand, argue that any increase in abortions as a result of federal funding, no matter how small, is unacceptable.

The opponent's position, however, seems inconsistent with their position on other policy issues in which there is a small risk that some lives will be lost. For example, they do not oppose public funding of new bridges and highways or FDA approval of new drugs, despite the clear statistical risk that some lives will be lost as a result. Nor do they oppose the sale of guns and knives, even though some unknown number of persons will intentionally kill others as a result. Rather than demand a zero level of risk of loss of life with regard to these policies, fetal tissue opponents tolerate the risks because they are so relatively small and important public purposes are served. With abortion and fetal tissue donation, however, the slight magnitude of the threat to fetuses counts not at all. For them even enormous benefits to long-suffering patients and families cannot justify a small risk that a few additional abortions might occur, despite careful efforts to insulate tissue donation from the decision to abort.

Conception and Abortion to Obtain Tissue

Despite these differences, both proponents and opponents of fetal tissue transplants share the view that abortion for the purpose of obtaining tissue is undesirable and should not be encouraged. As noted, the NIH Advisory Panel, like other advisory bodies, most ethical commentators, and federal law have built in safeguards to prevent abortion solely to obtain tissue for transplant.[48]

With 1.5 million abortions occurring annually in the United States, the question of aborting to get tissue for transplant is largely theoretic. However, several developments could change the situation. If fetal tissue transplants turn out to be successful for Parkinson's disease and diabetes, the demand could easily outstrip supply, especially if tissue from several fetuses is needed for one transplant. Also, reduction in the number of surgical abortions, whether due to the use of contragestive agents such as RU486 or other factors, could also reduce supply.[49] Or if histocompatibility made a related tissue donor necessary, pressure to abort to produce fetal tissue for a relative would mount. If any of these events occurred, the question of aborting or producing fetal tissue for transplant purposes would be a real and important issue, forcing us to consider whether one's reproductive capacity could be used for such a nonreproductive purpose.

To consider this issue, let us suppose that because of histocompatibility factors or supply problems, fetal tissue from a related donor was necessary to save the life of a spouse, child, parent, sibling, or the woman herself. Would it be wrong to abort an existing pregnancy to obtain the needed tissue for that person? Would it be wrong to conceive in order to produce a pregnancy that could be aborted to get needed tissue? Let us distinguish the situation where the woman is already pregnant from the situation where she conceives in order to procure tissue by abortion.

THE WOMAN IS ALREADY PREGNANT

If the woman is already pregnant, the right to avoid procreation by ending pregnancy to help a loved one is at issue. But for the family member's need, the woman would have gone to term with the pregnancy. She is now choosing to abort, not because she does not wish to parent, but because she finds the needs of the family member more pressing than her interest in having this particular offspring.

The ethical acceptability of such an act depends on the acceptability of abortion generally. If early abortion is ethically permissible, the particular reasons why the pregnancy is unwanted should not ordinarily affect the ethical acceptability of abortion. The woman's decision that the burdens of gestation and/or child rearing are too great is respected because she is in the best position to assess those burdens and because early fetuses are too neurologically immature to have interests in their own right.[50] As discussed in chapter 3, aborting previable fetuses does not harm or wrong them, since they are insufficiently developed to experience harm. The symbolic impact of abortion on respect for human life is outweighed by the pregnant woman's interests in avoiding the burdens of pregnancy.

If abortion is acceptable to avoid those burdens, it is difficult to see why abortion is any less acceptable when the pregnancy becomes unwanted because abortion will provide the opportunity to save a loved one in need.[51] Although a deliberate sacrifice of the fetus occurs, the sacrifice is occurring for a reason that is at least as strong, if not stronger, than abortion to avoid unplanned or unwanted motherhood.

On the other hand, if abortion is deemed morally impermissible, then abortion to procure tissue to save a life would be as well. However, if abortion is viewed as morally impermissible except in very exceptional circumstances, such as to protect the mother's life or health, in cases of rape or incest, or severe genetic deformity, the abortion to procure tissue could be supported. The need to save another's life seems to be equivalent in gravity to those exceptional circumstances.

Of course, aborting a wanted pregnancy to prevent severe neurologic disease in oneself or one's family poses an excruciating dilemma. An otherwise wanted fetus will be sacrificed to save a parent, spouse, sibling, or child who already exists. Such a tragic choice will engender loss or grief whatever the decision. However, unless one is against abortion in most or all circumstances, one cannot say that the choice to abort is ethically impermissible. There is no sound ethical basis for prohibiting this sacrifice of the fetus when its sacrifice to end an unwanted pregnancy or avoid other burdens is permitted.

Legally, the question of aborting to provide tissue for transplant to a family member or oneself would depend on the legality of abortion in the jurisdiction in question. Under *Roe v. Wade*, there is no limit on the reasons or motivations for previability abortion—the pregnant woman is the sole judge of the need. On this standard, there would be no barrier to aborting to get tissue for transplant, and a law restricting such abortions, such as the recently enacted federal law, would be presumptively invalid.[52]

If *Roe* is reversed or revised so that abortion in most circumstances or for particular reasons can be restricted, then a restriction on aborting to get tissue for transplant—for example, against designating the recipient of a tissue donation—might well be constitutional. However, its wisdom could be questioned. As noted, if the jurisdiction otherwise accepted abortion for compelling reasons, banning abortions to obtain tissue to save a family member's life would be difficult to justify independently. It would seem to be as compelling, if not more so, than other reasons for abortion. If the fear is that some women will be coerced or pressured into abortions by family members, ways to minimize that danger without preventing all abortions to procure tissue could be devised.

CONCEIVING AND ABORTING FOR TRANSPLANT PURPOSES

When a woman not yet pregnant seeks to conceive in order to abort and provide tissue for transplant, the issues raised are slightly different because the right to conceive, as well as the right to abort, is implicated.[53] It is a clearer case of using one's reproductive capacity for nonreproductive purposes than is aborting an existing pregnancy to obtain tissue. The right to procreate is not involved, because no intention to have and rear children exists.[54] Rather, the issue is whether one may take the first steps toward procreation when there is no intent to complete the process.

Would such a practice be ethical? Again, the question depends on the perceived acceptability of abortion. If abortion to obtain tissue for transplant is acceptable if a pregnancy otherwise existed, no greater harm occurs to the fetus conceived expressly to be aborted. Since there is no greater harm to the fetus, the difference seems to be a symbolic one, akin to the symbolic offense of creating embryos solely for research or creating and transferring many embryos to the uterus when selective reduction of a multifetal pregnancy is likely to ensue.

Deliberate creation with intent to abort may have greater symbolic significance, however, because it denotes a greater willingness to use fetuses as a means to serve other ends. However, aborting when already pregnant to procure tissue for transplant or because the pregnancy is unwanted also denotes a willingness to use the fetus as a means to other ends. As long as abortion of an existing pregnancy for transplant purposes is ethically accepted, people might reasonably conclude—as they could with creation of embryos solely for research—that the additional symbolic devaluation of human life through deliberate creation and destruction of prenatal life is negligible, and thus is insufficient to outweigh the substantial gain to transplant recipients that deliberate creation provides.[55]

In sum, deliberate creation of fetuses to be aborted for tissue procurement is more ethically complex and defensible than its current widespread dismissal would suggest. Such a practice is, of course, not in itself desirable, but in a specific situation of strong personal or familial need may be ethically justified. Persons who rationally compare the competing concerns may well conclude that in some circumstances, with safeguards to protect women from coercion or exploitation, the use of one's reproductive capacity to obtain fetal tissue for transplant should be ethically and legally acceptable.[56] When the need for such abortions arises, this issue should be fully debated and not dismissed out of hand as ethically unacceptable.

REPRODUCTION TO GET TISSUE FOR TRANSPLANT

Another variation on the theme of using reproductive capacity in nontraditional ways arises when a couple conceives a child to be a tissue donor. Unlike the previous discussion of conceiving and aborting to obtain tissue, no abortion occurs. Instead, the couple goes to term and delivers the child, who then serves as a bone marrow or organ donor for an existing child.

This issue received national attention with the Ayala case in 1990. The Ayalas are a Southern California couple in their early forties whose seventeen-year-old daughter Anissa had a virulent form of leukemia that was in remission. Her only hope for a permanent cure was a bone marrow transplant. Neither her nineteen-year-old brother nor her parents were a suitable match, and a nonrelated donor was not available.[57]

Faced with the prospect of losing their daughter when the leukemia recurred, the Ayalas decided to have another child who might serve as a donor for Anissa. Mr. Ayala's vasectomy first had to be reversed. Six months later his forty-two-year-old wife became pregnant. Prenatal tests indicated that the fetus, which had a one in four chance of having compatible tissue, was a match.[58] In April 1990 they gave birth to a daughter who had been conceived specifically to serve as a marrow donor.[59]

The Ayala case was widely reported in print and electronic media across the country. While some medical ethicists questioned the notion of having a child solely as a means to provide tissue, support was overwhelmingly in favor of the Ayalas. They were committed to rear their new child whether or not she was a suitable tissue match, and conveyed the impression of a warm, loving family devoted to the best interests of their children. Surprised by the questions that some ethicists raised, Ms. Ayala stated, "Our baby is going to have more love than she can probably put up with."[60] Daughter Anissa stated, "She's my baby sister, and we're going to love her for who she is, not for what she can give us."[61]

With wide and generally favorable publicity, we can expect more such cases to arise. Even though many doctors refuse to advise parents to adopt this approach, parents with a child needing bone marrow may have no other alternative.[62] Is such a practice an ethically appropriate exercise of procreative liberty? Or is it a morally objectionable practice that should be discouraged or prohibited?[63]

At first glance, having a child who will serve as a tissue donor for an existing child seems well within procreative liberty. After all, a child is conceived and carried to term, and will be reared by the parents as a member of the family. The difference is that the motivation for reproduction is having the child serve as a means—of being a tissue source—of treating an existing sick child.

Some ethicists have objected that conceiving a child to donate tissue treats the child as a mere means who is not being valued for himself, but solely as a source of tissue for another. They have noted that it risks turning the child into a mere thing—an organ farm or "medicine for an existing child."[64] Such attitudes have made physicians reluctant to recommend or encourage parents with sick children to pursue this alternative.

In cases in which the parents intend to rear the child who is conceived for donation, this charge seems greatly exaggerated and out of touch with the complex motivations that lead parents to have children. While unqualified love and wanting children for their own sake may be the ideal, conceiving a child to be a marrow donor is not any worse or less altruistic than the myriad of other reasons for which children are sought. These include narcissistic wishes to enhance parental glory, reassurance against death and mortality, a source of income, caretakers in old age, or even to replace a previous child who has died. A selfish motivation is but one of many factors, and should not detract from going forward with reproduction, if the child will be loved and respected as a person once born.

Thus having a child to be a tissue donor is not ethically disqualifying. In the Ayala and other cases, cord blood alone might provide the necessary ingredient, so no further intrusion on the child need occur. Even if a bone marrow transplant is necessary, the risks and burdens to the donor seem well within the range of parental discretion over a child, who is presumably benefited both by her existence and the chance to be a donor for a sibling. After all, parents are ordinarily free to have minor children serve as donors to siblings when they were not conceived for that purpose.[65] Thus having a child to be a donor should also be acceptable.

Perhaps the fear is that conceiving a child to be a tissue donor, though loving and admirable in the Ayala case, will lead to abuses in other cases. Suppose, for example, that the fetus will be aborted or the child given up for adoption if its tissue does not match. Would such practices independently be abuses that should not be permitted? Whatever their status, is permitting the Ayala situation likely to bring them about?

We have already discussed the implications of conceiving in order to abort to get tissue. In the scenario described here, the abortion would occur not to obtain tissue, but because the child will not be able to provide tissue that properly matches. Many people might find this to be an improper or unacceptable motive for abortion. Legally, however, if abortion is permissible for any reason, this reason would also suffice, even if many people would find it offensive. If abortion is illegal, this problem will not arise.

As an ethical matter, however, this case does appear less compelling than aborting to get tissue, because no one's life is directly aided. Rather, a fetus is being rejected because it lacks the proper genes when it was knowingly conceived with that risk. While we saw in chapter 7 that parents should have the right to select genes of offspring when the selection is tied up with having a normal child, here a normal fetus is being aborted because it will not be able to provide usable tissue to an existing child. But if a woman may abort normal fetuses when she is not able or interested in rearing offspring without an investigation into her reasons for that assessment, then she should be able to do so here as well.

Of course, some people would find it highly offensive that a woman would knowingly conceive when there was a known risk (in this case a 75 percent risk) that any fetus would be aborted. Yet such risks are acceptable when a couple has a 1:4 or 1:2 risk of having a fetus with a severe genetic abnormality which will lead to abortion. It also is acceptable when pergonal is used to stimulate the ovaries, thus running the risk of selective reduction. If one truly believes that fetuses lack rights, then abortion in this situation should also be permissible, even if it is symbolically less acceptable than other situations of unwanted pregnancy. In any event, the chance that some such abortions will occur is not a reason for banning conceptions for tissue where the pregnancy will go to term, no matter what the tissue match.[66]

Alternatively, the couple might go to term and if the child lacks the right tissue, give the child up for adoption. The couple is unwilling to rear simply because the child lacks the right tissue, not because they are unable to or unwilling to rear in general.[67] At first blush this action seems cruel and unfeeling toward their child's welfare. Many of us would morally condemn such action.

Yet this action may be more defensible than it first appears when it is compared with alternatives. For instance, the child in this case is clearly better off than the fetus with the wrong tissue that is aborted. At least here the parents are willing to go to term and give the child a life, albeit with adoptive parents. While crassly selfish, the parents' act gives the child a life that can turn out to be a happy and loving one. Their act also fulfills the needs of the adoptive couple who presumably will love and cherish the child. The case is troubling because it seems clearly preferable that the biologic parents raise their child.[68] Yet between being aborted and being born and then relinquished for adoption, the child is better off with adoptive parents than not being born at all.[69]

It is reasonable to conclude that neither aborting the deliberately conceived fetus with the wrong tissue or carrying it to term and giving it up for adoption is so clearly wrong that both actions should always be condemned, much less prohibited. Even if they were condemned or prohibited, their occurrence is not so inevitable that all conceptions of children to obtain tissue should be condemned. In most instances the child so conceived will be welcomed into the family and loved regardless of tissue status and success of the transplant.

In short, procreative liberty should include the right to have children for any motive, including to serve as a marrow donor, if such goals or uses of the child independently respect that child's interests. If postbirth organ or tissue donation in infancy is independently acceptable, then it should also be if the child was deliberately conceived and brought to term for that purpose.[70] That assessment should be made independently of the genesis of the child.

The choice to reproduce is complex and varied enough to accommodate many interests and motives. The important question is not what brought about conception and delivery, but what happens to these children afterwards. As long as parents will act for the best interests of the children once born, their motives in bringing them into the world should not matter.

CONCLUSION

This chapter has examined ways in which reproductive capacity is used to accomplish goals other than producing offspring for rearing. With three of the technologies examined, reproductive capacity is used to produce embryos or fetuses that will be discarded or destroyed to serve other needs. The fourth technology, producing children to serve as tissue or organ donors, may also lead to abortion (if the fetus is not the correct match), but more often will lead to the birth of children.

Controversies over these technologies concern what is proper use of reproductive capacity when birth of offspring is not planned or intended. Some persons will object to these practices as threats to the dignity of women precisely because reproductive capacity is alienated or disconnected from its usual procreative function, and because women bear the physical burdens of producing the embryos or fetuses involved. However, the main objections arise from the treatment of embryos and fetuses—their intentional creation and destruction to serve other ends.

Whether society will accept these uses depends on how embryos and fetuses are valued as compared to the interests being served by their deliberate creation and destruction. A key factor in evaluating these concerns is the realization that these do not substantially differ from other accepted practices. If embryo discard and embryo research are accepted, then creating and discarding embryos solely for research purposes, when necessary to conduct useful research, should also be accepted. Similarly, if early abortion for unwanted pregnancy may occur, how can early abortion to procure fetal tissue for transplant be deemed unacceptable? Again, the need for selective reduction of multifetal pregnancy arises because of infertility treatments that are themselves widely accepted. Nor is the Ayala situation of conceiving children to be tissue donors that distinct from the complex array of reasons of why people have children. In short, a closer look reveals that what at first blush seems so shocking is rather familiar and commonplace.

Although these controversies all involve use of reproductive capacity, they may not all represent exercise of reproductive freedom, at least not in the basic sense of freedom to have or not have offspring. Of course, many of the issues concern the interruption or termination of a reproductive process that could eventuate in offspring—a paradigm example of procreative choice. However, the interruption is either deliberately planned and contemplated prior to conception or the need for it arises for reasons other than the usual reasons that motivate the desire not to procreate.

How the conflicts are characterized, however, may be less important than their substance. Even if they do not fit neatly into the narrow rubric of procreative liberty, they involve personal decisions to use one's reproductive capacity in ways very important to the parties directly concerned. Embryos for research, fetal tissue for loved ones, increasing chances of a healthy pregnancy, and procuring marrow cells for sick children are themselves all worthy goals. They do not represent a cavalier or frivolous use of reproductive capacity, and do not denigrate or disrespect prenatal forms of human life more than other widely accepted practices. If embryos and fetuses do not have inherent moral claims to be protected, these uses of reproductive capacity should be permitted when they are freely chosen by the women directly involved.

CHAPTER 10

Class, Feminist, and Communitarian Critiques of Procreative Liberty

WITH PROCREATIVE liberty as a beacon, this book has visited the ethical, legal, and social conflicts presented by new reproductive technology. The journey has fleshed out the meaning of procreative liberty by arguing for presumptive moral and legal protection for reproductive technologies that expand procreative options. Those technologies that are not centrally connected to the values that underlie procreative liberty deserve less respect.

The resulting picture is a growing array of sophisticated technologies that can help individuals achieve their reproductive goals. As with many technologies, a bright, hopeful side coexists with dismay and distrust over how reproductive technologies might be used. For many people the technical ability to prevent or end pregnancy, to relieve infertility, to increase the chance of healthy offspring, or to obtain tissue for research and therapy is a great boon, and confirms one's faith in scientific progress.

Yet others feel profound discomfort with reproductive manipulations, and urge strict regulation or even prohibition. The source of their disquiet may be traced back to fears of manipulating nature and interfering with God's plans that have plagued science since its inception. Here the danger is even more ominous, because reproductive technologies manipulate the earliest stages of human life and potentially harm prenatal life, offspring, women, and the family.

In responding to this technology, individuals and society are both caught between autonomy and ambivalence—between the demands of personal choice and the disquiet that uses of autonomy causes them and society. One is damned either way—either overly technologizing the intimate, or losing the very real benefits that this technology provides.

The burden of this book has been to show the importance of procreative liberty in resolving these controversies. The lens of procreative liberty is essential because reproductive technologies are necessarily bound up with procreative choice. They are means to achieve or avoid the reproductive experiences that are central to personal conceptions of meaning and identity. To deny procreative choice is to deny or impose an all-encompassing reproductive experience on persons without their consent, thus denying them respect and dignity at the most basic level.

Although procreative liberty is a deeply held value, its scope and contours have never previously been fully elaborated. Past controversies have concerned contraception and abortion, and rarely, with the exception of eugenic sterilization and overpopulation in the Third World, dealt with limitations on procreation itself. The advent of new reproductive technologies has changed the landscape of conflict, and forced us to inquire into the meaning and scope of procreative liberty.

This book's discussion of seven controversial reproductive technologies has shown the intimate connection between procreative liberty and technology. Once this connection is made, the choice of individuals to use or not use these technologies should be presumptively respected because of the privileged position that procreative liberty occupies as a moral and legal right. Where only peripheral aspects of procreation are involved, the right to use those techniques must rest on some basis other than procreative liberty.

The invocation of procreative liberty as a dominant value is not intended to demolish opposition or end discussion. It is offered as a template to guide inquiry and evaluation, and to assure that moral inquiry and public policy do not ignore the importance of personal choice in these matters. No right is absolute. Even procreative liberty can be limited or restricted when adequate cause can be shown. Procreative choices that clearly harm the tangible interests of others are subject to regulation or even prohibition. Even if they cannot be prohibited, their use can be condemned as irresponsible or ill-advised, or not encouraged.

With this approach, however, we have seen that there are few instances in which the feared harms of the new technology are compelling enough to justify restrictive legal intervention (though the need for responsible use remains). Again and again the dire warnings of harm turn out to be baseless or speculative fears, or to reflect highly contested positions about fetal or embryo status, gestational motherhood, and the nature of families—positions that are usually insufficient to justify interference with procreation. In nearly every instance, public policy should keep the gateway to technology open, allowing individuals the freedom to enter as they will.

In the few instances in which choice could be limited, the core values of procreative liberty do not appear to be directly implicated, as with restrictions on pregnant women using drugs, Norplant for the retarded, and nontherapeutic genetic engineering. Even when a good case for restricting reproductive choice exists, the regulatory emphasis should be on counseling, education, notice, and noncoercive incentives, though criminal penalties or injunctions may in some cases be justified.

Some people, of course, will disagree with this analysis, either because they dispute the privileged position accorded procreative liberty or the assessment of harms from individual choice. For example, they may think that I have underestimated the impact of these technologies on women, children, and the family, or undervalued the moral status of embryos and fetuses. Or they may simply be more cautious. With technologies that have not yet been widely used, much less assimilated into the social fabric, it may be premature to pronounce them socially acceptable or even essential to procreative choice.

Yet even if one differs with the book's position in particular instances, the importance of procreative liberty in assessing other applications of technology should remain. For example, persons holding pro-life views will disagree with a biologically based, symbolic analysis of abortion and other prenatal conflicts. But this disagreement should affect only those situations in which embryos or fetuses are directly threatened, and not all other instances of procreative choice.

Even persons with pro-life beliefs might grant the importance of procreative liberty in deciding whether persons may or may not use technologies that do not destroy prenatal life. They may still recognize the right of infertile couples to use IVF, at least within certain limits, and may favor prenatal screening where therapeutic interventions are possible. They may also support uses of Norplant and other technologies when people are not equipped to raise children, as long as embryos and fetuses are not destroyed. Despite differences in some areas, considerable room remains for respecting procreative choice.

An additional advantage of a procreative liberty framework for assessing reproductive technology is the guidance that this approach provides in evaluating future innovations. The development of IVF, prenatal screening, contragestion, and other techniques marks a watershed in human reproduction from which there is no turning back. Future developments will push the envelope of technological control even further, as extracorporeal gestation, cloning, embryo splitting, genetic engineering, embryo tissue farms, posthumous birthing, and other variations come on line. Each of them will present the same dilemmas of individual choice and public policy that we now face.

Procreative liberty should provide a useful framework for evaluating those future developments as well. The effect of each new technlogy on procreative choice will have to be assessed. If procreative interests are centrally implicated, then only strong countervailing interests will justify limitation. As illustrated repeatedly throughout this book, many of the concerns and fears will, upon closer analysis, turn out to be speculative fears or symbolic perceptions that do not justify infringing core procreative interests. If we accept a strong version of procreative liberty, then public policy for those technologies, as for most of those surveyed in this book, may have to rely on education and persuasion rather than coercion.

THE PROBLEMS OF A RIGHTS-BASED APPROACH

The approach of this book has been explicitly and unswervingly rights based. Taking procreative liberty as a fundamental moral and legal right, it has assumed that the individual's procreative liberty should rule unless there are compelling reasons to the contrary.

While such an approach characterizes many social issues in the United States, a rights-based approach has been strongly critcized in recent years as overly individualistic and insufficiently sensitive to the needs of the community. In a recent book, for example, Professor Mary Ann Glendon has argued that rights talk is limiting because it is absolutist, individualist, and inimical to a sense of social responsibility.[1] Others have argued that rights talk is too private and individualistic, ignoring how public claims interpenetrate the private sphere.[2] It also exposes a social blindness to the claims of interdependence and mutual responsibility that are at the heart of social living.[3]

These criticisms of rights talk are especially applicable to reproduction. A rights-based perspective tends to view reproduction as an isolated, individual act without effects on others. The determinative consideration is whether an individual thinks that a particular technology will serve his or her personal reproductive goals. Except for the rare case of compelling harm, the effects of reproductive choices on offspring, on women, on family, on society, and on the general tone and fabric of life are treated as irrelevant to moral analysis or public policy.[4]

Yet reproduction is the act that most clearly implicates community and other persons. Reproduction is never solipsistic. It always occurs with a partner, even if that partner is an anonymous egg or sperm donor, and usually requires the collaboration of physicians and nurses. Its occurrence also directly affects others by creating a new person who in turn affects them and society in various ways. Reproduction is never exclusively a private matter and cannot be completely accounted for in the language of individual rights. Emphasizing procreative rights thus risks denying the central, social dimensions of reproduction.

Critics of rights talk point particularly to the abortion debate, where the pro-choice claim ignores both the interests of fetuses and the interests of fathers and potential grandparents.[5] This criticism might also be leveled against other reproductive technologies, from IVF and collaborative reproduction to genetic screening and fetal tissue transplants. Emphasizing procreative rights necessarily deemphasizes the effects of these technologies on prenatal life, offspring, handicapped children, the family, women, and collaborators.

Although powerful and important, however, this critique of rights does not defeat the priority assigned to procreative rights anymore than it defeats the priority of free speech, due process, travel, and other important rights. To begin with, the critique does not always prove the ill effects that it claims. Glendon, for example, overlooks the fact that many rights "encourage precisely the forms of deliberation and communal interaction" that Glendon herself favors.[6] This is true of political and social rights, which make communal deliberation and democracy possible.[7] It is also true of rights to use procreative technologies. Thus IVF encourages the formation of families and the cooperative, dependent relationships that inhere therein. The use of donors and surrogates requires a special kind of cooperation, often among strangers, that leads to new forms of community. Even aborting to get fetal tissue for a loved one can be a sacrifice that binds rather than divides.

Second, rights-based approaches to reproduction or other issues do not ignore other interests so much as judge them, after careful scrutiny, as inadequate to sustain interference with individual choice. If harmful effects are clearly established or the action in question does not implicate central features of fundamental liberty, public concerns may take priority over private choice. In many cases, however, the state is relegated to exhortation and noncoercive sanctions to protect communal interests because it cannot satisfy the burden of serious harm necessary to justify overriding fundamental rights.

A third problem with the critique of rights is that the alternative it offers is weak and thin, even less desirable than whatever excesses rights might breed. Without the protection of rights, important aspects of individual dignity and integrity have no protection from legislative majorities or policymakers. Elizabeth Kingdom's hope that getting beyond rights will enable public policy to make "a wider calculation of the proper distribution of social benefits" overlooks the need for rights to protect us from the policy calculations of zealous administrators.[8] Indeed, the emergence of rights is due to the failure of the community and public officials to give due regard to the needs of affected individuals.

This is especially clear in the case of abortion, which Glendon and Elizabeth Fox-Genovese claim shows the divisive, individualistic vices of a rights approach. The claim for a right to abortion comes out of a failed collective responsibility toward motherhood, which makes abortion an essential option. If pro-life groups were truly concerned with the weak and vulnerable, as their concern with the fetus claims, they would make greater efforts to rectify the social and economic conditions that make abortion a necessary option for women. Their failure in this regard suggests rather an interest in controlling "women's reproductive capacities ... (in order) ... to continue a system of discrimination that is based on sex."[9] Rights are essential precisely to guard against discriminatory agendas that deny dignity and integrity to women and men. They are responses to failures of social responsibility, not the causes of them.[10]

To be convincing, however, a rights-based approach must acknowledge its defects even while proclaiming its strengths. It cannot ignore the social dimension, even if social claims are seldom sufficient to limit procreative choice. To assure that full credence is given to these dimensions, three specific criticisms of a rights-based approach are discussed. In each case we will see that procreative liberty, despite some qualifications, emerges alive and well.

MONEY AND CLASS

A major problem with a rights-based approach is that it ignores the social and economic context in which exercise of rights is embedded. Procreative rights are negative in protecting against private or state interference, but they give no positive assistance to someone who lacks the resources essential to exercise the right. A rights-based approach to reproductive choice thus has no way to take the effects of money and class into account. As Rhonda Copeland has noted:

> The negative theory of privacy is . . . profoundly inadequate as a basis for reproductive and sexual freedom because it perpetuates the myth that the ability to effectuate one's choices rests exclusively on the individual, rather than acknowledging that choices are facilitated, hindered or entirely frustrated by social conditions. In doing so negative privacy theory exempts the state from responsibility for contributing to the material conditions and social relations that impede, and conversely, could encourage autonomous decision-making.[11]

The truth of this statement is evident in how the distribution of wealth operates as a prime determinant of who exercises reproductive rights. The most obvious wealth effect concerns access to reproductive technology. For example, women who lack the money to pay for Norplant or abortions are much less able to avoid reproduction than those who can pay. Yet the Supreme Court has held that the state's failure to fund abortions for indigent women does not violate their right to terminate pregnancy because it places no obstacle in their path that was not already there.[12] It is also the poor who feel the brunt of 24-hour waiting periods for abortion, and who would be most acutely affected if *Roe v. Wade* were ever reversed.

Lack of resources also affect one's ability to undergo IVF and related assisted reproductive techniques. At a cost of $7,000 per cycle, only middle- and upper-class couples can afford this treatment. Since several cycles may be needed to establish pregnancy, this is a technique that will clearly be wealth-based. Similarly, egg donation and surrogacy, which have equivalent or higher costs, will also be distributed according to wealth. Nor will prenatal screening and genetic manipulation be widely available to those who cannot pay for them.

There is irony in the financial disparities that determine differential access here. Poor and minorities have greater rates of infertility than middle and upper classes, yet only the latter can afford the high costs of IVF and other assisted reproductive treatments. Given the current crisis of access to health care for poor people, the idea of Medicaid payments for infertility treatment is politically unlikely, so these disparities are likely to continue.

Allocating reproductive technologies and other essential goods and services according to ability to pay raises profound questions of social justice. Because infertility impairs a basic aspect of species-typical functioning, a strong argument for including it in any basic health-care package can be made.[13] Yet it does not follow that society's failure to assure access to reproductive technologies for all who would benefit justifies denying access to those who have the means to pay. Such a principle has not been followed with other medical procedures, even life-saving procedures such as heart transplants. As troubled as we might be by differential access, the demands of equality should not bar access for those fortunate enough to have the means.

Class and money may also influence the roles individuals play in the collaborative reproductive process. Under the theory of procreative liberty proposed in this book, individuals have the right to hire or engage donors and surrogates, or to serve as donors and surrogates themselves.[14] Since donors and surrogates are usually paid for their contribution, the danger is that only the middle class and wealthy will have the resources to hire them, while only the lower classes will be inclined to assume these roles. If this is so, money and class will greatly skew the distribution of roles and services in collaborative reproduction.

The latter concern, however, may be most acute for surrogacy. Although lack of funds may prevent poor people from obtaining gamete donations, poverty has not been a determinant of who provides sperm and egg donations. Proximity, reliability, health, and fertility have been the main factors physicians have sought in gamete donors. While egg donors are paid as much as $1,500 to $2,000 per cycle, it is unlikely that only poor women in need of money will choose to be donors.

Class, however, may be a stronger factor in the selection of surrogate mothers. Again, poor people will not usually be able to buy surrogate services, if a willing family member is not available. However, they are more likely to be recruited as surrogates because of the $10,000 or more that they will be paid. It is not surprising that Mary Beth Whitehead, the surrogate in the *Baby M* case, was of a lower social class and less educated than the recipient couple. Similarly, in the *Anna C. v. Mark J.* gestational surrogate case, the surrogate was black, while the hiring couple was white/Asian.[15] Although many surrogates have gone to high school or college, there is a danger that class bias and financial need will determine the supply of surrogates. Carried to extremes, a breeder class of poor, minority women whose reproductive capacity is exploited by wealthier people could emerge.

But what is to be done about this practice? Denying poorer women that opportunity by prohibiting payment or by allowing payment only to middle-class surrogates denies them a reproductive role which they find meaningful. Given that poorer women serve as nannies, babysitters, housekeepers, and factory workers, gestational services might also be sold, even though it will offend the respect that some persons have for maternal gestation. Should couples be denied access to surrogacy because of the risk of class bias, when the surrogate is freely and intelligently choosing that role? Whatever our qualms about such a practice, it may have to be tolerated because the procreative liberty of all the parties is so intimately involved.

A final area in which class and money will make itself felt is in state interventions to protect offspring from harmful prenatal conduct or to limit irresponsible reproduction by compulsory contraception. Punishing women for prenatal child abuse or ordering cesarean sections against their will appears to have a disproportionate racial and class impact. For example, a Florida study showed that while the same percentage of white and black women have signs of illegal drugs in their blood at birth, the state refers black women disproportionately to the criminal justice system or to child welfare agencies.[16] Other studies have shown that mandatory cesarean sections are most commonly sought for black and poor women, not for whites who also refuse the operation.[17] Similarly, compulsory contraception for child abusers or HIV women seems to target the poor and minorities more than other groups. Although an invidious discriminatory purpose has not been shown to underlie these disparities, the danger that wealth, class, and race will be factors in the state's coercive use of reproductive technology cannot be ignored.

These points about the role of money and class in distributing reproductive technologies and procreative choice show the limits of a negative rights-based approach to procreative liberty. It is another example of the disparities that differential distribution of wealth in a liberal society inevitably bring. One can decry the disparities that exist and urge that society correct distributive inequities, however, without denying all persons the right to make these choices. In the end, the need for social justice is not a compelling reason for limiting the procreative choice of those who can pay.

THE FEMINIST CRITIQUE

A strong emphasis on procreative liberty has also been questioned by feminists who fear that technology will lessen women's control over reproduction and further oppression of women. Feminist critics have usually focused on the dangers to women in surrogate motherhood or objected to prenatal interventions for the sake of offspring. However, the feminist critique goes deeper than a challenge to these techniques, and calls into question all reproductive technologies that redound to the benefit of a male-dominated society at the expense of women.[18]

The feminist critique of a rights-based approach to reproductive technology has several strands. Sometimes the objections go to the very idea of subjecting the natural reproductive process to technological control, because such control is viewed as a male-driven violation of the natural order. The more central fear, however, is that because of men's greater access to wealth and power, they will use reproductive technologies to control and oppress women. Indeed, some feminists assert that men devised these techniques in order to control female reproduction just when women began gaining social and economic power. They fear that a rights-based approach to reproductive technology will further patriarchal domination of women by reinforcing the traditional identification of women with childbearing and child rearing. At the very least, it will result in women taking on additional reproductive burdens to serve male procreative agendas.

Given the long history of sexism in medicine, the feminist critique must be taken seriously. A long tradition exists of men controlling female reproduction. Male doctors wrested control of the birth process from female midwives in the eighteenth and nineteenth centuries. In the early twentieth century they developed techniques of twilight sleep and anesthesia to further that control, which the natural childbirth movement of the 1960s and 1970s fought hard to overcome.[19] Hysterectomy, involuntary sterilization, and mastectomy reflect further assaults on female sexuality and reproduction. Electronic fetal monitoring and high rates for cesarean births may also be seen as further examples of male control.[20]

Some developments in reproductive technology seem to be cut from the same cloth. Forced cesarean section or jail for drug use discovered by doctors during pregnancy strikes some people as a form of medical violence against women. Forced contraception to limit "irresponsible reproduction" could be viewed as a way to bring untrammeled female sexuality under control. Restrictions on abortion often seem more concerned with imposing sexual and reproductive orthodoxy than on protecting fetuses.

Noncoital treatments of infertility can also be seen in this light. Women undergo the burdensome roller-coaster ride of IVF treatment to please their husbands. IVF technologies assault the woman's body with powerful hormones to coax out eggs and make the uterus receptive to embryos. Women may also feel compelled to screen out defective embryos and fetuses to make sure that they deliver a "good baby."

Because women bear the brunt of reproductive work, injustice in the distribution of reproductive burdens and benefits is inescapable. However, the view that a rights-based view of reproductive technology places power increasingly in the hands of men to the detriment of women overlooks the many ways in which technology offers options that expand the freedom of women. It also overlooks how a rights-based approach, despite its contextual limitations, assures women a large measure of control over their reproductive lives.

Consider how several technologies discussed in this book help women to avoid unwanted pregnancy or to have healthy offspring. Norplant is a safe, effective, and reversible long-lasting contraception that many women will welcome. When RU486 becomes available in the United States, it will allow unwanted pregnancies to be terminated at early stages without surgery, and thus increase access to abortion. IVF and the other assisted reproductive techniques enable women to rear offspring when they previously would have had to remain childless or adopt. Earlier and less invasive prenatal diagnosis allows a woman to avoid giving birth to handicapped children. Tissue production techniques may eventually allow a woman to save the life of a child, a parent, or even herself. Given these possibilities, reproductive technologies would appear to advance the interests of women.

Although a rights-based approach to reproduction cannot eliminate the inherent inequalities in male and female procreation, it can provide substantial protection for women. It is the best guarantee of a woman's control over the options these technologies offer. Legal recognition of procreative liberty will protect women from public sector impositions on their procreative choice. Respecting this liberty will stop the state from outlawing early abortion. Respect for this right will also protect women against forced sterilization, forced abortion, or forced contraception to prevent harm to offspring or taxpayers. Some limits on reproductively related conduct, such as drug use during pregnancy, might still be possible, but the threat here is not to procreative liberty and neither men nor women have the right to harm offspring by egregious or irresponsible prenatal conduct. When everything is considered, a strong commitment to procreative liberty will protect more than it will harm the interests of women.

Of course this is not to deny the ways in which technology can be used to harm women, nor the barriers that stand in the way of women having the means and the situational power to exercise free choice in decisions about technology. However, the most common target of feminist attacks is the argument that procreative liberty leads to the enforcement of surrogate mother contracts against the wishes of the gestational mother. Although much less common than other assisted reproductive techniques, surrogacy has come to symbolize the struggle of women to gain control of pregnancy and reproduction.[21]

Many feminists always favor the gestational mother in these disputes, as do most of the courts and legislatures that have addressed the issue.[22] Yet which solution is most protective of women is debatable—the woman who provides the egg for gestational surrogacy also has important reproductive interests at stake, as do women who wish to serve as surrogates who are denied the opportunity because of the legal unenforceability of their preconception promise. Many liberal feminists now argue that the intentions of the contracting parties should control rearing.[23] In their view, such a solution puts women in ultimate control, even though it requires that they be bound by surrogacy contracts just as they are by their contracts in other settings. It also undercuts traditional notions of reproductive orthodoxy that identify women with gestation and child rearing.

In the private sphere, the main issue for women will be whether they will be free to use—to have access to—the technologies they desire. Procreative liberty will protect them against state restrictions that are based on speculative harms or particular moral views of proper reproductive behavior, a major threat in this area. They will thus be free to use or not use IVF, egg and embryo donation, gestational surrogacy, genetic screening, embryo biopsy, and fetal therapy to treat infertility or to have healthy children.

Of course, a right against the state to use these techniques will not overcome contextual constraints on a woman's freedom. It does not help her if she lacks the funds to purchase the services in question. Nor will it remove the financial pressures that might lead her to choose to be an egg donor or a surrogate. It also does not protect her from her partner's, her family's, or her own internally generated demands—the product of socialization in a patriarchal society—to have children, despite the physical, social, or psychological burdens to her of doing so. Yet these limitations do not diminish the importance of the negative protections that a recognition of procreative liberty establishes, even if women do end up carrying a heavier reproductive load then men.

Some philosophers argue that more reproductive choices are not always better for women because new options do not always leave all of a woman's previous alternatives unchanged.[24] As evidence they cite how the development of IVF leads to pressure on women to undergo several burdensome cycles of treatment, and how prenatal sex determination might lead to pressure to abort. They also point to how prenatal genetic testing now makes a woman responsible for having handicapped offspring if she rejects amniocentesis, when previously she would have been seen as a victim of the natural lottery.[25]

One cannot deny that that reproductive choices will not increase self-determination for all women, because some will be pressured to make choices that they previously would not have had to face, or will lack the resources to take advantage of the opportunities presented. On balance, however, there is no reason to think that women do not end up with more rather than less reproductive freedom as a result of technological innovation. If so, procreative liberty is an important bulwark that helps women achieve the greater freedom that reproductive advances make possible. The more important lesson for social policy is the need to protect women from new forms of private sector coercion that arise because of these techniques, and to support their efforts to exercise procreative autonomy.

One need only imagine a world without procreative liberty to appreciate its contribution to the well-being of women. Although procreative liberty gives little protection from family or internal pressures to procreate or from lack of resources, it does prevent arbitrary, moralistic, or speculative governmental impositions on a woman's procreative choice. Even in a world without the technological options now available, recognition of negative procreative liberty would be an important achievement.

THE COMMUNITARIAN CRITIQUE: RIGHTS AND RESPONSIBILITY

Rights-based approaches are also criticized for their disregard of the needs of community. An emphasis on rights is necessarily individualist. It reflects a "do your own thing" mentality that ignores the impact of exercising rights on the shape, the tone, and the overall well-being of communities, and may obstruct the resolution of pressing economic and social problems.[26] Responsibility in the exercise of rights is essential if communities are to survive and be vital, yet rights talk invariably slights one's responsibility to the community.

This criticism is especially applicable to reproductive rights. Procreative liberty emphasizes individual satisfaction and deemphasizes the social consequences of procreative choice. It respects individual desire but denigrates duty and responsibility in how desire is fulfilled. Yet responsibility in procreation is essential because of its effects on resulting offspring. Indeed, many persons would argue that no one should reproduce unless they are able and willing to care and nurture the children they produce. Yet this book, except for the argument in chapter 8 for prenatal responsibility, largely rejects that conception of procreative liberty, as do feminists and others who want strict walls against any governmental intervention in reproductive choice.

Procreative liberty arguments for use of new reproductive technologies are vulnerable to the communitarian critique on several grounds. Many consumers of these techniques—and professionals who profit from offering them—rush to use them with little thought of their impact on offspring, family, and society. One may ask whether it is socially responsible to spend a billion dollars a year on assisted reproduction when so many other health needs are unmet, and when so many children await in foster homes for adoption.[27] Couples who spend thousands of dollars on such treatments may be less concerned about their child's welfare than their own selfish desires. Cumulatively, such practices could undermine the bonds on which the welfare of children and the community depend.

The community also suffers from routinization of prenatal screening practices. Embryos and fetuses become objects to be discarded or destroyed if they do not meet standards of quality or convenience, thus diminishing respect for the first stages of human life and the well-being of children who are born simply ordinary or with minor handicaps. The willingness to employ gamete donors and surrogates as reproductive collaborators also undermines community. Infertile couples might view donors and surrogates not as equals in a mutually collaborative enterprise, but as depersonalized cogs in the production of children. Written contracts distance the infertile couple and surrogate from the emotional reality of their joint endeavor.[28] Disaggregation and recombination of reproductive components also undermine the traditional importance of genetic and gestational bonds in defining families, and may leave children and parents confused about their lineage and social responsibilities. Finally, couples who harvest the uterus for transplant and research material contribute, like slash-and-burn farmers in the rain forest, to the increasing erosion of community conceptions of the sanctity of human life.

These concerns should be taken seriously, but the assumption that a rights-based approach to reproductive technology will inevitably diminish community greatly overstates the case. Procreative liberty does entitle women on welfare, convicted child abusers, and those with HIV to procreate, but as we saw in chapter 4, it is not clear that such reproduction is always irresponsible. We have also seen, in chapter 8, that procreative liberty does not give women or men the right to engage in prenatal conduct that will harm offspring. The expense and burdens of assisted reproduction is as likely to make the child loved and cherished as it is to commodify it as a product to satisfy parental selfishness. Prenatal genetic interventions to enhance the health of offspring may be more rooted in love than in narcissism.

Nor will the use of surrogates and donors necessarily be depersonalized and adversarial. Couples usually meet the surrogate, have frequent contact during pregnancy, and may correspond or meet in later years. Often egg donors are friends or family, and are increasingly sought out even when they are strangers. Written contracts, by providing certainty and understanding of mutual obligations, bring parties together more often than they divide. Contrary to rights critics, the use of donors and surrogates is as likely to be truly collaborative and cooperative as it is to be adversarial and antagonistic. Rather than undermine family, these practices present new variations of family and community that could help fill the void left by flux in the shape of the American family.

If this is so, an emphasis on reproductive rights is not inconsistent with reproductive responsibility and the needs of community, and is unlikely to damage individuals, families or larger social concerns more than it benefits them. The fears raised, however, do remind us of the possible reverberations of reproductive decisions on individuals and the community and thus the need for sensitivity and respect for others in their use.

Efforts to assure responsible use of reproductive technologies could take several forms. One is for both providers and consumers to resist the seductive urge to use a technology because it is there and might work. A technological solution for infertility is a powerful temptation, as the readiness of couples to try IVF and related procedures shows. Because the technology may be more onerous and less effective than at first appears, couples should be accurately informed of their prospects and counseled about the complications that could arise.[29]

A second approach is to ask potential users to think carefully about the social and psychological ramifications of collaborative reproduction for themselves, the children, and the donors and surrogates who assist them. Infertile couples, donors, and surrogates should explore the social and emotional uncertainties they face before embarking on such a weighty venture. They should be especially careful before undertaking truly novel procedures, such as splitting embryos to create twins born years apart, using related or intergenerational surrogates, creating embryos for tissue, and the like.[30]

A third approach is to develop guidelines or canons of ethical behavior. A legal right to use reproductive technologies does not necessarily entitle one to private-sector access. Health professionals are gatekeepers who ultimately determine who will use these technologies. They should use discretion in accepting patients and in acceding to their demands for technological help, yet not exclude persons on the basis of sexual preference, disability, or life-style alone. Above all, they should treat their patients with dignity and respect, and not mislead or exploit their desire to reproduce merely to make a profit. Regulatory measures to protect consumers from provider overreaching, as discussed in chapter 5, are clearly justified.

Finally, a rights approach to reproductive technology is not an imprimatur on all uses of that technology. It does not require that the state subsidize or otherwise encourage the use of all reproductive techniques, and provides no immunity from moral condemnation, persuasion, or noncoercive instruction in how that technology should be used. Thus not all forms of collaborative reproduction need be subsidized, even if health insurance should or does cover some infertility treatment. States may also refuse to enact laws that facilitate collaborative reproduction, though that approach might cause more problems than it prevents.[31] In short, there is ample room for protecting the community while also respecting individual choice. How to encourage responsible use without infringing procreative liberty will remain a major challenge for public policy.

CONCLUSION: AUTONOMY AND AMBIVALENCE

Resort to technology is a powerful temptation to persons who wish to have or to avoid having offspring. Reliance on technology, however, has both a bright and a dark side. It can be used in a caring, supportive, and communal way, or it can be used to oppress, dominate, and alienate. The ultimate challenge is to use it well.

Despite the problems of a rights-based approach, I have argued that procreative liberty should be presumptively protected in moral analysis and in public policy determinations about new reproductive technology. Procreation is central to individual meaning and dignity, and respect for procreative liberty best resolves the many controversies surveyed. A commitment to autonomy, however, does not eliminate the ambivalence that use of these techniques creates at both the individual and societal level.

At the individual level, persons may be ambivalent about the manipulations and social uncertainties that technologized means of reproduction entail, yet feel that they have few alternatives if they are to overcome infertility, avoid handicapped children, or save a loved one. At the societal level, ambivalence arises from the unknown social effects of permitting individuals to engineer offspring and to alter traditional understandings of family. Yet restricting individual efforts to find reproductive meaning through technology engenders further ambivalence, for it violates procreative freedom and implicates the state in intimate decisions best left to personal choice.

As science produces more technologies to control reproduction, public response will oscillate between attraction and repulsion, between respect for autonomy and concern for how that freedom is used. In the end, the reception of individual reproductive technologies will depend on their efficacy, the goals they serve, and their real and symbolic effects. Ambivalence will dissipate only when a clear verdict on the desirability or undesirability of a particular technology is possible. Given normative differences and uncertain empirical effects, that will not quickly occur.

There is no stopping the desire for greater control of the reproductive process. Since this is so value-laden an area, ethical, legal, and social conflicts over reproductive technology are likely to continue for many years. In confronting those conflicts, we must not deny the importance of procreative liberty just to escape the discomfort that its use often engenders. There is no better alternative than leaving procreative decisions to the individuals whose procreative desires are most directly involved.

Notes

Chapter 1
Introduction

1. The estimate of 30,000 to 40,000 is based on estimates of the number of persons who have children by donor insemination every year (estimated as 20,000 to 30,000) and the number of in vitro fertilization cycles (19,079 in 1990). See United States Congress, Office of Technology Assessment, *Infertility: Medical and Social Choices* (Washington: Government Printing Office, 1988). Thus 30,000 to 40,000 is a rough estimate of the persons who have sought noncoital assistance in the past year.

2. Office of Technology Assessment, *Infertility: Medical and Social Choices.*

3. Robert F. Howe, "Jacobson Guilty on All 52 Counts of Fraud, Perjury," *The Washington Post*, 5 March 1992, A1.

4. Daniel J. Wikler and Norma J. Wikler, "Turkey-Baster Babies: The Demedicalization of Artificial Insemination," *Milbank Quarterly* 69(1991):5.

5. Society for Assisted Reproductive Technology, The American Society for Reproductive Medicine, "Assisted Reproductive Technology in the United States and Canada: 1993 Results Generated from the American Society of Reproductive Medicine/Society for Assisted Reproductive Technology Registry, *Fertility and Sterility* 64(1995):13–17. This study reports 5,103 deliveries from IVF for 1993.

6. John F. Meany, Susan F. Riggle, and George C. Cunningham, "Providers as Consumers of Prenatal Genetic Testing Services: What Do the National Data Tell Us?" *Fetal Diagnosis and Therapy*, spec. supp. 8 (Spring 1993).

7. The emphasis on profit is evident in the planned public offering of stock in a chain of IVF clinics. The goal was for this group to become "the McDonald's of the babymaking business." Alison Leigh Cowan, "Can a Baby-Making Venture Deliver," *New York Times*, 1 June 1992.

8. However, as the analysis presented in chapters 7, 8, and 9 will show, not all claims to use or not to use a reproductive technology will turn out to involve procreative liberty.

9. One exception is Michael Bayles's *Reproductive Ethics* (Englewood Cliffs, N.J.: Prentice Hall, 1984).

Chapter 2
The Presumptive Primacy of Procreative Liberty

1. Whether labeled reproductive or not, gestation is a central experience for women and should enjoy the special respect or protected status accorded reproductive activities. On this view, a woman who receives an embryo donation or who serves as a gestational surrogate is having a reproductive experience, whether or not she also rears.

2. The distinction between liberty and claim right follows Joel Feinberg's account of those terms in his "Voluntary Euthanasia and the Inalienable Right to Life," *Philosophy and Public Affairs* 7(1978):93–95.

3. Constitutional rights are generally negative rather than positive. With the exception of counsel in criminal trials, there is no obligation on the government to provide the means necessary to exercise constitutional rights.

4. Dan Brock has argued that contraceptive services are so cheap and their lack has such a substantial impact on persons that the state has a moral obligation to provide contraceptives to poor persons. Dan Brock, "Reproductive Freedom: Its Nature, Bases, and Limits" (unpublished paper, 1992).

5. Sonnet 12 ("When I do count the clock that tells the time/And see the brave day sunk in hideous night"). Sonnet 2 ("When forty winters shall besiege thy brow/And dig deep trenches in thy beauty's field") also sings the praises of reproduction as an answer to death and old age.

6. Margaret Atwood, *The Handmaid's Tale* (Boston: Houghton Mifflin, 1986).

7. "Where Death and Fear Went Forth and Multiplied," *New York Times*, 14 January 1990.

8. B. Meredith Burke, "Ceaucescu's Main Victims: Women and Children," *New York Times*, 25 January 1990.

9. Sheryl WuDunn, "China, with Ever More to Feed, Pushes Anew for Small Families," *New York Times*, 2 June 1991.

10. The 1977 sterilization campaign plays a key role in the denouement of Salmon Rushdie's *Midnight's Children: A Novel* (New York: Knopf, 1981). The narrator cries, just before he too is sterilized: "They are doing nashendi—sterilization is being performed. Save our women and children. And a riot is beginning" (p. 414).

11. Phillip Reilly, *The Surgical Solution* (Baltimore: Johns Hopkins University Press, 1991).

12. Paul A. Lombardo, "Three Generations, No Imbeciles: New Light on *Buck v. Bell*," *New York University Law Review* 60(1985):30.

13. With abortion a heated issue, this is the aspect that most readily comes to mind when "procreative liberty" is asserted.

14. Thus such questions as the parental right to have treatment withheld from severely handicapped newborns is not discussed. See John A. Robertson, "Procreative Liberty and the Control of Conception, Pregnancy, and Childbirth," *Virginia Law Review* 69(1983):405, 458–462.

15. This issue is discussed in chapter 4.

16. However, Congress, under Title X of the 1970 Public Health Service Act, 42 U.S.C. 300-300a-41a, provides federal funding for family planning services.

17. See Kizer v. Commonwealth, 228 Va. 256, 321 S.E.2d 291 (1984)(reversing conviction for marital rape), North Carolina General Statutes S. 14-27-8.

18. Griswold v. Connecticut, 381 U.S. 479 (1965).

19. Eisenstadt v. Baird, 405 U.S. 438 (1972); Carey v. Population Services Int'l, 431 U.S. 678 (1977).

20. The marital bedroom is not a sanctuary for activities that can otherwise be made criminal. Also, the same right would be recognized if the law only penalized sale of contraceptives, and not their use, thus obviating the need to search the

bedroom. See Ronald Dworkin, "Unenumerated Rights: Whether and How Roe Should be Overruled," *University of Chicago Law Review* 59(1992):381.

21. See Davis v. Davis, 842 S.W.2d 588 (Tenn. 1992). However, state laws that mandated embryo donation in lieu of discard would limit this right. See chapter 5.

22. Roe, 410 U.S. 113 (1973); Casey, 112 S.Ct. 2791 (1992).

23. Casey, 112 S.Ct. 2791.

24. Baird v. Bellotti, 443 U.S. 622 (1979).

25. Maher v. Roe, 432 U.S. 464 (1977); Harris v. McCrae, 448 U.S. 297 (1980).

26. This question affects only a small number of abortions, but becomes significant with late second and third trimester abortions.

27. In this case the liberty interest in avoiding reproduction is not at stake because the woman is choosing to go to term and thus have offspring. See chapter 8.

28. Planned Parenthood v. Danforth, 428 U.S. 52, 96 S.Ct. 2831 (1976). Nor can a state require that a woman notify her husband before receiving an abortion. Planned Parenthood v. Casey, 112 S.Ct. 2791 (1992).

29. For the imposition of child support obligations on men who had been assured by the woman that pregnancy could not result from their act of intercourse, see Hughes v. Hutt, 500 Pa. 209, 455 A.2d 623 (1982); Stephen K. v. Roni L., 105 Cal. App. 3d 604, 164 Cal. Rptr. 618 (1980); In re Pamela P., 443 N.Y.S.2d 343, 100 Misc. 2d 978 (1981).

30. Davis v. Davis, 842 S.W.2d 588 (Tenn. 1992).

31. This right has received explicit recognition in the United Nations' 1978 Universal Declaration of Human Rights ("men and women of full age . . . [have the right] to marry and found a family"), the International Covenant of Civil and Political Rights (Art. 23, 1976), and the European Convention on Human Rights (Art. 12, 1953).

32. See chapters 4 and 7 for further discussion.

33. The low marginal value of additional reproduction would ordinarily be relevant only when one has already had a large number of children, and thus may not be important for many of the issues discussed in this book.

34. In a technical sense, genetic reproduction is not partial at all but an instance of complete reproduction. However, it is partial when separated from the gestation or rearing that usually attends reproduction.

35. In resolving this question, we will have to determine the importance to people of the knowledge that a biologic descendant will come into being and live after one has died. Is the sense of possible continuity with nature from knowing that posthumous reproduction might occur so meaningful to people that it should be respected? Could not posthumous reproduction become as important to some individuals as the prospect of the posthumous use of one's ideas or philanthropic contributions? See John Robertson, "Posthumous Reproduction," *Indiana Law Journal* 69(1994):1027–66.

36. See chapter 7.

37. Catholic Church, Congregation for the Doctrine of the Faith, "Instruction on Respect for Human Life in Its Origin and on the Dignity of Procreation," *Origins* 16(1987):698–711.

38. They are also concerned that women will be exploited or pressured by circumstances into arrangements that turn out to harm their interests. See chapter 6.

39. In 1928 in Buck v. Bell, 274 U.S. 200, 47 S.Ct. 584 (1927), the Supreme Court did uphold a law permitting the involuntary sterilization of an allegedly retarded woman, but this is not a precedent for restricting marital reproduction.

40. Skinner v. Oklahoma, 316 U.S. 535, 541 (1942).

41. Meyer v. Nebraska, 262 U.S. 390, 393 (1923).

42. Stanley v. Illinois, 405 U.S. 645, 651 (1972) (citations omitted).

43. Cleveland Bd. of Education v. LaFleur, 414 U.S. 632, 639–40, (1973) (citations omitted).

44. Eisenstadt v. Baird, 405 U.S. 438, 453 (1972). See also Bowers v. Hardwick, 478 U.S. 186, 204, 106 S.Ct. 2841, 2851 (1986) (Blackmun, J., dissenting) ("We protect the decision whether to have a child because parenthood alters so dramatically an individual's self-definition, not because of demographic considerations or the Bible's command to be fruitful and multiply").

45. Casey, 112 S.Ct. 2791 (1992).

46. The traditional connection of marital intimacy and reproduction should appeal to Justice Scalia, who requires a well-established tradition to recognize an unenumerated fundamental right. See Michael H. v. Gerald D., 491 U.S. 110, 109 S.Ct. 2333 (1989); Turner v. Safley, 482 U.S. 78, 107 S.Ct. 2254 (1987).

47. This would be true whether the married couple suffers from disabilities, poverty, or even past criminal convictions for child abuse. See chapter 4.

48. In Dandridge v. Williams, 397 U.S. 471, 90 S.Ct. 1153(1970), the Supreme Court held that not increasing welfare benefits for additional children was not a penalty for reproducing, but the denial of a benefit that the state was not otherwise obligated to provide.

49. Statutes in Illinois and Missouri that appear to punish knowing transmission of HIV to another are thus unconstitutional to the extent that they apply to transmission to offspring as a result of reproduction. Ill. Ann. Stat. Sec. ch.720, para. 5/12–16.2 (Smith-Hurd 1992); Mo. Ann. Stat. Sec. 191.677 (Vernon 1992).

50. Goodwin v. Turner, 908 F.2d 1395 (8th Cir. 1990). See also Katherine Bishop, "14 Prisoners Sue to Have Right to Save Sperm," New York Times, 5 January 1992, p. 11.

51. The court assumed that women prisoners would have to be given access to artificial insemination if the right of male prisoners to reproduce in this way was recognized. Yet the greater burdens that pregnancy and childbirth impose on the prison system would appear to distinguish the claims of female prisoners to have sperm provided to them for artificial insemination, and justify different treatment of each group.

52. See Carey v. Population Services Int'l, 431 U.S. 678 (1977); Bowers v. Hardwick, 478 U.S. 186 (1986).

53. National Center for Health Statistics, "Advance Report of Final Natality Statistics, 1995," Vital Statistics of the United States, 1993, in preparation. See Appendix, Table I-3.

54. These measures would interfere with bodily integrity, deprive a woman of the chance to reproduce in the future, or infringe the right to rear one's children.

55. Their negative right to reproduce would protect them against interference with their efforts to reproduce with the willing assistance of physicians and collaborators. However, this right does not give them a right to demand from the state or others the services or funds that they need to achieve their reproductive goals.

56. Turner v. Goodwin, 908 F.2d 1395 (8th Cir. 1990).

57. Carried to an extreme this reasoning would entitle fertile or infertile couples to contract for another woman to conceive and carry a child, which she then relinquishes for adoption, to term for them. Such an extension would call into question current adoption laws, which do not enforce prenatal agreements to relinquish a child for adoption. See chapter 6 for elaboration of this point.

58. Such extreme cases are dealt with in chapter 7.

Chapter 3
Abortion, Contragestion, and the Rususcitation of *Roe v. Wade*

1. Casey v. Planned Parenthood, 112 S.Ct. 2791 (1992).

2. Their loss of power was highlighted when two days after inauguration on the twentieth anniversary of *Roe v. Wade*, President Clinton issued executive orders that overturned the gag rule, restored federal funding for fetal tissue research, and permitted abortions in military hospitals abroad, all of which had been hotly contested restrictions imposed by Presidents Reagan and Bush. Robin Toner, "Clinton Orders Reversal of Abortion Restrictions Left by Reagan and Bush," *New York Times*, 23 January 1992

3. Questions of fetal status and embryo protection are also discussed in chapters 5, 7, and 9.

4. A poll conducted 29–30 January 1992 surveyed one thousand adults and found that although only 11 percent described themselves as supporting abortions in all circumstances, only 6 percent described themselves as advocating the prohibition of abortion in all circumstances. There was a margin of error of plus or minus 3.1 percent. Public Opinion Strategies poll, reprinted in "Poll: Majority Do Not Support 24 Wk. Allowance of Roe," *Abortion Report*, 11 February 1992, Spotlight Story.

A poll commissioned jointly by the Wirthlin Group, the National Right to Life Committee, and the U.S. Catholic Conference, surveyed one thousand adults from 17 June to 19 June 1992 and found that although only 10 percent were in favor of prohibiting abortion in all circumstances, only 11 percent felt abortion should be allowed at any time during a woman's pregnancy for any reason. The margin of error was plus or minus 3.9 percent. Wirthlin poll, reprinted in "Poll: Shows America Split on Overturning Rust," *Abortion Report*, 25 June 1991, Spotlight Story.

An earlier poll indicating the failure of the majority of Americans to support the options on the extreme ends of the abortion spectrum was commissioned by the *Boston Globe* and conducted by KRC/Communications Research of Cambridge, Mass. It found that 37 percent of one thousand registered voters supported legal abortions "in all circumstances," while only about one in ten said abortions should be legal "in no circumstances." The margin of error was plus or minus 3 percent. Bronner, "Poll Shows Shift Toward Support of Abortion Rights," *Boston Globe*, 17 December 1989, Nat'l/Foreign section.

Summaries of various abortion polls and a discussion of poll contradictions can be found in Karen L. Bell, "Toward a New Analysis of the Abortion Debate," *Arizona Law Review* 33(1991):907, 909–913. The issue of poll inconsistency is also addressed in Roger Rosenblatt, *Life Itself* (New York: Random House, 1992), 183–189.

5. A survey conducted by pollster Mark Clements found that 88 percent of those questioned supported abortion in cases of rape or incest. If there was a chance that the baby was to be born severely deformed, 78 percent felt that the mother should have the right to have an abortion. "Results from a National Survey: Should Abortion Remain Legal?" *Houston Chronicle*, 17 May 1992, *Parade*. Another poll showing majority support for allowing abortion in the "hard cases" was commissioned by Americans United for Life and conducted by the Gallup organization in May 1990. In this poll 80 percent of the respondents said abortion was acceptable in the first trimester if the mother's life were in danger. Seventy percent said first-trimester abortions should be legal in cases of rape or incest and 58 percent said abortion was acceptable in the first-trimester if there was a strong chance of fetal deformity. The margin of error was plus or minus 3 percent. "Americans Oppose Most Abortions," *AUL Insights*, May 1991, 3.

Similar views were uncovered by a *Boston Globe*/WBZ-TV poll of one thousand registered voters conducted by KRC/Communications Research of Cambridge in December 1989. About 85 percent thought abortion should be legal where pregnancy results from rape, incest, or endangers the woman's life. About 70 percent also thought that abortion should be permitted in cases of genetic deformity. The margin of error was plus or minus 3 percent. Bronner, "Poll Shows Shift toward Support of Abortion Rights," *Boston Globe*, 17 December 1989, Nat'l/Foreign section.

6. See Larry Rhoter, "Doctor Is Slain during Protest over Abortions, *New York Times*, 11 March 1993. An anti-abortion activist has also been charged with attempted murder of a Wichita, Kansas, abortion provider. Dirk Johnson, "Abortion, Bibles, and Bullets: Making of a Militant," *New York Times*, 28 August 1993. As this article shows, the most extreme members of such groups think that such killings are justified.

7. However, European requirements include longer waiting periods and in some cases that the abortion is necessary for mental health. See Mary Ann Glendon, *Abortion and Divorce in Western Law* (Cambridge, Mass.: Harvard University Press, 1987).

8. This sentence borrows from the title of Laurence Tribe's insightful and comprehensive book, *Abortion: The Clash of Absolutes* (New York: W. W. Norton, 1991).

9. As long as informed consent and waiting-period requirements do not effectively prevent them from aborting when that is their decision. See Ronald Dworkin, Life's Dominion: An Argument about Abortion and Euthanasia (New York: Alfred Knopf, 1993).

10. Abortion was not defined as murder at common law. When it became criminal, it could be committed only after quickening, which was evidence that

the woman was in fact pregnant. See Marvin Olashky, *Abortion Rights: A Social History of Abortion in America* (Wheaton, Ill.: Crossways Books, 1992).

11. The ability to delay marriage or practice abstinence are ways to avoid reproduction that are taken for granted in the Western world, but which may not be real options for millions of women in non-western and Third World societies.

12. Indeed, the burdens of unwanted pregnancy and childbirth are so great that many women, when abortion is prohibited, risk their life and health to have illegal abortions. It is estimated that 200,000 women die each year throughout the world as a result of illegal abortion. If abortion becomes illegal in the United States again, we may expect many more cases of septic abortion, hemorrhaging, and even deaths, a pre-*Roe* common occurrence that is now unknown to most physicians.

13. Justice Blackmun noted in his concurring opinion in *Casey*:

> A state's restrictions on a woman's right to terminate her pregnancy also implicate constitutional guarantees of gender equality. State restrictions on abortion compel women to continue pregnancies they otherwise might terminate. By restricting the right to terminate pregnancies, the State conscripts women's bodies into its service, forcing women to continue their pregnancies, suffer the pains of childbirth, and in most instances, provide years of maternal care. The State does not compensate women for their services; instead, it assumes that they owe this duty as a matter of course. *Casey*, 112 S.Ct. at 2486–87.

14. Because one's position on prenatal status is so closely tied to one's moral and religious beliefs, attempts at rational persuasion and analysis might seem irrelevant. However, to the extent that rational debate is welcome, the following replies to both the strong and the weak version of the duty to protect embryos and fetuses must be considered.

15. For a fuller account of the biological development of preimplantation embryos, see chapter 5.

16. As Judith Jarvis Thomson has noted, an acorn is not an oak tree, even though it has the potential to become one. Similarly, the potential of an embryo or fetus to become a person does not mean that it already is one. "A Defense of Abortion," *Philosophy and Public Affairs* 1(1971):47.

17. Ibid. See also Regan, "Rewriting Roe v. Wade," *Michigan Law Review* 77(1979):1569.

18. It would also require that women be treated equally with men if persons responsible for the needs of others are required to lend the use of their bodies.

19. This statement assumes that the fetus is being valued on symbolic grounds because of its potential rather than its actual characteristics. Only when it has interests in its own right does it become a subject of moral rights and duties.

20. Roe v. Wade, 410 U.S. 113 (1973).

21. Indeed, the Supreme Court in defining viability as a limit on abortion did not say that at viability the fetus becomes a person within the Fourteenth Amendment.

22. If technological advances pushed viability back to the first trimester, the Court's rule would then prohibit termination of pregnancy at that early stage,

even though the viable fetus could survive after expulsion and the woman could be freed of further gestation. If so, what would be the point of burdening the woman with months of gestation if unnecessary to protect the life of the fetus?

23. Jane Brody, "A Quality of Life Determined by a Baby's Size," *New York Times*, 1 October 1991.

24. It must also overcome our usual reluctance to impose bodily burdens on one person to serve the needs of others.

25. Saying that the fetus is alive or human omits the important question of whether it is also an alive, human person. Humanness alone is not the same as personhood, or else any piece of living human tissue would also be a person.

26. Robertson, "In the Beginning: The Legal Status of Early Embryos," *Virginia Law Review* 76(1990):437, 444–450.

27. Indeed, such judgments are so intensely personal that it is a violation of liberty to have the state prescribe them. Dworkin, "Are There Unenumerated Rights: Whether and How Roe v. Wade Should Be Overruled," *University of Chicago Law Review* 59(1992):381. See also Dworkin, *Life's Dominion*.

28. Robertson, "In the Beginning."

29. Feinberg, "The Mistreatment of Dead Bodies," *Hastings Center Report* 15 (February 1985). See also Merryman, "Thinking about the Elgin Marbles," *Michigan Law Review* 83(1985):1881. A very similar analysis using different terms is made by Ronald Dworkin in *Life's Dominion*. He calls what I refer to as symbolic interests "detached" interests in human life, because they are detached from a judgment that the human entity involved is a person. He argues in this elegantly written book that detached judgments about the sanctity of human life are essentially religious opinions, and therefore cannot be legitimately imposed by the state on persons who hold differing views.

30. Roe v. Wade, 410 U.S. 113 (1973).

31. Indeed, even if Fourteenth Amendment personhood were accorded fetuses, it would not automatically follow that a state was obligated to outlaw abortion, as the Thomson approach suggests. The question would be whether the lack of protection for fetal persons was justified. Protecting the procreative liberty of the pregnant woman might be an acceptable, noninvidious ground for not extending protection to fetuses.

32. Griswold v. Connecticut, 381 U.S. 479 (1965).

33. Andrew Koppelman, "Forced Labor: A Thirteenth Amendment Defense of Abortion," *Northwestern Law Review* 84(1990):480.

34. This is the best way to understand the Court's statement that "when those trained in medicine, philosophy, and theology are unable to arrive at any consensus" about "the difficult question of when life begins," "the judiciary, at this point in the development of man's knowledge, is not in a position to speculate about the answer." *Roe*, 410 U.S at 159.

35. Although the Court in *Roe v. Wade* did not explain the reason for viability line, this is the best reason that can be given.

36. John Hart Ely, "The Wages of Crying Wolf: A Comment on Roe v. Wade," *Yale Law Review* 82(1973):920; Robert Bork, "Again, a Struggle for the Soul of the Court," *New York Times*, 8 July 1992.

37. Webster v. Reproductive Health Services, 492 U.S. 490 (1989).

38. Even if the Court required that the state interest be "important" or "legitimate," a wide range of state interests, including protection of prenatal life, would then suffice to justify restrictive state abortion legislation.

39. A state that banned early abortion in order to protect prenatal human life would be hard pressed not to ban postfertilization methods of birth control as well. Neurological development of the implanted embryo is not so different from that of preimplantation embryos to justify the distinction. Yet Utah, a pro-life state, did precisely that in a statute passed in 1991 when it appeared that *Roe v. Wade* might be reversed. It defined abortion as "the intentional termination . . . of human pregnancy after *implantation of a fertilized ovum*." Utah Code Ann. Sec. 76–7-302 (Michie 1991). One might legitimately wonder why the early embryo should be protected just after implantation if it need not be protected just before.

40. A reversal of *Roe v. Wade* would have opened the door to other state intrusions on reproductive choice. If contragestives can be banned on the theory either that one does not have a fundamental right to avoid carrying an unwanted pregnancy to term, or that the state's interest in protecting prenatal life at any stage trumps that interest, then the state could require that women take progesterone to assure implantation or to prevent spontaneous miscarriage. On the other hand, if a legal duty requiring women to take drugs that will maintain pregnancy cannot be imposed, why would a law that prohibits the use of contragestive agents to remove the endometrial support for maintaining pregnancy be any more valid?

41. *Casey*, 112 S.Ct. 2791 (1992).

42. Indeed, Justices Kennedy and O'Connor changed their position from previous statements about the state's ability to protect prenatal life at the expense of the woman.

43. *Casey* at 2807.

44. Id. at 2807–2808.

45. Id. at 2817, citing Roe v. Wade, 410 U.S. 113 (1973).

46. Id.

47. Id. at 2807. Indeed, the dissenting justices (Chief Justice Rehnquist and Justices White, Scalia, and Thomas) did not challenge the line of precedent on which the Court relied, but simply asserted that it does not extend to ending pregnancy, because most states outlawed abortion at the time of enactment of the Fourteenth Amendment and because abortion destroys fetuses.

48. Id. at 2818, 2820.

49. Akron v. Akron Center for Reproductive Health, 462 U.S. 416 (1983); Thornburgh v. American College of Obstetricians and Gynecologists, 476 U.S. 474 (1986).

50. *Casey* at 2818.

51. See Barnes v. Moore, 970 F.2d 12 (5th Cir. 1992), *cert. denied*, 113 S.Ct. 656 (1992). Another question is whether the undue burden test will permit previously invalidated restrictions, such as that all second-trimester abortions occur in hospitals, to be imposed now. See Akron v. Akron Center for Reproductive Health, 462 U.S. 416 (1983).

52. "U.S. Abortion Law: Still the Most Permissive on Earth," *The Wall Street Journal*, 1 July 1992.

53. Glendon, *Abortion and Divorce in Western Law* (Cambrige, Mass.: Harvard University Press, 1987).

54. "Government Parliament Votes to Liberalize Statute on Abortion," *New York Times*, 26 June 1992.

55. This issue is discussed in chapter 5.

56. See chapter 9.

57. See chapters 7 and 9.

58. When taken with a synthetic prostaglandin within forty-nine days of the last period (within a month of fertilization), RU486 is effective in ending 98 percent of pregnancies. L. Silvestre, C. Dubois, M. Renault, Y. Rezvani, E. Baulieu, and A. Ulmann, "Voluntary Interruption of Pregnancy with Mifepristone (RU486) and a Prostaglandin Analogue," *New England Journal of Medicine* 322(1990):645.

59. Indeed, the embryo is not yet even truly individual at this stage, because up until implantation spontaneous twinning could occur. See Robertson, "In the Beginning" 442–443.

60. Some observers claim that Roussel Uclaf engineered these events in order to place the onus of introducing RU486 on the government and away from Roussel Uclaf. See R. Alta Charo, "A Political History of RU-486," *Biomedical Politics* (Washington, D.C.: National Academy Press, 1991), 62–69.

61. Philip J. Hilts, "Door May Be Open for Abortion Pill to Be Sold in the United States," *New York Times*, 25 February 1993.

62. Because the need for tissue and organ donation to one's own children seldom arises, this may not be a major inconsistency.

63. Kristen Luker, *Abortion and the Politics of Motherhood* (Berkeley: University of California Press, 1984).

Chapter 4
Norplant, Forced Contraception, and Irresponsible Reproduction

1. Norplant illustrates well the theme of autonomy and ambivalence that arises with new reproductive technologies. The ambivalence is strong because it involves the state in mandating a particular reproductive outcome, and directly interfering with choice. Even if justified in particular circumstances, state involvement sets a dangerous precedent that could lead to instances of forced contraception and other interventions that are less compelling.

2. This approval culminated twenty years of research and development sponsored by the Population Council, and made available to American women a contraceptive that, since 1966, has been used by more than 55,000 women in forty-six countries.

3. The drug is contained in the silastic capsules in dry, crystalline form. Stacey Arthur, "The Norplant Prescription: Birth Control, Woman Control or Crime Control," *UCLA Law Review* 40(1993):1.

4. P. D. Darney et al., "Acceptance and Perceptions of Norplant among Users in San Francisco, USA," *Studies in Family Planning* 21(1990): 152; D. Shoupe et al., "The Signficance of Bleeding Patterns in Norplant Users," *Obstetrics and Gynecology* 77(1991):256.

5. Easy removal assumes that a physician is available and willing to do the procedure. Finding a physician to remove Norplant is a problem in some Third World settings and in situations in which the physician disagrees with the woman's decision to stop the contraceptive. There may also be a cost barrier to removal.

6. Norplant, like other contraceptives, is not usually covered by health insurance policies. Tamar Lewin, "Wide Use Seen For an Implant in Birth Control," *New York Times*, 29 November 1991.

7. Other contraceptives, such as Depo-Provera, which lasts three months, and Orvil, the "morning after pill," should also be made available to those unable to pay the cost.

8. State of Washington, 52nd Legislature, 1992 Regular Session, House Bill 2909.

9. Editorial, "Poverty and Norplant: Can Contraception Reduce the Underclass?" *Philadelphia Inquirer*, 12 December 1990. A vehement protest from black journalists and the black community led to an apology. "Apology: The Editorial on 'Norplant and Poverty' Was Misguided and Wrongheaded," *Philadelphia Inquirer*, 23 December 1990.

10. "Governor's Welfare Plan Pushes Free Birth Control," *New York Times*, 17 January 1993.

11. Tamar Lewin, "Baltimore School Clinics to Offer Birth Control by Surgical Implant," *New York Times*, 4 December 1992.

12. Matthew Rees, "Shot in the Arm," *The New Republic*, 9 December 1991.

13. There is more willingness to impose limitations on noncoital reproduction, usually because the connection with the freedom to procreate is not recognized. See chapters 2, 5, and 6.

14. Phillip Reilly, *The Surgical Solution* (Baltimore: Johns Hopkins University Press, 1991).

15. Relf v. Weinberger, 386 F. Supp. 1384 (D.C. D.Ct. 1974). As a result of the Relf litigation, informed consent and a thirty-day waiting period are now required for sterilization in federally funded programs. Note, "Coerced Sterilization under Federally Funded Family Planning Programs," *New England Law Review* 11(1976):589–614. See also Reilly, *The Surgical Solution*, 150–52.

16. One could also talk about the reproductive responsibility of society—its obligation to make sure that safe and healthy means of reproduction or its avoidance are available, including resources that children brought into the world need to have a healthy and productive life.

17. Here we must distinguish between prenatal harm that is unavoidable with their birth and prenatal or postnatal harm that is avoidable but which in the circumstances may not be avoided. See chapter 8.

18. See Smith v. Cote, 128 N.H. 231, 513 A.2d 341 (1986); Becker v. Schwartz, 46 N.Y.2d 401, 386 N.E.2d 807, 413 N.Y.S.2d 895 (1978); Nelson v. Krusen, 678 S.W.2d 918 (Tx. 1984).

19. Of course, there is no guarantee that the remedial action that will mitigate the harm of wrongful life will occur.

20. Derek Parfit, "On Doing the Best for Our Children," in *Ethics and Population*, ed. M. D. Bayles (Cambridge, Mass.: Schenkman, 1976).

21. In this example, unlike most of the situations discussed in this chapter, the woman has an alternative way to have a healthy child. She can simply wait a month.

22. Derek Parfit, *Reason and Persons* (New York: Oxford University Press, 1984); David Heyd, *Genethics: The Moral Issues in the Creation of People* (Berkeley: University of California Press, 1992).

23. Although not enumerated in the text of the Constitution, such a belief doubtlessly has constitutional status. Reproduction is so basic to human life and meaning that deprivation without consent would be widely acknowledged as a violation of a fundamental liberty. Indeed, the Supreme Court has acknowledged the existence of such a right in dicta in several cases. See chapter 2.

24. Whether it will be determinative that they have reproduced already, or could reproduce in the future in more felicitous circumstances, is unclear.

25. See discussion of this point in chapter 2. Note that the issue is whether unmarried persons have the right to engage in coitus or have access to noncoital means of reproduction, such as IVF. Once conception occurs, they clearly have a right to go to term, and once birth occurs, to rear offspring. But it does not follow that they have a constitutional right to conceive in the first place, even though they cannot be denied the right to gestate a formed fetus or rear a born child.

26. Because Norplant is easily monitored and requires a one-time intervention, it is preferable to a general condition to use birth control or to avoid pregnancy.

27. Tamar Lewin, "Implanted Birth Control Device Renews Debate over Forced Contraception," *New York Times*, 10 January 1991.

28. Michael Lev, "Judge Firm on Forced Contraception," *New York Times*, 11 January 1991.

29. Id. See Arthur, "The Norplant Prescription."

30. At least one court has struck down such a condition on this ground. See ibid.

31. A major limitation with this point, however, is that most child welfare agencies are so overworked and underfunded that they may not be a reliable monitor of the offender's behavior with future children. Also, adequate foster care to protect the child may not be available. The less restrictive alternative of monitoring and removal to foster care may be more a theoretical than real protection of future children from convicted child abusers.

32. The claim that contraception is justified to protect unborn offspring has cogency only if the offspring would have a life so burdened with suffering that its life, from its own perspective, were not worth living. But even serious child abuse does not appear to cause a life of such unremitting suffering that its life is wrongful, e.g., that the child would have preferred no life at all and would commit suicide at the first available opportunity. For example, from the perspective of the child, even a life in which one has been abused by parents would seem preferable to no life at all.

33. For example, offspring of cocaine-addicted women cost the medical care system many times what other babies do.

34. Of course, if the woman is pregnant when she enters prison or manages to

get pregnant while there, she cannot be forced nor prevented from having an abortion.

35. Goodwin v. Turner, 908 F.2d 1395 (8th Cir. 1990).

36. It may be that loss of the greater power to imprison and prevent reproduction while in prison is based on an essential feature of prison administration, and is not an inherent or necessary part of punishment.

37. Gregg v. Georgia, 428 U.S. 153 (1976); Rummel v. Estelle, 445 U.S. 263 (1980).

38. If Norplant as a condition of probation surmounted previous hurdles, it would still face equal protection problems. All of the mandatory contraception cases to date have involved women, even though men also are convicted of child abuse. Perhaps this is because women are more likely to care for children, and thus are more likely to be in a position to repeat their abusive behavior. But men sentenced to prison for child abuse could claim a violation of equal protection if they are not given the same option of temporary contraception that women are. This challenge would be especially powerful if both a husband and wife were convicted of child abuse, and the woman were offered the option of Norplant and the husband sent to prison.

39. John Arras, "AIDS and Reproductive Decisions: Having Children in Fear and Trembling," *Milbank Quarterly* 68(1990):353, 367.

40. David Michaels and Carol Levine, "Estimates of the Number of Motherless Youth Orphaned by AIDS in the United States," *Journal of the American Medical Association* 268(24)(1992):3456. The authors argue that ignoring this problem "invites a social catastrophe of the greatest magnitude" because the "death of a parent . . . is one of the most traumatic experiences any child can suffer. When that death is accompanied by stigma and isolation and is followed by instability and insecurity, as it is in AIDS, the potential for trouble, both immediately and in the future, is magnified." Id. at 3460.

41. C. Levine and N. Dubler, "Uncertain Risks and Bitter Realities: The Reproductive Choices of HIV-Infected Women," *Milbank Quarterly* 68(1990):321, 323. For women trapped in poverty, illness, crime, and other humiliations, "A baby is the chance to have something concrete to love, or, as important, to be loved by. It is proof of fertility and the visible sign of having been loved or at least touched by another." Id. at 334. The importance of reproducing is even greater if the woman will die of her disease, because of her need to "leave someone behind for a mother or husband to care for in the future . . . the link to immortality that genealogy presents." Id. at 335.

42. This case is thus to be contrasted with the Bladerunner problem in chapter 7, where the procreator could make offspring healthy and whole but chooses, out of perverse malice or narcissism, to make the child worse than she need be.

43. The strongest case for such a claim might be Tay-Sachs disease, but that disease would also present a strong case for nontreatment early in the onset of the disease, so that any harm to the child from mere existence could be mitigated.

44. Such persons may still have a substantial interest in reproducing. For example, HIV women who will die in a short time may still find great meaning in having a child whom they will not rear for long. See Levine and Dubler, "Uncertain Risks."

45. While the state could require that providers inform at-risk persons of the availability of such tests, it is less clear whether the state could require that such testing occur. It may be that minimally intrusive tests that leave the person free to act on the results would not interfere with procreative choice, and would serve a useful function. By contrast, requiring that known carriers of genetic disease use birth control or that they abort affected fetuses would clearly interfere with procreative liberty.

46. Arras, "AIDS and Reproductive Decisions," 353.

47. "Apology," *Philadelphia Inquirer*, 23 December 1990.

48. Nancy Cates, *Buying Time: The Dollar-a-Day Program* (Case Program prepared for the Kennedy School of Government, Harvard University, 1990). See also Lucy Williams, "The Ideology of Division: Behavior Modification Welfare Reform Proposals," *Yale Law Journal* 102(1992):719, 737.

49. The philosophical literature on coercion is complex, and only rarely would find that an offer of a benefit to which the person is not otherwise entitled is coercive. However, see David Zimmerman, "Coercive Wage Offers," *Philosophy and Public Affairs* 10(1981):121.

50. Note here the Wisconsin and New Jersey plans and other attempts to get people off welfare by such conditions. See Isabel Wilkerson, "Wisconsin Welfare Plan: To Reward the Married," *New York Times*, 2 February 1991.

51. Maher v. Roe, 432 U.S. 464 (1977); Harris v. McCrae, 448 U.S. 297 (1980); Dandridge v. Williams, 397 U.S. 471 (1970).

52. Kathleen Sullivan, "Unconstitutional Constitutions," *Harvard Law Review* 102(1989):1413.

53. Buck v. Bell, 274 U.S. 200 (1927).

54. Paul A. Lombardo, "Three Generations, No Imbeciles: New Light on *Buck v. Bell*," *New York University Law Review* 60(1985):30, is an insightful and intriguing historical analysis of the deficiencies in the factual basis of that decision.

55. In re Guardianship of Eberhardy, 102 Wis.2d 539, 307 N.W.2d 881 (1981).

56. See, e.g., In re Grady, 85 N.J. 235, 426 A.2d 467 (1981); In re Moe, 385 Mass. 555, 432 N.E.2d 712 (1982); In re Guardianship of Hayes, 93 Wash.2d 228, 608 P.2d 635 (1980).

57. This argument is developed in Robertson, "Procreative Liberty and the Control of Conception, Pregnancy and Childbirth," *Virginia Law Review* 69(1983):405, 411–413.

58. Lewin, "Baltimore School Clinics to Offer Birth Control by Surgical Implant," *New York Times*, 4 December 1992.

59. An antifertility vaccine has not yet been developed, though it is an important area of future research. To be acceptable, it would also have to have a limited duration of efficacy and be reversible when one wished to restore fertility. See Carl Dejerassi, "The Bitter Pill," *Science* 245(1989):356, 359.

60. One may disagree with this assessment, particularly because of the side effects that many young women would experience.

61. Even though there is a high rate of teenage pregnancy, only a very small percentage of female adolescents become pregnant.

Chapter 5
IVF, Infertility, and the Status of Embryos

1. The focus is on married couples because most women seeking IVF are married, and most IVF programs treat only married couples. Whether the state could prohibit single persons access to IVF is discussed later in the chapter.

2. United States Congress, Office of Technology Assessment, *Infertility: Medical and Social Choices* (Washington, D.C.: Government Printing Office, 1988).

3. The American Fertility Society, the professional organization of infertility providers, increased its membership from 4000 members in 1970 to 11,237 members in 1993. Telephone conversation with Louella Watkins, Membership Secretary, American Fertility Society, 11 February 1993.

4. Society for Assisted Reproductive Technology, The American Society for Reproductive Medicine, "Assisted Reproductive Technology in the United States and Canada: 1993 Results Generated from the American Society of Reproductive Medicine/Society for Assisted Reproductive Technology Registry," *Fertility and Sterility* 64(1995):13–17. This study reports 5,103 deliveries from IVF for 1993. By extrapolation the number of births over the last four years is over 15,000.

5. Success here is measured by take-home baby rate per stimulation or egg retrieval cycle, and not clinical pregnancy rate, which many programs use to improve their statistics.

6. Eventually egg retrieval will occur in the physician's office, which will reduce the costs of the procedure. Retrieving eggs during a natural cycle without stimulation will also reduce costs, though it may also reduce efficacy.

7. Elizabeth Bartholet vividly expresses concerns about infertile women feeling compelled by their own sense of inadequacy to try IVF and to keep trying because there "is often no logical stopping point." *Family Bonds: Adoption and the Politics of Parenting* (Boston: Houghton Mifflin, 1993), 202.

8. Catholic Church, Congregation for the Doctrine of the Faith, "Instruction on Respect for Human Life in Its Origin and on the Dignity of Procreation," *Origins* 16(1987):698–711.

9. Results from the Assisted Reproductive Technology Registry, 1993, note 4 above.

10. See chapter 2, where the argument for infertile married couples having the same right to reproduce that fertile married couples have is developed.

11. For the sake of convenience, the term "embryo" is used throughout this chapter and book rather than the technically more accurate "preembryo." Embryo thus refers to all postfertilization, preimplantation stages of development.

12. Grobstein, "The Early Development of Human Embryos," *Journal of Medicine and Philosophy* 10(1985):213, 214. Much of the ensuing description is based on Grobstein's excellent survey of early human and mammalian development.

13. However, the fertilized egg is not yet individual, as only at implantation can a single new individual be identified. Also, recent studies suggest that a new genome is not expressed until the four- to eight-cell stage of development. See Braude, Bolton, and Moore, "Human Gene Expression First Occurs between the

Four- and Eight-Cell Stages of Preimplantation Development," *Nature* 332(1988):459, 460.

14. Grobstein, "Early Development," 216–17.

15. Ibid., 219, 232.

16. Ibid., 219–220.

17. Ibid., 223.

18. Ibid.

19. Ibid., 223–225.

20. This view parallels the view described in chapter 3 of respecting fetuses because of their symbolic value. Although not persons or entities which themselves have rights, embryos are potent symbols of human life and deserve some degree of respect on that basis alone.

21. Department of Health and Human Services, the Ethical Advisory Board in the United States, U.S. Department of Health, Education and Welfare, Ethics Advisory Board, HEW Support of Research Involving Human In Vitro Fertilization and Embryo Transfer, 44 Fed.Reg. 35,033 (1979).

22. The Warnock Committee Report in Great Britain, United Kingdom, Department of Health and Social Security, Report of the Committee of Inquiring into Human Fertilisation and Embryology (1984).

23. Ontario Law Reform Commission, Report on Human Artificial Reproduction and Related Matters (1985).

24. Davis v. Davis, 842 S.W.2d 588 (Tenn. 1992). In reaching that conclusion, the Court relied heavily on the American Fertility Society's report "Ethical Considerations of the New Reproductive Technologies," which articulated a view similar to that set forth in the text. *Fertility and Sterility* 46, (supp. 1 (1986):295–305.

25. "Who or What is a Preembryo," *Kennedy Institute of Bioethics Journal* 1(1991):1–15.

26. John A. Robertson, "In the Beginning: The Legal Status of Early Embryos," *Virginia Law Review* 76(1990):437, 452.

27. It follows then that an IVF program must have the consent of both partners before thawing, transferring, implanting, discarding, or donating embryos.

28. No. 71-3588 (S.D.N.Y. 1978) (memorandum decision); see Fleming, "New Frontiers in Conception: Medical Breakthroughs and Moral Dilemmas," *New York Times Magazine*, 20 July 1987, describing case and fertility issues in general.

29. A solution here would be to have the couple and program agree on a liquadated schedule of damages to be paid if embryos are inadvertently destroyed. The damages should be calibrated to the cost of creating the embryos.

30. 717 F.Supp. 421 (E.D. Va. 1989).

31. Letter from Dr. Howard W. Jones to Dr. Richard P. Marrs (9 August 1988), exhibit H to Plaintiff's Brief in Support of Petition for Temporary Restraining Order and Preliminary Injunction.

32. Advance instructions may be issued at a time relatively early in the process of seeking pregnancy through IVF, when a person's needs and interests may not be fully understood or envisaged. See John A. Robertson, "Prior Agreements for Disposition of Frozen Embryos," *Ohio State Law Journal* 51(1990):407, 418–423.

33. In Davis v. Davis, the Tennessee Supreme Court did say that a prior agreement between the couple for disposition of the frozen embryos in the case of divorce would have been enforced. In Davis v. Davis, 842 S.W.2d 588, 597 (Tenn. 1992).

34. Elizabeth Rosenthal, "Cost of High-Tech Fertility: Too Many Tiny Babies," *New York Times*, 26 May 1992, discusses some of the problems of the higher rate of multigestational pregnancies that occurs when more than two embryos are placed in a woman's uterus. See also chapter 9, where selective reduction of multifetal pregnancies is discussed.

35. See note 24.

36. Some programs will not permit discard of fresh embryos, but will allow embryos that have been frozen for a period of time to be discarded.

37. Although the issue raises questions of the couple's right to avoid genetic reproduction, the embryo discard policy might also influence their willingness to use IVF in the first place, thus implicating their right to reproduce as well.

38. Roe v. Wade, 410 U.S. 113 (1973); Planned Parenthood v. Casey, 112 S.Ct. 2791 (1992).

39. Medical Research International, 15, 21.

40. Of course, it would not harm children to be born to older mothers, even if younger mothers are more desirable rearers of offspring, if the children in question had no alternative way of being born. See chapters 4 and 8.

41. For further discussion of this issue, see J. Robertson, "Posthumous Reproduction," *Indiana Law Journal* 69(1994):1027–66.

42. Professor Walter Wadlington deserves credit for this witty variation on the old rule.

43. 842 S.W.2d 588 (Tenn. 1992).

44. "When weighed against the interests of the individuals and the burdens inherent in parenthood, the state's interest in the potential life of these preembryos is not sufficient to justify any infringement upon the freedom of these individuals to make their own decisions as to whether to allow a process to continue that may result in such a dramatic change in their lives as becoming parents." Davis v. Davis, 842 S.W.2d 588, 602–03 (Tenn. 1992).

45. In cases where there is no prior agreement on disposition, the courts should, as the Tennessee court recommended, resolve such disputes according to whether the party wishing to preserve the embryos has a realistic possibility of achieving his or her reproductive goals by other means. If there are no alternative opportunities to reproduce, or if going through IVF again would be unduly burdensome, it may be fairer to award the embryos to the party for whom they represent the last chance to have offspring, as might occur if the wife has lost ovarian function since the embryos were preserved. In that case, the unconsenting party should also be relieved of child support obligations. In most cases, however, the party wishing the embryos to be destroyed should prevail. See Robertson, "Resolving Disputes over Frozen Embryos," *Hastings Center Report*, November/December 1989; Robertson, "In the Beginning," 473–483.

46. Robert Pear, "Fertility Clinics Face Crackdown," *New York Times*, 26 October 1992.

47. Public Law 102-493 (H.R.4773), 24 October 1992. The act calls for reporting of the live birth rate for IVF and other assisted reproductive techniques,

defined as the ratio of live births divided (1) by the number of ovarian stimulation procedures attempted at each program, and (2) by the number of successful oocyte retrieval procedures performed by each program. Section 2(b)(2)(A) and (B). Virginia now also requires clinic-specific disclosure of success rates to patients before IVF treatments occur. Va. Code Ann. Sec. 54.1-2971.1 (Michie 1991).

48. Alison Leigh Cowan, "Can a Baby-Making Venture Deliver?" *New York Times*, 1 June 1992. However, the public offering was never made.

49. Ark. Code Ann. Sec. 23-85-137 (Michie 1992); Haw. Rev. Stat. Ann. Sec. 431:10A-116.5 (1992); Md. Ann. Code art. 48A, Sec. 354DD (1992); Tex. Ins. Code Ann. art. 3.51-6, Sec. 3A (West 1993).

50. Egert v. Connecticut General Life Ins. Co., 900 F.2d 1032 (7th Cir.)(infertility an illness and IVF necessary to treat it); Kinzie v. Physician's Liability Insur. Co., 750 P.2d 1140 (Okl. App. 1987) (IVF not a medically necessary procedure under the insurance contract).

51. David C. Hadorn, "Setting Health Care Priorities in Oregon: Cost Effectiveness Meets the Rule of Rescue," *Journal of the American Medical Association* 265(1991):2218.

52. Such discrimination against persons with HIV may be a violation of the Americans with Disabilities Act, because HIV status qualifies as a disability within the meaning of that law and an infertility clinic may be considered a place of public accommodation. 42 U.S.C. 12182 (1990).

53. The patient groups in question may have a right against a state that denies them access to IVF or other reproductive services, but they would not have the same right to services from private actors unless civil rights or antidiscrimination laws apply. See chapters 2 and 4.

54. Persons who view the fertilized egg and embryo as persons from the time of fertilization may differ over the extent to which IVF should be permitted at all. Some may permit it with no freezing, or with freezing but no embryo discard.

Chapter 6
Collaborative Reproduction

1. One has to turn to mythological events such as Athena springing full-blown from the head of Zeus for examples of truly noncollaborative reproduction. Even the Immaculate Conception of the Virgin Mary was collaborative (though noncoital), for it required divine infusion by the Godhead.

2. Only egg and embryo donation and gestational surrogacy are truly high-tech procedures. The most widely used collaborative technique, donor sperm, involves only a syringe. It is estimated that 20,000 to 30,000 children are born each year through donor sperm. United States Congress, Office of Technology Assessment, *Infertility: Medical and Social Choices* (Washington, D.C.: Government Printing Office, 1988). Egg donation, a product of IVF, is now increasingly practiced, with over fifty clinics providing the service. Embryo donation and surrogacy are occurring to a lesser extent.

3. The term "biologic" is used in this chapter to refer to either a genetic or gestational relationship with the child who is reared. For the man, the biologic connection in reproduction is always genetic. The biologic connection for the

woman may be either genetic or gestational or both, depending on the particular technique used.

4. Collaborative reproduction involves varying degrees of deviance from the two-person model of biologically related parentage. Egg donation is closest to the model, because each rearing partner has a biologic connection with offspring. Gestational surrogacy provides both with a genetic connection, though the gestational tie is missing. Sperm donation allows the woman the full connection and the man none, while embryo donation gives only the woman a biological (gestational) tie. Full surrogacy, on the other hand, gives the man a genetic connection and his wife none (the surrogate presumably being out of the picture). In contrast to adoption, each technique allows at least one, and sometimes both of the partners, a biologic connection with offspring.

5. The situation becomes even more complicated if the surrogate is the sister or mother of the husband or wife, or if any of the parties divorces and remarries a person with children from a previous marriage. In practice, however, most collaborative reproduction will involve sperm or egg donation and occasionally surrogacy, thus falling short of the five-parent combination often alluded to as a danger of collaborative reproductive practices.

6. National Center for Health Statistics, "Advance Report of Final Natality Statistics, 1990," *Monthly Vital Statistics Report* 41, no. 9 supp. (1993):33, table 16.

7. R. Snowden, G. Mitchell, and E. Snowden, *Artificial Reproduction: A Social Investigation* (London, Boston: G. Allen and Unwin, 1983), 50–54, 71–82, 97–104.

8. Physicians need to be very sensitive to these aspects of treatment, for the psychological and social dimensions may be as important as the medical.

9. Preventing harm to offspring would thus not constitute the compelling state interest necessary to justify a governmental ban on use of these techniques. See chapter 4 for further discussion of this point.

10. Commerical sperm banks now distribute lists of donors identified by height, weight, hair and eye color, race or ethnic background, education, and even hobbies, from which couples choose.

11. Family members who know each other may also serve as egg donors or surrogates.

12. Mahlstedt and Greenfield, "Assisted Reproductive Technology with Donor Gametes: The Need for Patient Preparation," *Fertility and Sterility* 52(1989):908.

13. Since adopted children have no constitutional right to learn the identity of their birth parents, it is unlikely that a constitutional right of collaborative offspring to identify their genetic or gestational parents would be recognized. At the very least, the state should protect collaborative offspring by requiring that identifying information be confidentially maintained so that it could be provided if later deemed essential. See John A. Robertson, "Embryos, Families and Procreative Liberty: The Legal Structure of the New Reproduction," *Southern California Law Review* 59(1986):939, 1015–1018.

14. Laws that privileged disclosure of identity over the collaborators' desire for privacy would not violate their procreative liberty. If a state determines that

adopted or collaborative offspring have a substantial interest in having identifying information about their biologic parents, this interest should be sufficient to justify regulations that burden the procreative or privacy rights of collaborators. For further discussion of this issue and the paradoxes it presents, see Robertson, "Embryos, Families, and Procreative Liberty."

15. The operative standard should require clear and convincing evidence that the intended parents will abuse or neglect the child—the same standard for interfering with rearing of children produced coitally.

16. It also deprives donors and surrogates of playing a more limited reproductive role, because couples might be unwilling to go forward without the assurance of a binding contract.

17. A contract model assumes some means for assuring that the parties are aware of the legal, binding implications of their agreement, and that agreements are freely made. Public policies to assure intelligent, noncoerced contract formation, such as review by a judge or review panel, may be appropriate in some cases.

18. Office of Technology Assessment, *Infertility: Medical and Social Choices*.

19. See Cal. Civ. Code Sec. 7005 (West 1990).

20. In re Pamela P., 443 N.Y.S.2d 343, 110 Micsc.2d 978 (1981).

21. Jhordan C. v. Mary K., No. AO27810 (Cal. Ct. of App. Apr. 25, 1986).

22. See Daniel Wikler and Norma J. Wikler, "Turkey-Baster Babies: The Demedicalization of Artificial Insemination," *Milbank Quarterly* 65(1991):5, for an interesting account of the issues that such practices present.

23. In 1993, 135 clinics reported performing IVF-ET with donated oocytes, with 2,446 transfers of oocytes donated by known and anonymous donors. Seven hundred and eighty-one children were born as a result. About 35 percent of these births were twins, and 5 percent triplets. Society for Assisted Reproductive Technology, The American Society for Reproductive Medicine, "Assisted Reproductive Technology in the United States and Canada: 1993 Results Generated from the American Society of Reproductive Medicine/Society for Assisted Reproductive Technology Registry," *Fertility and Sterility* 64(1995):17–18.

24. Egg donors may be other women going through IVF, women undergoing abdominal surgery for other reasons, or women recruited specifically to be egg donors. In some cases the recipient recruits the donor herself, who may be a friend or even a family member. Often they are paid. Egg donation may also occur by artificial insemination and uterine lavage, so that the recipient receives the embryo at the blastocyst stage. See John A. Robertson, "Ethical and Legal Issues in Human Egg Donation," *Fertility and Sterility* 52(1989):353.

25. Okla. Stat. Ann. tit. 10, Sec. 544 (1991); Tex. S.B. 512, 73rd Leg., R.S. (1993); S. 2082, 1993 Reg. Sess., 1993 Florida Laws.

26. The presence of a female rearer distinguishes this situation from sperm donation to a single woman, where no rearing male is present. Of course, the gestational mother and her husband could die, leaving the child of egg donation without financial support, but this contingency could also occur with sperm donation to a married couple.

27. Their claim for contact with the child, however, might have special poi-

gnancy if their own efforts at IVF, which led to the donated embryo, have not resulted in offspring.

28. The surrogate could be a sister, a mother, or a stranger hired directly or through a broker for this purpose.

29. Many persons object to use of the term "surrogate" to describe this relationship. In their view, the "surrogate" is the actual mother of the child and should be referred to as such. The wife of the hiring couple is thus a surrogate rearer for the biologic mother. However, because of the wide currency of the term "surrogate," I will continue to use it here.

30. Both forms of surrogacy are products of the 1980s. Full surrogacy dates from around 1980, when Noel Keane began a surrogacy brokerage operation in Michigan. It has been the most widely publicized of these procedures due to the Baby M case. Several hundred surrogate births now occur annually, and several brokers function to meet demand. For couples in which the wife's fertility cannot be achieved by other treatments, this might be the only method for that couple to have a child. Gestational surrogacy, on the other hand, is a product of more recent advances in IVF. The first births began appearing in the late 1980s. Its use is likely to grow, and may involve sisters or even mothers of the couple who need gestational services in order to reproduce.

31. Maura Ryan, "The Argument for Unlimited Procreative Liberty: A Feminist Critique," *Hastings Center Report*, July/August 1990, 6.

32. Many feminist writers also share this view. See Lori Andrews, *New Conceptions* (New York: St. Martin's Press, 1984); M. Shultz, "Reproductive Technology and Intent-Based Patenthood: An Opportunity for Gender Neutrality," *Wisconsin Law Review* 1990(1990):298.

33. The claim that the child is bonded to the gestational mother and thus will be hurt by relinquishment is highly contestable. See Hill, "What Does It Mean to Be a 'Parent'? The Claims of Biology As the Basis for Parental Rights," *New York University Law Review* 66(1991):353, 394–400. He also refutes the claim that only a gestational parent can nurture and love a child. Id. at 400–405.

34. See Robertson, "Embryos, Families, and Procreative Liberty." John A. Robertson, "Procreative Liberty and the State's Burden of Proof in Regulating Noncoital Reproduction," *Law, Medicine and Health Care* 16(1988):27.

35. Ironically, this view of gestation reflects attitudes toward childbearing and women that underlies much gender discrimination. Privileging the gestational role also undermines the notion that women are free, autonomous actors who can, like others, be bound by promises on which others have relied.

36. In the Matter of Baby M, 537 A.2d 1227, 1234 (N.J. 1988). For a critique of this holding, see Robertson, "Procreative Liberty and the State's Burden of Proof," 27.

37. State statutes making all surrogate contracts void and unenforceable: Ariz. Rev. Stat. Ann. Sec. 25-218 (West 1991); Ind. Code Ann. Sec. 31-8-2-2 (West Supp. 1991); Mich. Comp. Laws Ann. Sec. 722.855 (West Supp. 1991); 1992 N.Y. Laws Sec. 308; N.D. Cent. Code Sec. 14-18-05 (1991); Utah Code Ann. Sec. 76-7-204 (Michie Supp. 1992). Statutes making surrogate contracts unenforceable when they involve compensation: La. Rev. Stat. Ann. Sec. 9:2713 (West 1991); Neb. Rev. Stat. Sec. 25-21,200 (1989); Wash. Rev. Code Ann. Secs.

26.26.230-26.26.240 (West Supp. 1992). See also Ky. Rev. Stat. Ann. Sec. 199.590 (Michie 1991). However, Arkansas will enforce the agreement to have the hiring couple rear the child. AR ST sec. 9-10-201.

38. Anna J. v. Mark C., 822 P.2d 1317, 4 Cal. Rptr. 2nd 170 (1992).

39. Professor Martha Field sees no difference between the two and would allow the birth mother in either case to assert a rearing role for some period after birth. "Surrogacy Contracts—Gestational and Traditional: The Argument for Nonenforcement," *Washburn Law Journal* 31(1992):433.

40. These arrangements are most likely when relatives or friends act as donors or surrogates. It may also arise with same-sex couples who wish to have and rear children, but only one partner has a biological tie with offspring.

41. A law against a donor or surrogate having contact with rearing parents and offspring would interfere with rights to rear one's biologic offspring and other rights of intimate association. Although the Supreme Court in Michael H. v. Gerald D., 491 U.S. 110 (1989) upheld a California law that denied the genetic father the right to visit his daughter, the situations envisaged here, where all parties agree in advance, are distinguishable. However, one cannot reliably predict what the ultimate legal outcome of such a case would be.

42. Lehr v. Robertson, 436 U.S. 248 (1983). For a fuller account of this issue, see Janet L. Dolgin, "Just a Gene: Judicial Assumptions about Parenthood," *UCLA Law Review* 40(1993):637.

43. Thus a sperm or egg donor who insists on visitation or limited custody of a child resulting from a donation to a married couple will have more difficulty in getting the agreement recognized than a donation to a single woman. But see Crouch v. McIntyre, 780 P.2d 239 (Or. App. 1989).

44. C.M. v. C.C., 152 N.J. Super. 160, 377 A.2d 821 (Cumberland County Ct. 1977).

45. In the Matter of Alison D. v. Virginia M., 572 N.E.2d 27, 77 N.Y.2d 651, 569 N.Y.Supp.2d 586 (1991).

46. Strictly speaking, the party seeking to rear in this case has not reproduced, because she has no biologic tie with the child. However, one could argue for recognition of such arrangements because of the important interest of the nonbiologic parent, his or her role in making conception and birth possible, the previous relation with the child, and the need for reliance on such agreements if parties are to go forward with these instances of collaborative reproduction. Whether the interest at stake is labeled procreative, it may independently be worth protecting. The implications of such a view for adoption law are discussed below.

47. R. Alta Charo has argued that "having several parents to love you" can never be a bad thing, and thus should count in favor of the excluded biologic parent who wishes to rear. "And Baby Makes Three . . . Or Four, Or Five: Defining the Family after the Reprotech Revolution" (*Texas Journal of Women and the Law*, Spring 1994, 3).

48. The assumption is that the courts would recognize both genetic and gestational mothers as parents within the family code—a result that has not yet occurred. In addition, this method of forming a family—a form of egg donation—is more expensive and onerous than is artificial insemination of one partner. But it will appeal to lesbian couples who wish to protect their rights to rear collaboratively produced children or who each wish to have biologic offspring. Alterna-

tively, and less onerously, the nonbiologic rearing partner could seek to adopt the child to protect her rearing rights. Such co-parent or second-parent adoptions have occurred in Texas, Vermont, Alaska, Massachusetts, and other states, but are not available in all states.

49. In Stiver v. Parker, 975 F.2d 261 (6th Cir. 1992), a surrogate mother sued the lawyer and doctors involved in arranging her surrogacy because she allegedly contracted cytomegalovirus infection during insemination with the contracting husband's sperm. She claimed that they failed to test his sperm for the virus before the insemination.

50. However, some persons would reject any active state encouragement of collaborative reproduction, particularly of surrogacy.

51. However, limits on the number of times one could be a egg or sperm donor might be acceptable.

52. Donors are now routinely screened—or should be—for HIV.

53. Egg donors who are themselves going through IVF (and who donate extra eggs) may be especially invested in these issues, particularly if their own IVF efforts do not succeed.

54. Phillip Parker, "Surrogate Mothers' Motivations: Initial Findings," *American Journal of Psychiatry* 140(January 1983):1.

55. Va. Code. Ann. Sec. 20-162(A)(Supp. 1991); N.H. Rev. Stat. Ann. Sec. 168-B:25(V)(Supp. 1991).

56. Surrogate brokers have been sued by surrogates disappointed in the experience for failure to inform them adequately or for other breaches of duties alleged to be owed them.

57. See *Stiver v. Parker*.

58. Would state laws requiring the exclusion of certain women as surrogates violate their procreative liberty? Arguably not, because their reproductive role is partial, and infertile couples can select other surrogates.

59. There is some controversy over whether egg donors should be paid for their eggs or for the "time, risk and associated inconvenience" of donation, as the American Fertility Society recommends.

60. See National Organ Transplantation Act, 42 U.S.C.A. No. 274(e); Note, "Regulating the Sale of Human Organs," *Virginia Law Review* 71(1985):1015. For an analysis of the application of these laws to egg donation, see John Robertson, "Legal Uncertainties in Human Egg Donation" (1993) (forthcoming).

61. Mich. Comp. Laws Ann. Sec. 722.855 (West Supp. 1991); 1992 N.Y. Laws 308; Utah Code Ann. Sec. 76-7-204 (Michie Supp. 1992); Va. Code Ann. Sec. 20-162(A) (Supp. 1991).

62. It is unclear how the New Jersey court would consider paid gestational surrogacy, since adoption by the infertile couple, who are biologic parents, may not be necessary.

63. The best discussion of exploitation in the surrogacy context is Alan Wertheimer, "Two Questions about Surrogacy and Exploitation," *Philosophy and Public Affairs* 21(1992):211. He concludes that "Surrogacy may be exploitive and exploitation may be wrong, but it does not follow that such exploitation is a reason for prohibiting surrogacy or refusing to enforce surrogacy contracts." Id. at 239.

64. Virginia Held, "Coercion and Coercive Offers," in *Nomos XIV: Coercion*, ed. J. Roland Pennock (Boston: Aldine-Atherton, 1972). David Zimmerman argues that some offers can be coercive. See "Coercive Wage Offers," *Philosophy and Public Affairs* 10(1981):121–145.

65. Radin, "Market-Inalienability," *Harvard Law Review*, 100(1987):1849, 1921–1936.

66. Scott Altman effectively counters her arguments in "(Com)Modifying Experience," *Southern California Law Review* 65(1992):293.

67. Radin, "Market-Inalienability," 1921–1936.

68. Debra Satz, for example, has argued that the wrong of paid surrogacy is the unequal treatment of women that arises from creating markets for their reproductive labor. "Markets in Women's Reproductive Labor," *Philosophy and Public Affairs* 21(1992):107. See also Christine Overall, *Ethics and Human Reproduction: A Feminist Analysis* (Boston: Allen and Unwin, 1987), 111–137.

69. Such an implication may not, however, be what the feminist critics of surrogacy have in mind, for it could lead to contracting with women for reproductive services in situations where the hiring male or couple will have no biologic relation with children they seek to rear.

70. In such arrangements, persons who contribute egg, sperm, and gestation to produce the child to be reared by others would have to agree in advance to the arrangement, thus avoiding the problems that arose in the 1993 Baby Jessica case, where the mother but not the father had relinquished parental rights to a couple desiring to adopt her baby.

71. John Hill has presented an elegant argument for this result in "What Does It Mean to Be a Parent."

72. Ibid.

73. In addition to the infertile couple organizing donors and surrogates to produce a child for them, one could imagine scenarios involving single men who hire a surrogate, or an egg donor and gestational surrogate, to produce a child.

74. Although she is not in favor of assisted collaborative reproduction, Elizabeth Bartholet presents a powerful critique of the current adoption system's emphasis on genetic ties in *Family Bonds: Adoption and the Politics of Parenting* (Boston: Houghton Mifflin, 1993).

Chapter 7
Selection and Shaping of Offspring Characteristics

1. John F. Meany, Susan F. Riggle, and George C. Cunningham, "Providers as Consumers of Prenatal Genetic Testing Services: What Do the National Data Tell Us?" *Fetal Diagnosis and Therapy*, Special Supp. 8 (Spring 1993).

2. Barbara Katz Rothman, *The Tentative Pregnancy* (New York: Viking, 1986).

3. The claim of access is not to government resources to make selection techniques available, but to freedom from interference by government with private decisions to use them.

4. In the few cases where the life did appear wrongful, a right to avoid prolonging that life should then exist. See chapter 4 for discussion of this issue.

5. Even if they did impose medical or other costs on taxpayers, those costs are

ordinarily not sufficient to justify restricting a person's interest in procreation. See chapter 4.

6. However, pressure to screen may come from a private sector that fears malpractice liability or sees the chance for further profit.

7. Of course, a problem here is that one would be making this assessment prospectively, and thus might lack information or know intimately how the burdens and benefits would feel. But that is true whether the offspring is normal or affected, because in neither case can one tell in advance how later child rearing will be experienced.

8. If the abortion right is grounded in the fetus's lack of interests due to its rudimentary stage of biological development, then there would be no greater duty to preserve its life in some cases over others. Abortion for any reason would not violate a moral duty because prior to viability there is no moral subject to be harmed. However, the symbolic costs of abortion might vary with the reason for it.

9. This argument would be hard pressed to justify birth control, which might also be viewed as treating children as objects of parental pleasure by postponing their arrival to an opportune time. Similarly, the large investments of time and money in treatment of infertility might be viewed as placing an undue emphasis on producing children for the sake of parents.

10. While one could argue that parents have an obligation to care for handicapped children once born, it does not follow that they are obligated to have such children in the first place. Indeed, one could argue not only that couples have the right to avoid handicapped births, but that they have a moral duty to do so, at least where they will not bear the costs of rearing. See chapter 4.

11. B. E. Wilfond and N. C. Fost, "The Cystic Fibrosis Gene: Medical and Social Implications for Heterozygote Detection," *Journal of the American Medical Association* 263(1990):2777; John A. Robertson, "Procreative Liberty and Human Genetics," *Emory Law Journal* 39(1990):697.

12. See Robertson, "Procreative Liberty and Human Genetics."

13. Philip Reilly, *Genetics, Law and Society* (Cambridge, Mass.: Harvard University Press, 1977).

14. Wilfond and Fost, "Cystic Fibrosis Gene."

15. John A. Robertson, "Ethical and Legal Issues in Preimplantation Genetic Screening," *Fertility and Sterility* 57(1)(1992):1.

16. Slippery slope arguments are discussed in the context of germline genetic therapy later in this chapter.

17. There are other concerns as well, including a moral sense that it is simply wrong to take any action to have one's offspring be one sex or another. See Mary Ann Warren, *Gendercide: The Implications of Sex Selection* (Totowa, N.J.: Rowan and Allanheld, 1985).

18. S. Elias and J. L. Simpson, eds., *Maternal Serum Screening for Fetal Genetic Disorders* (New York: Church Livingstone, 1992).

19. Privately imposed restrictions, such as doctors who refuse to inform of prenatal tests, may also be a barrier. However, tort law should protect persons from this barrier, unless the physician has informed the patient of his personal beliefs and given her an opportunity to seek other medical care, or the medical care is offered in a state that does not recognize wrongful birth claims. See, e.g.,

Hickman v. Group Health Plan, Inc., 396 N.W.2d 10 (Minn. 1986); Note, "Wrongful Birth Actions: The Case against Legislative Curtailment," *Harvard Law Review* 100(1987):2017.

20. This argument is developed in chapter 3. Even if this premise is rejected, it still would not follow that a woman has a moral obligation to carry a fetus to term. See chapter 3.

21. Of course, abortion for trivial reasons or gender may be symbolically distasteful and may cause us to view the woman who so aborts as callous or unfeeling even if she has violated no moral duty to the fetus.

22. If some indications for genetic diagnosis were deemed too trivial to permit abortion, then the reasons for abortion where the fetus is normal could also be scrutinized for their acceptability. If we do not generally subject those decisions to moral scrutiny, then abortions for genetic reasons should also be exempt from scrutiny.

23. The Pennsylvania statute at issue in *Casey v. Planned Parenthood* also contained a provision prohibiting abortion on the basis of gender. 18 Pa. Cons. Stat. Ann. Sec. 3204(c) (West Supp. 1992). The parties attacking the abortion statute chose not to attack that provision. Under *Roe*, such a provision would appear to be invalid.

24. Utah Code Ann. Sec. 76-7-302 (Michie 1991); Egan, "Idaho Governor Vetoes Measure Intended to Test Abortion Ruling," *New York Times*, 31 March 1990.

25. See chapter 3, note 5.

26. Dorothy Wertz and John Fletcher, "Fatal Knowledge? Prenatal Diagnosis and Sex Selection," *Hastings Center Report* 19(1989):21.

27. See note 19 supra. In states that recognize a broad scope for wrongful birth, physicians who object to prenatal screening of fetuses can avoid liability by informing the patient of their beliefs and giving them an opportunity to seek services elsewhere.

28. Positive preconception interventions are also possible. Selection of donors for egg or sperm donation has a positive side to it. With sperm donation, couples pick the donor they desire from catalogs that commercial sperm banks distribute listing the donor's height, hair and eye color, ethnic background, education, and interests. Positive preconception efforts to determine the gender of offspring by sperm separation techniques also occurs. By spinning sperm in a centrifuge, the heavier XX or female sperm can be separated from the lighter XY male sperm. Insemination then occurs with the sperm of choice, in the hope of increasing the chances that a child of the desired gender will result. Since these techniques will not be widely sought and may have little efficacy, they will have little effect on overall gender balance, and should be within the couple's procreative discretion.

29. See M. Harrison et al., "Successful Repair In Utero of a Fetal Diaphragmatic Hernia after Removal of Herniated Viscera from the Left Thorax," *New England Journal of Medicine* 322(1990):1582, 1584.

30. If the condition is treatable in utero and the woman is going to term, she may have a duty to accept prenatal in utero treatment as an aspect of her prenatal duty to prevent avoidable harm to offspring. John A. Robertson, "The Right to Procreate and In Utero Fetal Therapy," *Journal of Legal Medicine* 3(1982):438–439. See also chapter 8.

31. Issues such as will it lead to a duty to intervene, will it treat the fetus as a patient, and will it lead to other forms of engineering are not sufficient reasons to stop efforts to correct defects for the benefit of the child who will be born.

32. Of course, such a result would not be a wrong to the child who, but for the procedure, never would have been born.

33. It would not follow, however, that state subsidies or even insurance coverage of therapeutic gene therapy should be provided, especially if the couple has alternative ways to have healthy offspring.

34. How much of an alteration in DNA is necessary to change personal identity and thus produce a different person than would exist if the gene therapy had not occurred? See Noam J. Zohar, "Prospects for 'Genetic Therapy'—Can a Person Benefit from Being Altered," *Bioethics* 5(1991):275.

35. U.S. National Institutes of Health, Recombinant DNA Advisory Committee, *Federal Register* 55(1990):7743.

36. Enhancement interventions could also occur in utero on fetuses, but because of the greater power of earlier interventions, I discuss the issue in the embryo context only.

37. The most likely candidate at present might be the gene for perfect pitch, which is thought to correlate with musical ability. A single gene with this effect has been identified. Sandra Blakeslee, "Perfect Pitch: The Key May Lie in the Genes," *New York Times*, 20 November 1990.

38. Meyer v. Nebraska, 262 U.S. 390 (1923); Pierce v. Society of Sisters, 266 U.S. 510 (1925); Wisconsin v. Yoder, 406 U.S. 205 (1972) are cases that recognize the fundamental right of parents to rear offspring as they wish.

39. I will put aside for the moment whether a genetically enhanced child could ever be harmed because, but for the enhancement, a different child would exist.

40. Of course, one might ask why only the interest in raising "normal" children should be protected, if individuals find the same or greater meaning in raising supernormal children. At some point a constitutive notion of why reproduction is important has to inform the debate, or else there are no limits to shaping offspring characteristics at all, not even when cloning or intentional diminishment is involved.

41. Thus instead of painful Growth Hormone (GH) shots every day to add height, a GH gene would be added in vitro to produce the same effect.

42. If a woman who can produce very few eggs produced one egg, it could be split at the four-cell stage into four separate embryos, each of which would have the same genome. See John A. Robertson, "Ethical and Policy Issues in Cloning by Blastomere Separation," *The Hastings Center Report*, March 1994.

43. The question of government or corporations cloning individuals is beyond the scope of the discussion. The assumption is that any individual clone is a person with rights, and once born cannot be treated like property. Thus even if a single person hired a surrogate to produce a clone, the resulting child would still be a person with all the rights of persons, whatever the impetus for his creation or the intellectual property rights in the cloning procedure.

44. If getting a healthy child is the dominant motive, there would seem to be other ways to achieve that end, such as preimplantation screening. Of course, there is always some risk in those cases, but the risk is so small that cloning could not easily be defended as the most reasonable way to assure healthy offspring. In

contrast, cloning to produce less than a healthy child raises the Bladerunner scenario discussed below.

45. Cloning is negative to the extent that it rejects or excludes other genomes.

46. Frank Pizzuli, "Asexual Reproduction and Genetic Engineering: A Constitutional Assessment of the Technology of Cloning," *Southern California Law Review* 47(1974):476.

47. Indeed, multiple clones from one genome could be made so that any clone would have numerous genetically identical copies, though of course the phenotypes might then vary. Questions of intellectual property or ownership of the desired genome and limits on the multiple run would also have to be addressed.

48. Identical twins gain support from each other and have a special bond that lasts throughout life. Whether that comes from sharing the womb or sharing genes or both is unclear. Since a clone will not have shared the womb but only genes, the support that identical twins or even fraternal twins share may be missing, unless that bond is based on genes alone.

49. Derek Parfit, *Reason and Persons* (Oxford: Clarendon Press, 1984). See also note 26 supra and David Heyd, *Genethics* (Berkeley: University of California Press, 1992), for a more complete discussion of this issue.

50. See chapter 2 and note 40 supra.

51. Assuming that they would still be the same person.

52. This statement still has problems. What if the fabricator truly loved his creations and cared for them after they were born? This situation is different than that of persons who have no way to reproduce other than by producing an unavoidably handicapped child.

53. The counterargument would be that the child will be even less prepared to function well in the world if the parents are so uncomfortable with a taller or nondeaf child that they feel that they cannot rear her well. In that case, however, would they not have a duty to seek foster care or assistance in rearing?

54. They would still have the right to abort fetuses or discard embryos that are not deaf or extremely short, choosing instead to carry to term only those who have the disability the parents share. I am indebted to R. Alta Charo for helpful discussion of this issue.

Chapter 8
Preventing Prenatal Harm to Offspring

1. Typically, courts find that the legislature did not intend to cover prenatal conduct in the statute that is being applied, thus leaving it to legislatures to pass laws that specifically apply to prenatal conduct they wish to criminalize as harmful prenatal conduct. See Johnson v. State, 602 So.2d 1288 (Fla. 1992).

2. Attitudes toward abortion also affect this issue, since the parties often mistakenly think that recognizing prenatal duties recognizes the fetus as an independent entity with rights, which could lead to more restrictive abortion policies.

3. My own involvment with this issue began with an investigation of legal and ethical duties in use of fetal therapy. See John A. Robertson, "The Right to Procreate and In Utero Fetal Therapy," *Journal of Legal Medicine* 3(1982):333.

4. C. S. Phibbs, D. A. Bateman, and R. M. Schwartz, "The Neonatal Costs of

Maternal Cocaine Use," *Journal of the American Medical Association* 266(1991):1521, 1525.

5. J. Fielding, "Smoking and Health," *New England Journal of Medicine* 313(1985):491–496.

6. (New York: Harper and Row, 1989).

7. Robb London, "2 Waiters Lose Jobs for Liquor Warning to Women," *New York Times*, 30 March 1991.

8. Oil, Chemical and Atomic Workers International Union v. American Cyanamid Company, 741 F.2d 444 (1984); Haynes v. Shelby Memorial Hospital, 726 F.2d 1543 (11th Cir. 1984); Wright v. Olin Corp., 697 F.2d 1172 (4th Cir. 1982).

9. United Auto Workers v. Johnson's Controls, 111 S.Ct. 1196 (1991).

10. For example, Congress could change Title VII to permit employers to discriminate in these cases. If evidence of effects on both men and women are shown, the obligation of companies to invest in making the workplace safer in order to protect offspring would then have to be resolved.

11. In some of the cases discussed in chapter 4 the child can be conceived and even be born healthy, but postnatal or even prenatal actions that cause harm are in fact unavoidable in the circumstances in which the parties are acting.

12. Although the discussion focuses on the rights and duties of pregnant women, the analysis applies to any person in a position to cause prenatal harm to offspring. The father's duties are discussed in greater detail later.

13. As noted in chapter 7, mandatory carrier or prenatal screening that did not require contraception or abortion would not infringe procreative liberty.

14. At a certain point, when such behavior has caused the harm that offspring, if born, will experience, the birth of an unhealthy child is then unavoidable. However, prior to the behavior, the child could have been born healthy.

15. In that case, a choice not to procreate is being made at a point too late in the pregnancy to be honored. After viability, moral and legal duties to the viable fetus may take priority over the desire to avoid reproduction.

16. Even if the woman has not definitively decided to go to term, as long as there is a chance that she will she may be held morally accountable for prenatal actions that unreasonably harm offspring.

17. A basic question is whether the woman or some other decision maker—physician, employer, the state—should have authority to determine the most desirable balance.

18. See Renslow v. Mennonite Hospital, 67 Ill.2d 348, 367 N.E.2d 1250 (1977), where medical providers who negligently transfused a woman with Rh-positive blood were found liable for the injuries suffered by a subsequently conceived child who was injured by the preconception transfusion.

19. While infant mortality rates in the United States are dropping, they are still very high for poor and minority women, mainly due to their lack of access to prenatal care.

20. Kevin Sack, "Unlikely Union in Albany: Feminists and Liquor Sellers," *New York Times*, 5 April 1991.

21. This point is phrased in gender-neutral terms because there could be situations in which males are more at risk for causing prenatal harm to offspring

than females, though in many cases women would be the target of selective exclusion.

22. The paradox of preventing the birth of the very persons that one is trying to protect arises with workplace issues. If excluded from the workplace, the children sought to be protected would never be born. Other, healthier children would be. See chapter 4.

23. Civil sanctions as a result of tort suits brought by injured children against negligent parents are also possible, though are not likely to be a major factor. See Grodin v. Grodin, 102 Mich. App. 396, 301 N.W.2d 869 (1980), and John A. Robertson, "Procreative Liberty and the Control of Conception, Pregnancy and Childbirth," *Virginia Law Review* 69(1983):405, 437–442.

24. Tamar Lewin, "When Courts Take Charge of the Unborn," *New York Times*, 9 January 1989; idem, "Drug Use during Pregnancy: New Issue before the Courts," *New York Times*, 6 February 1990.

25. Robertson and Shulman, "Pregnancy and Prenatal Harm: The Case of Mothers with PKU," *Hastings Center Report* 17(1987):23.

26. Johnson v. State, 602 So.2d 1288 (Fla. 1992).

27. Ibid.

28. Lewin, "Drug Use during Pregnancy."

29. Isabel Wilkerson, "Jury in Illinois Refuses to Charge Mother in Drug Death of Newborn," *New York Times*, 27 May 1989.

30. Lewin, "When Courts Take Charge."

31. Report of the American Medical Association Board of Trustees, Legal Interventions during Pregnancy, *Journal of the American Medical Association* 264(1990):2663; Committee on Ethics, American College of Obstetrics and Gynecology, "Patient Choice: Maternal-Fetal Conflict," no. 55 (October 1987), reprinted in *Woman's Health Issues* 1 (Fall 1990):13–15.

32. Since a legal person would not exist until live birth, in utero transmission of drugs would not violate the drug delivery statute. Nor would there be delivery once the cord is cut. The two-minute window after delivery and before cutting the cord was crucial for the prosecution's claim of delivery of drugs to a minor in State v. Johnson.

33. This emphasis on prenatal actions harming offspring provides an opening wedge for greater state intervention in families. Smoking by one parent has already been used to assign child custody in divorce cases.

34. (Boston: Houghton Mifflin, 1986). Although Atwood's novel was inspired by the strict laws against abortion imposed by Ceauşescu, there is an obvious parallel to criminal sanctions for prenatal conduct.

35. Ira J. Chasoff, "The Prevalence of Illicit Drug Use during Pregnancy and Discrepancies in Reporting in Pinellas County, Fla.," *New England Journal of Medicine* 322(1990):1202. The difference in reporting, however, might be explained in part by the fact that evidence of marijuana was more likely to be found in white women while cocaine was more likely to be found in black women, and evidence is lacking that prenatal use of marijuana is as harmful to offspring as cocaine.

36. The principle is clearest when a third party, who may often be the father, attacks a pregnant woman and the newborn dies as a result of the attack sometime

after birth. It has also been applied against a woman who through a prenatal assault on twin fetuses caused them to die postnatally. See E. Coke, *Institutes* 50 (1648), for the common law origins of this distinction.

37. See Dorothy Roberts, "Punishing Drug Addicts Who Have Babies: Women of Color, Equality, and the Right of Privacy," *Harvard Law Review* 104 (1990): 1419.

38. A policy that prefers children not be born at all rather than that they be born avoidably damaged in order to protect other children from being born damaged is not unreasonable. See discussion in chapter 7.

39. Two related issues concern the role or duty of physicians and nurses to report suspected prenatal child abuse, and whether the harmful effects of drugs or other conduct are as clearly established as asserted.

40. As previously noted, coercive policies to prevent the birth of unavoidably handicapped children raise different issues, and are much more difficult to justify. See chapter 4.

41. Jefferson v. Griffin Spalding Memorial Hospital, 247 Ga. 86, 274 S.E.2d 457 (1981).

42. In re A.C., 537 A.2d 1235 (D.C. Ct. Appeals 1990).

43. Randall S. Stafford, "Alternative Strategies for Controlling Rising Cesarean Section Rates," *Journal of the American Medical Association* 263(1990): 683.

44. Of course, postnatal sanctions also interfere with liberty, but after an adjudication of culpability and statutory violation. Here the body is seized prior to occurrence of harm. While courts have not gone so far as to literally require an actual seizure and performance of surgery, they do issue an order to which the woman usually submits. If she does not, she would presumably be incarcerated for contempt.

45. V. E. Kolder, J. Gallagher, and M. T. Parsons, "Court-Ordered Obstetrical Interventions," *New England Journal of Medicine* 316(1987):1192–1196.

46. The right to be free of state-imposed bodily intrusions is not absolute. Compulsory vaccination was upheld in Jacobsen v. Massachusetts, 197 U.S. 11 (1905). Blood tests for evidence of drunk driving are constitutionally permitted, though major surgery for recovery of a bullet as evidence is not. Compare Schmerber v. California, 384 U.S. 757 (1966), with Winston v. Lee, 470 U.S. 753 (1985). Under *Roe v. Wade* states can require that women undergo the physical burdens of three months of gestation for the sake of a child. Blood transfusions have also been imposed on pregnant women who had religious objections for the sake of the child-to-be. Raleigh Fitkin-Paul Morgan Memorial Hospital v. Anderson, 42 N.J. 421, 201 A.2d 537 (1964), *cert. denied*, 377 U.S. 985, 84 S.Ct. 1894, 12 L.Ed.2d 1032 (1964).

47. On the other hand, if the frequency of the need to intervene is so slight, perhaps it is not wise to authorize a mechanism that can be abused in other circumstances.

48. The statute should not authorize the actual seizure of the woman, but permit her to be punished for disobeying an order to submit to the treatment in question, as occurs with prior restraints of the press in the rare circumstances in which they are authorized.

49. See M. Harrison et al., "Successful Repair In Utero of a Fetal Diaphragmatic Hernia after Removal of Herniated Viscera from the Left Thorax," *New England Journal of Medicine* 322(1990):1582, 1584.

50. The situation of women with phenylketonuria who refuse to resume the diet that protected their health raises the possibility of prenatal incarceration in order to impose a special diet. In most instances, such incarceration would not be justified. See Robertson and Shulman, "Pregnancy and Prenatal Harm," 23.

51. Obviously there are exceptions to this point based on lack of resources to prevent pregnancy or to obtain abortion.

52. The male obligation in such cases is not dependent on the male being the father, but rather in engaging in conduct that foreseeably risks serious harm to offspring.

53. Or both could be held accountable if they both refused.

54. I will assume in this hypothetical situation that the child was intentionally conceived by the father. However, as long as the father voluntarily had sexual intercourse, he might still be held to have an obligation—because he is the father—to provide needed blood products on the same theory that he can be held for child support. This is true even if he objects to the woman continuing the pregnancy, and requests that she abort. However, this duty might not apply to a sperm donor who agreed in donating sperm to relinquish all rearing rights and duties in offspring.

55. A partial liver donation is highly intrusive and carries the medical risks of major abdominal surgery, but does not pose a major risk to the donor of loss of liver function. Singer, Siegler, et al., "Ethics of Liver Transplantation with Living Donors," *New England Journal of Medicine* 321(1989):620.

56. In that case, her spleen was nicked in the course of the surgery, which necessitated removal of her spleen.

57. See chapter 3 for a discussion of a woman's duty not to abort after viability.

Chapter 9
Farming the Uterus

1. An exception is the case discussed below of producing children to serve as organ donors.

2. The dissenting justices made this point in Young v. American Mini-Theaters, 427 U.S. 50 (1976), a case in which the Court upheld a zoning law that tried to disperse adult bookstores throughout the city of Detroit. The decision appeared to give protected nonobscene speech that was sexually explicit less protection than nonsexually explicit speech, despite the usual rule that no distinctions can be made about the content of protected speech.

3. In 1975 federal regulations required that any research involving IVF or embryos must first be approved by an Ethics Advisory Board. 45 C.F.R. Sec. 46.209(d). In 1980 the existing EAB was disbanded and never reconstituted, thus effectively ending any federal support of such research. In addition, many states had laws that prohibited or greatly restricted embryo research. In 1993 Congress overruled this regulation, thus opening the door to federal funding of IVF and

embryo research. National Institutes of Health Revitalization Act of 1993, Pub.L.No. 103–43, Sec. 121, 107 Stat. 133.

4. These issues are discussed in greater detail in John A. Robertson, "Embryo Research," *Western Ontario Law Review* 24(1986):15.

5. Whether nonreproductive studies may occur has not been definitively resolved. However, if the research will contribute to the relief of disease and suffering, there is no reason why it should not occur with embryos on which reproductive research would otherwise be acceptable.

6. This position is at odds with the policy adopted for fetal research that no research should be done on fetuses going to be aborted that would not be done on fetuses going to term. However, the equality principle recognized for fetal research erroneously assumed that fetuses going to term and those going to be aborted have the same status, overlooking the fact that research on fetuses going to term could affect the resulting child. Fortunately, the same claim has not been made for embryos.

7. Yet such a strict position against embryo research overlooks the extent to which minimally risky research occurs on infants, children, and other incompetent human subjects. A truly parallel position with embryo research would allow research that does not harm embryos. Depending on how one views the possibility of harm to embryos that are going to be discarded, a great deal of research could then be permitted.

8. See Robertson, "Embryo Research," for citations.

9. See G. Annas and M. Grodin, ed., *The Nazi Doctors and the Nuremberg Code: Human Rights in Human Experimentation* (New York: Oxford University Press, 1992).

10. See Robertson, "Embryo Research."

11. 18 Pa.C.S.A. Sec. 3216 (West Supp. 1992).

12. The rationale for such laws appear to be a view that embryos are human subjects or symbols thereof. But one can question the symbolic gains of banning research on embryos that can be discarded when they are too rudimentary to be harmed. Thus such legislation may be attacked on grounds of vagueness (what is therapeutic vs. nontherapeutic, what is an individual, etc.) as well as on substantive grounds of irrationality and interference with procreative liberty. See Lifchez v. Hartigan, 735 F. Supp. 1361 (N.D. Ill. 1990); Margaret S. Edwards, 794 F.2d 994 (5th Cir. 1986).

13. Embryos could be created for research and then transferred to the uterus to see the effects on resulting offspring, but ordinarily embryos created for research are intended to be discarded after the research procedure.

14. Germany, for example, permits no embryo research at all. Gesetz zum Schutz von Embryonen (Embryonenschutzgesetz-ESchG) vom 13. Dezember 1990. See also David Dickson, "Europe Split on Embryo Research," *Science* 242(1988):1117.

15. This exception thus allows researchers to determine whether frozen and thawed eggs or micromanipulated eggs and sperm will fertilize, without requiring that the resulting embryos also be placed in a uterus before more is known about the effects of the experimental procedure. See Buckle, Dawson, and Singer, "The Syngamy Debate: When Does a Human Life Begin?" *Law, Medicine, and Health Care* 17(1989):174.

16. Until more demand for research embryos occurs, however, it will not be possible to determine the extent to which excess embryos from IVF will meet researchers' demands, and thus the extent of the need to create embryos solely for research purposes.

17. The line between research with embryos created solely for that purpose and with discarded excess embryos cannot always be easily drawn. Whenever more eggs than can safely be implanted are inseminated, with the excess to be donated for research, embryos for research and no intention to transfer will be deliberately created.

18. The case where many more embryos will be created than can be safely transferred, with the excess then donated for research prior to discard, is more easily included in procreative liberty. Although there is a risk that more embryos will be created than can be safely placed in the uterus, the embryos are created with the purpose of producing offspring and thus might reasonably be considered part of procreative liberty. However, one might question whether the practice is so essential to initiating pregnancy that it should receive the protection accorded procreative liberty. If it is not, then policies designed to protect excess embryos, such as requiring that all embryos be transferred or donated, or limiting the number of eggs that can be inseminated, could be adopted without infringing procreative liberty.

19. At this point one is in the realm of moral and symbolic judgment, where personal moral intuitions may hold more sway than rational arguments.

20. Infertility (Medical Procedures) Act Sec. 6(5) (Victoria, Australia, 1984).

21. Indeed, recognition of this line shows an inherent contradiction in the right-to-life position of a new person existing from the moment of fertilization. The syngamy line shows that fertilization is not a moment, but a long series of continuous events. If not all moments or aspects are to be valued, then one has to confront the basis for the point picked. Once this issue is opened and logically developed, it may be hard to justify any line before sentience. Such implications could lead right-to-life groups in the United States to reject even the syngamy line as a marker of permissible embryo research.

22. See chapter 5.

23. See chapter 2.

24. Selective termination of twins due to the genetic abnormality or deformity of one raises somewhat different issues. The situation usually arises in a naturally occurring pregnancy and not in an infertile couple, so it is unlikely to be iatrogenically caused. Also, it may not be discovered until the second trimester, making termination more difficult. Finally, the couple might be more willing to terminate both if selective termination is not available.

25. The problems this causes for families are described in Elizabeth Rosenthal, "Cost of High-Tech Fertility: Too Many Babies," *New York Times*, 26 May 1992.

26. A more complete account of the procedure is as follows:

The technique . . . involves the transabdominal insertion under ultrasound guidance, of a spinal needle (usually a 22 gauge). The abdomen is prepped and draped as for an amniocentesis procedure. The insertion site is carefully chosen for each embryo to attempt a direct, vertical, downward approach. It has been our experience that it is far less painful to go straight down than to maneuver through the abdomen at a significant angle from vertical. When the position right over the fetal heart is confirmed in both longitudinal and transverse . . . planes, the needle is sharply thrust into the thorax. If the thrust is too gentle, the embryo will reflexively move or roll away, and the alignment process has to be completely redone. Even if one "misses" with an attempt, it is usually not necessary to completely remove the needle. It can be repositioned for a new attempt. Once the needle is thrust into the embryo, it is important to make sure of proper placement. While one aims for the heart, it is a very small target in the first trimester. Anywhere completely within the fetal thorax is acceptable. . . .

Once the needle is properly positioned, the inner stylet of the needle is removed. A 3cc syringe is attached and the plunger pulled back gently. There should be negative pressure just as one expects from the same maneuver at laparoscopy. There may be but usually is not any cardiac home, but there should not be any amniotic fluid. . . .

Once the operator is sure of the position, a small dose of potassium chloride is injected. The KCL injection (about .5 cc) results in cardiac standstill usually within 1–2 minutes of the injection with ultimate reabsorption of the sac. On occasion, cardiac motion will continue for a longer time, but a definite slowing which appears 'pre-terminal' will be apparent. A pleural or cardiac effusion can often be appreciated.

Mark Evans, Marlene May, and John Fletcher, "Multifetal Pregnancy Reduction and Selective Termination," in L. Iff, J. J. Apuzzio, and A. N. Vintzileos, *Textbook of Operative Obstetrics*, 2d ed. (New York: Pergamon Press, 1992).

27. Id.

28. Because the issue has not been widely debated, it is not clear how persons holding strict right-to-life views would view killing some fetuses to save others.

29. Difficult questions about how serious to the mother the incremental risk is would have to be resolved.

30. In Great Britain, "No more than three fertilized eggs or embryos shall be placed in a woman in any one cycle, regardless of the procedure used." Code of Practice, Human Fertilization and Embryology Authority, p.7.i.

31. See Evans, May, and Fletcher, "Multifetal Pregnancy Reduction."

32. The substantial nigra cells seemed to produce the dopamine, whose absence was the cause of Parkinson's disease.

33. Consultants to the Advisory Committee to the Director, National Institutes of Health, *Report of the Human Fetal Tissue Transplantation Research Panel*, December 1988.

34. He also doubted whether the recommended separation between the abortion decision and the decision to donate fetal tissue could be maintained, because consent would have to be obtained before the abortion is actually performed. Letter from Secretary Louis Sullivan to Dr. William Raub, Acting Director, NIH, 2 November 1989.

35. The House bill required women donating tissue to sign a consent form that stated that they had not restricted the recipient of the donation, that the recipient's identity was unknown to them, and that the decision to donate was indepen-

dent of the decision to abort. They also had to sign an additional statement that they were not undergoing the abortion in order to make tissue available for transplant.

36. Warren Leary, "Bush to Set Up Fetal Tissue Bank with Restrictions over Abortion," *New York Times*, 20 May 1992. Most tissue from these sources would not be usable because of defective genetic material or infection that made it unsuitable for transplant in humans. Also, it appears that the administration greatly overestimated the amount of tissue that could be collected from these sources. Philip J. Hilts, "Fetal Tissue Bank Not a Viable Option, Agency Memo Says," *New York Times*, 27 July 1993.

37. Robin Toner, "Clinton Orders Reversal of Abortion Restrictions Left by Reagan and Bush," *New York Times*, 23 January 1993.

38. National Institutes of Health Revitalization Act of 1993, Pub.L.No. 103-43, Sect. 111, 107 Stat. 129 (to be codified at 42 U.S.C. Sec. 498A).

39. Gina Kolata, "Transplants of Fetal Tissue Seen Easing a Brain Disease," *New York Times*, 7 May 1992.

40. They also argue that the woman who aborts cannot give valid proxy consent for use of the tissue that she chose to abort, and that no one else is situated to give consent. James Burtchaell, "Case Study: University Policy on Experimental Use of Aborted Fetal Tissue," *IRB: A Journal of Human Subject Research*, July/August 1988, 7.

41. Of course, it is possible that the proponents of fetal tissue use take that position because it is not now necessary to go to such sources, and might view the matter differently if it did become necessary.

42. The British Medical Association adopted guidelines very similar to the NIH Advisory Panel, including a ban on designated donations and against any conception or abortion solely to provide material for transplantation. As part of the legislation codifying federal authority to fund fetal tissue transplantation research, Congress also made it a federal crime punishable by up to ten years in prison to abort or participate in abortion solely to get tissue for transplant. National Institutes of Health Revitalization Act of 1993, Pub.L.No. 103-43, Sec. 112, 107 Stat. 131 (to be codified at 42 U.S.C. Sec. 498 B(b)).

43. Unless the effect were so small as to be de minimis, as it appears to be. See the discussion below.

44. He also doubted whether the recommended separation between the abortion decision and the decision to donate fetal tissue could be maintained, because consent would have to be obtained before the abortion is actually performed. "This will potentially influence the decisionmaking process, despite the safeguards recommended by the NIH Advisory Panels. In addition, should the research efforts in question prove successful, a demand for aborted fetuses could be created. Pressure would then be created to produce more tissue." Letter from Secretary Louis Sullivan to Dr. William Raub, Acting Director, NIH, 2 November 1989.

45. Sullivan letter, ibid.

46. Asking for consent after the abortion procedure is not practical, because of the condition of the woman who has just undergone the abortion and the need to procure the fetal tissue immediately after the abortion.

47. Many women considering abortion will not be aware of the practice, unless the practice becomes so widespread and successful that abortion becomes associated with tissue donation. In any event, will not the desire to end an unwanted pregnancy still be the key factor in the abortion decision?

48. See notes 38 and 41. Under these provisions women who donate must sign a statement that they were given no inducements to abort and donate, and it is a federal crime punishable by ten years in prison to designate the recipient of fetal tissue or otherwise abort to get tissue.

49. In that case the actual abortion would occur at home, and it would not be possible to salvage tissue for transplant.

50. Obviously persons who are pro-life would disagree. See chapter 3.

51. As this brief discussion shows, the reasons one wishes to avoid reproduction by terminating pregnancy should not matter in this case, nor perhaps in others. Ordinarily we allow the woman to decide whether the physical, social, and psychological burdens of pregnancy and gestation are for her. An inquiry into why she finds those burdens unacceptable, and a determination of which are acceptable and which are not, is too difficult, intrusive of privacy, and potentially arbitrary, for it will be difficult to say which impacts on her life justify abortion and which ones do not. In either case, the right or interest in avoiding reproduction is at stake.

Here the desire to avoid reproduction is to save or treat another sick person. But that desire could lead to abortion in other situations. Suppose her child or spouse needed so much attention that continuing a pregnancy would interfere with their care. If a woman could abort in that case, she should be free to abort to get tissue to treat that same family member.

52. For analysis of the constitutionality of bans on abortion to procure tissue, see Robertson, "Fetal Tissue Transplants," *Washington University Law Quarterly* 66(1988):443, 480–491.

53. The same issue arises with creating embryos to grow into salvageable organs outside the body. Creating embryos to be farmed for tissue or organs is akin to creating embryos for research purposes, though they would be kept alive longer and would reach a later stage of development. If they were kept alive in the laboratory for more than fourteen days, when implantation in the uterus occurs and the primitive streak—the first rudiments of the nervous system—appears, the question would be whether removing organs and destroying embryos at that point harms them or has otherwise high symbolic costs. In such cases, procreative liberty would not be directly involved because there is no intention or likelihood of producing offspring.

54. Change of mind is always possible, so in some cases conceptions undertaken to procure tissue could end up with live children. If procreative liberty is not directly involved, should the activity—the use of reproductive capacity—nevertheless be protected? Here conceptions of bodily autonomy, as well as an interest in helping family members or others, comes into play. One might argue that this is as basic a right as procreative liberty (though the interests justifying it are different). Also, if one has a right to be a living kidney or bone marrow donor to a family member, then one should be able to give gametes or conceive and abort for a similar beneficent purpose. The main issue then becomes whether there is a

sufficient countervailing interest to justify limitation of that liberty interest. In this instance, the balancing of interests should not be affected by whether the liberty interest is designated as procreative.

55. Some people, no doubt, will resist this conclusion, even if they accept abortion to procure tissue when the woman is already pregnant. Whether rational or not, they assign moral or symbolic significance to deliberate creation.

56. Another concern with conception for the purpose of procuring fetal tissue is that it risks dehumanizing women by viewing their bodies and reproductive capacity as tissue factories. Such an effect would be even more likely if unrelated women were recruited for pay to serve as tissue producers for sick persons who had no female relative capable of serving that need. It has also been raised in recommendations that women not be permitted to postpone abortion a few days or change the abortion method to enhance the likelihood of procuring better tissue.

57. Some nine thousand people are awaiting unrelated bone marrow donors at any one time. The task of finding an unrelated donor is costly, onerous, and often unsuccessful, since there is only a 1:20,000 chance that any one person would be a match. Thousands of blood tests are thus necessary to find a suitable donor.

58. The total chance that their efforts would be successful was 6.4 percent. See *Time*, 5 March 1990, 56.

59. Her umbilical-cord fluid, which contained stem cells similar to those found in bone marrow, was immediately frozen for later use. If additional stem cells are needed, they can be obtained from the baby when it is six months or older, and the complications of donation are reduced. As of this writing, no marrow transplant has yet occurred, and the leukemic daughter is still alive.

60. *New York Times*, 16 February 1990.

61. "Creating a Child to Save Another," *Time*, 5 March 1990, 56.

62. Anissa's pediatric oncologist advised against having a child for this purpose. She stated, "I thought that it was a peculiar reason to have a baby. It made me uncomfortable. It didn't sit well, if that was the only reason, to have child to help another child." "Woman Is Willing to Have Baby to Save Her Ailing Daughter," *Los Angeles Times*, 16 February 1990.

63. Ethical commentary on the Ayala case included such comments as: "It's outrageous that people would go to this length" (Boyle); "It's the classic nightmare of using people as tissue and organ banks. . . . There's a revulsion that has to kick in" (Wolfe); "This represents thingification of a child. . . . It assaults some very deeply held values" (Fletcher). Other ethicists, however, found it understandable and acceptable.

64. Id.

65. While there is some question whether enough benefit to the nonconsenting minor can be shown in all cases, the courts seem to approve them as properly within parental discretion. See discussion below.

66. For discussion of slippery slope arguments, see chapter 7.

67. The case can also be imagined in which the tissue donation is made and then the couple gives up the child for adoption.

68. Here the injury will be felt by a live-born individual, and not merely by an embryo or fetus discarded or destroyed before it has interests that can be harmed.

69. Compare couples that carry a handicapped child to term rather than abort and then relinquish for adoption.

70. If having a child to serve as a tissue donor is praiseworthy, it is because the child will be loved in his own right, and will not be subjected to abuse or treated as a mere means once born. This depends on whether their use of the child as a donor is itself defensible. In a series of cases involving minor kidney and bone marrow donors (that helped define or create modern bioethics), courts have ruled that such procedures could be done when there was minimal risk to the minor or when the benefits to him outweighed the risks of the procedure. In cases of tissue donation to a sibling, especially to a twin, benefit was found in the companionship of the recipient, who would be enabled to survive by the donation. See Baron, Botsford, and Cole, "Live Organs and Tissue Transplants from Minor Donors in Massachusetts," *Boston University Law Review* 55(1975):159.

In an Ayala-type case, the question of benefit may not be as clear as one assumes. If marrow is taken soon after birth or in the first year or two, it may be difficult to show the actual benefit to the donor that justifies the procedure, other than being born in the first place. Avoidance of family grief alone might not be sufficient benefit to justify such an intrusive procedure on an unconsenting minor. Indeed, the need to show benefit to the source would bar the donation if the recipient were unrelated and unknown to the minor. Even if it were a known friend, there might be a serious question of whether benefits to the source outweighed the harm of the procedure.

Chapter 10
Class, Feminist, and Communitarian Critiques of Procreative Liberty

1. *Rights Talk: The Impoverishment of Political Discourse* (New York: Free Press, 1991).

2. Elizabeth Fox-Genovese, "Society's Child" (Review of *Life Itself: Abortion in the American Mind* by Roger Rosenblatt), *The New Republic*, 18 May 1992, 40–41.

3. This is one of Elizabeth Kingdom's criticisms of rights in *What's Wrong with Rights: Problems for Feminist Politics of Law* (Edinburgh, U.K.: Edinburgh University Press, 1991), 79–84.

4. I am grateful to Daniel and Sidney Callahan for first making me aware of this aspect of reproductive rights.

5. See Fox-Genovese, "Society's Child"; Daniel Callahan, "Bioethics and Fatherhood," *Utah Law Review* 1992(3):735.

6. Cass Sunstein, "Righttalk," *The New Republic*, 2 September 1991, 34.

7. As Sunstein notes, rights of speech and association, jury trial and antidiscrimination, are basic preconditions for social involvement, thus enhancing rather than dividing community. In addition, rights and duties are correlative, thereby creating an implicit sense of social responsibility. Id. at 35.

8. Kingdom, *What's Wrong with Rights*, 83.

9. Sunstein, "Righttalk," 36. Sunstein further notes: "If one looks at the context in which restrictions on abortion take place, at their real purposes and real effects, then the abortion right is most plausibly rooted not in privacy but in the

right to equality on the basis of sex. Current law nowhere compels men to devote their bodies to the protection of other people, even if life is at stake, and even if men are responsible for the very existence of those people. . . . Such restrictions are an important means of reasserting traditional gender roles." Id. See also chapter 3.

10. If the social vision of reproduction is to claim our allegiance, then society's commitment to the sanctity of life must be reflected in a social commitment to support it at all stages, including in those pregnant women who desire an abortion because they lack the resources to care for a child.

11. "Losing the Negative Right of Privacy: Building Sexual and Reproductive Freedom," *New York University Review of Law and Social Change* 18 (1991):46.

12. Maher v. Roe, 432 U.S. 464 (1977); Harris v. McCrae, 448 U.S. 297 (1980).

13. Norman Daniels, *Just Health Care* (New York: Cambridge University Press, 1985), 26–28.

14. Either directly or as a derivative right of the recipient. See chapters 2 and 6.

15. 822 P.2d 1317, 4 Cal. Rptr.2nd 170 (1992).

16. Ira J. Chasnoff, "The Prevalence of Illicit Drug Use during Pregnancy and Discrepancies in Mandatory Reporting in Pinellas County, Florida," *New England Journal of Medicine* 322(1990):1202. However, the differential treatment could be explained by the fact that the white women were more likely to have evidence of marijuana in their blood, while the black women had evidence of cocaine.

17. V. E. Kolder, J. Gallagher, and M. T. Parsons, "Court-Ordered Obstetrical Interventions," *New England Journal of Medicine* 316(1987):1192–1196.

18. Almost any issue of *Issues in Reproductive and Genetic Engineering: Journal of International Feminist Analysis* contains criticism of the dangers of new reproductive technologies, including IVF. See, for example, Bette Vanderwater, "Meanings and Strategies of Reproductive Control: Current Feminist Approaches to Reproductive Technology," 5(1992):215.

Part of the feminist objection to the medicalization of pregnancy through ultrasound, amniocentesis, cesarean sections, and IVF, to name but a few examples, is that women lose control over their own pregnancies and childbirths. Martha Field, "Surrogacy Contracts—Gestational and Traditional: The Argument for Nonenforcement," *Washburn Law Journal* 31(1991):1, 16. It is usually men who then control the process.

19. Judith Leavitt, "Birthing and Anesthesia: The Debate Over Twilight Sleep," *Signs* 6(1980):147.

20. Adrienne Rich, *Of Woman Born: Motherhood as Experience and Institution* (New York: W. W. Norton, 1976). 117–148; Bottoms, Rosen, and Sokol, "The Increase in the Cesarean Birth Rate," *New England Journal of Medicine* 302(1980):559; Banta, "Benefits and Risks of Electronic Fetal Monitoring," in *Birth Control and Controlling Birth*, ed., H. Holmes, B. Hoskins, and M. Gross (Atlantic Highlands, N.J.: Humanities Press, 1980), 147.

21. Martha Field notes: "A final thing about surrogacy is allocation of power between the sexes. Seen through one lens surrogacy concerns who will control